theclinics.com

CLINICS IN OCCUPATIONAL AND ENVIRONMENTAL MEDICINE

Occupational Injuries and Diseases of the Upper Extremity

GUEST EDITORS
Jane Derebery, MD
Morton L. Kasdan, MD
Roberto Gonzalez, MD

Volume 5 • Number 2

SAUNDERS

An Imprint of Elsevier, Inc.
PHILADELPHIA LONDON TORONTO MONTREAL SYDNEY TOKYO

W.B. SAUNDERS COMPANY
A Division of Elsevier Inc.

Elsevier Inc., 1600 John F. Kennedy Blvd., Suite 1800, Philadelphia, PA 19103-2899

http://www.occmed.theclinics.com

CLINICS IN OCCUPATIONAL AND ENVIRONMENTAL MEDICINE
Editor: Catherine Bewick

Volume 5, Number 2
ISSN 1526-0046
ISBN 1-4160-3616-4

Clinics in Occupational and Environmental Medicine (ISSN 1526-0046) is published quarterly in February, May, August, and November by W.B. Saunders Company, 360 Park Avenue South, New York, NY 10010. Business and editorial offices: 1600 John F. Kennedy Blvd., Suite 1800, Philadelphia, PA 19103-2899. Accounting and circulation offices: 6277 Sea Harbor Drive, Orlando, FL 32887-4800. Subscription prices are $120.00 per year for US individuals, $166.00 per year for US institutions, $60.00 per year for US students and residents, $135.00 per year for Canadian individuals, $204.00 per year for Canadian institutions, $155.00 per year for international individuals, $204.00 per year for international institutions and $78.00 per year for Canadian and foreign students/residents. Foreign air speed delivery is included in all *Clinics* subscription prices. All prices are subject to change without notice. **Customer Service: 1-800-654-2452 (US). From outside of the US, call 1-407-345-4000. E-mail: hhspcs@wbsaunders.com**. **POSTMASTER:** Send address changes to *Clinics in Occupational and Environmental Medicine,* Elsevier Periodicals Customer Service, 6277 Sea Harbor Drive, Orlando, FL 32887-4800.

Clinics in Occupational and Environmental Medicine is indexed in Index Medicus.

Printed in the United States of America.

GUEST EDITORS

JANE DEREBERY, MD, FACOEM, Vice President of Medical Affairs, Concentra Health Services, San Antonio, Texas

MORTON L. KASDAN, MD, FACS, Clinical Professor Department of Surgery, Division of Plastic Surgery, University of Louisville, Louisville, Kentucky

ROBERTO GONZALEZ, MD, Chief Resident, Division of Plastic Surgery, University of Louisville, Louisville, Kentucky

CONTRIBUTORS

JOHNNY CHANG, MD, Department of Plastic and Reconstructive Surgery, Lahey Clinic Foundation, Burlington, Massachusetts

HAL M. CORWIN, MD, Assistant Clinical Professor of Medicine, Division of Physical Medicine and Rehabilitation, School of Medicine, University of Louisville Health Sciences Center, Louisville, Kentucky

JANE DEREBERY, MD, FACOEM, Vice President of Medical Affairs, Concentra Health Services, San Antonio, Texas

HARI DHIR, MD, MPH, MBA, Associate Clinical Professor, Adjunct Professor, Department of Occupational and Environmental Medicine, University of Texas Health Center Tyler; Concentra Health Services, Austin, Texas

CHRISTOPHER DORO, MD, Resident Physician, Department of Orthopaedic Surgery, University of Michigan Medical Center, Ann Arbor, Michigan

DENNIS F. DRIVER, PT, DPT, MS, OCS, MTC, Regional Therapy Director, Houston/Louisiana/South Texas, Concentra Health Services, Houston, Texas

EARL GAAR, MD, FACS, Professor of Surgery, University of Louisville School of Medicine, Louisville Kentucky

GENEVA M. GIANG, MBA, Vice President, Data Analytics, Concentra Health Services, Addison, Texas

ROBERTO GONZALEZ, MD, Chief Resident, Division of Plastic Surgery, University of Louisville, Louisville, Kentucky

WALTER E. HARDING, JD, Partner, Boehl Stopher and Graves, LLP, Louisville, Kentucky

ROBERT G. HASSETT, DO, MPH, Assistant Vice President, Concentra Health Services, Addison, Texas

RADFORD J. HAYDEN, PA-C, Staff Physician Assistant, Orthopaedic Hand Service, Division of Hand Elbow and Microsurgery, Department of Orthopaedic Surgery, University of Michigan Medical Center, Ann Arbor; Affiliate Associate Professor, College of Health Professions, Physician Assistant Studies, University of Detroit Mercy, Detroit, Michigan

BRUCE F. HERMANN, MD, Resident, Department of Surgery, University of Louisville, Louisville, Kentucky

LISA JUNE, MD, Fellow, American College of Rheumatology, Private Practice, Rheumatology Associates, Louisville, Kentucky

MORTON L. KASDAN, MD, FACS, Clinical Professor Department of Surgery, Division of Plastic Surgery, University of Louisville, Louisville, Kentucky

DEAN S. LOUIS, MD, Professor of Surgery, Orthopaedic Hand Service, Division of Hand Elbow and Microsurgery, Department of Orthopaedic Surgery, University of Michigan Medical Center, Ann Arbor, Michigan

W. THOMAS MCCLELLAN, MD, Chief Resident, Department of Plastic and Reconstructive Surgery, Lahey Clinic Foundation Burlington, Massachusetts

TERRY M. MCCURRY, JR, MD, Department of Surgery, Division of Plastic Surgery, University of Louisville, Louisville, Kentucky

TRACY E. NAILOR, MD, Center Medical Director, Concentra Medical Centers, Atlanta, Georgia

BRIAN PEARCE, MSc, Consultant Ergonomist, Humane Technology Ltd., Rothley, Leicestershire, United Kingdom

VALERIE M. PRUITT, MD, MAJ, USAF, MC, General/Trauma Surgery, Surgical Critical Care, Assistant Program Director, General Surgery Residency, Keesler USAF Medical Center, Keesler Air Force Base, Mississippi

ROBERT M. SZABO, MD, MPH, Professor of Orthopaedics and Plastic Surgery, Chief, Hand and Upper Extremity Service, University of California, Davis, School of Medicine, Sacramento, California

WILLIAM H. TULLIS, MD, FAPA, Neuropsychiatric Associates of Austin, Austin, Texas

ADAM J. VERNADAKIS, MD, Assistant Professor, Department of Plastic and Reconstructive Surgery, Lahey Clinic Foundation Burlington, Massachusetts

JEFFREY L. WAINSTEIN, MD, Regional Medical Director, Concentra Medical Centers, Atlanta, Georgia

CONTENTS

FORTHCOMING ISSUES

Volume 5:3

Low Back Pain
Gerard Malanga, MD, *Guest Editor*

Volume 5:4

Exposure to Airbone Particles
Mark W. Frampton, MD, and
Mark J. Utell, MD, *Guest Editors*

RECENT ISSUES

Volume 5:1 (published February 2006)

Tobacco's Impact on Industry
Virginia Cullen Reichert, NP,
Arunabh Talwar, MD, and
Alan M. Fein, MD, *Guest Editors*

Volume 4:4

Industrial Solvents and Human Health, Part II
Scott D. Phillips, MD, and
Gary R. Krieger, MD, MPH, *Guest Editors*

Volume 4:3

Industrial Solvents and Human Health, Part I
Scott D. Phillips, MD, and
Gary R. Krieger, MD, MPH, *Guest Editors*

Volume 4:2

Managing Workers' Competition Costs
Judith Green-McKenzie, MD, MPH, *Guest Editor*

ELSEVIER
SAUNDERS

Clin Occup Environ Med
5 (2) xiii–xiv

CLINICS IN
OCCUPATIONAL AND
ENVIRONMENTAL
MEDICINE

Preface

Occupational Injuries and Diseases of the Upper Extremity

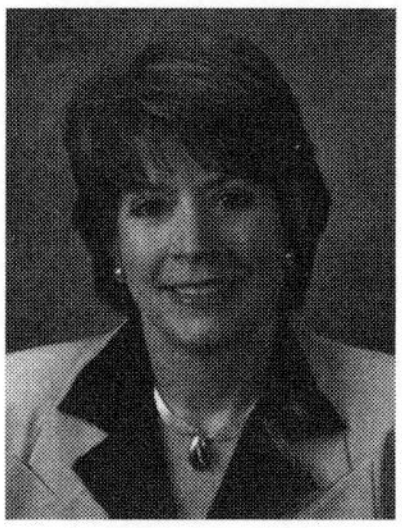

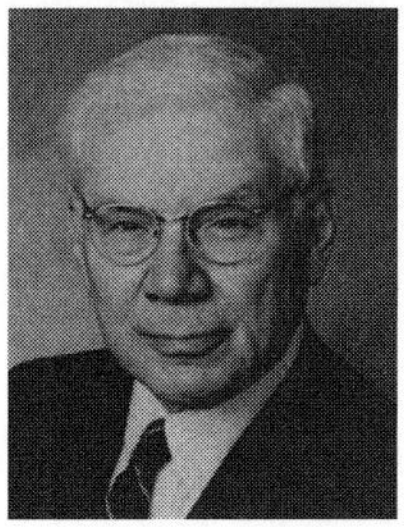

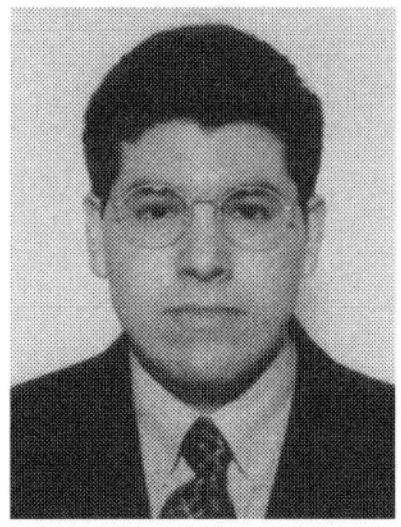

Jane Derebery, MD, FACOEM
Morton L. Kasdan, MD, FACS
Roberto Gonzalez, MD
Guest Editors

The goal of the authors has been to provide a practical, up-to-date clinical text on work-related upper-extremity disorders, encompassing the most recent scientific data on clinical efficacy in regard to management. Additionally, the issue's content draws from our own experiences as practitioners in the specialty area of occupational medicine.

Our emphasis is on promoting a biopsychosocial management approach, in conjunction with evidence-based practice, in regard to upper-extremity disorders. The biopsychosocial model promotes assessment of injured or ailing workers within the context of their specific environments, including both their work and personal life, inasmuch as these will significantly influence both illness and recovery. Although psychosocial components have been well recognized as critical issues in the clinical assessment of hand and arm pain and disability, this has traditionally been a neglected area of clinical focus.

Our sincere desire is that the considerable time, work, and collaboration that went into preparation of this text will speed the recovery and alleviate the suffering of our patients.

doi:10.1016/j.coem.2006.02.001
occmed.theclinics.com

Jane Derebery, MD, FACOEM
Concentra Health Services
10200 Broadway Boulevard, Suite 201
San Antonio, TX 78217, USA
E-mail address: Jane_Derebery@Concentra.com

Morton L. Kasdan, MD, FACS
Division of Plastic Surgery
University of Louisville
PO Box 6048
Louisville, KY 40206-6048, USA
E-mail address: m.kasdan@insightbb.com

Roberto Gonzalez, MD
Blair Plastic Surgery
3107 Fairway Drive
Altoona, PA 16602, USA
E-mail address: betoglez@hotmail.com

ELSEVIER
SAUNDERS

Clin Occup Environ Med
5 (2) 217–223

CLINICS IN OCCUPATIONAL AND ENVIRONMENTAL MEDICINE

Patient Selection

Terry M. McCurry, Jr, MD, Morton L. Kasdan, MD, FACS*

Department of Surgery, Division of Plastic Surgery, University of Louisville, PO Box 6048, Louisville, KY 40206, USA

To begin the discussion on patient selection we first must step back and clarify. The patient is the individual who seeks advice or treatment for a medical or surgical condition. The physician is the qualified medical professional who evaluates and, if deemed appropriate, renders medical or surgical care. This term does not refer to the decision of the patient as to whom he or she will consult, as in "patient's selection." How a patient comes to a specific physician can be as traditional as a direct referral from a primary care provider or as superfluous as persuasive advertising. In some communities, this referral pattern may be largely dictated by third-party payors.

Patient selection refers to the process by which the evaluating physician decides that the potential patient meets the proper criteria for him or her to accept responsibility for care. Many of the points we offer are not scientifically proven fact. Rather, they are the culmination of experience of the senior author (MLK) and others [1–10]. Because of its vagaries, patient selection is an inexact science. The goal of this discussion is to educate younger physicians and other health care professionals as to how to evaluate potential patients effectively.

Early in one's career, often the goal is to be as busy as possible. The inexperienced physician may equate activity with productivity and assume that both lead to a successful career. Poorly selected patients, for many reasons, tend to become unhappy patients and, subsequently, a large drain on a physician's time and resources. What follows is a cycle in which the physician and office staff spend more time with a small number of patients. In turn, this attention allows less time to pursue new referrals or devote time to family or avocations. The activity involved in dealing with an unhappy patient is not pleasant. Un-

* Corresponding author.
E-mail address: m.kasdan@insightbb.com (M.L. Kasdan).

doi:10.1016/j.coem.2005.11.009 ***occmed.theclinics.com***

happy patients become negative advertisements for a physician, and if matters turn to litigation, the costs of time and money to defend lawsuits quickly can become a major drain. Proper patient selection is paramount to a thriving and viable practice.

Patient selection encompasses two general considerations. According to Dr. Robert Goldwyn, these considerations are the "soma" and the "psyche" [1]. The soma refers to the actual pathologic condition that may be addressed through surgical means. The psyche refers to the mental and emotional well-being of the potential patient. Both of these considerations must be evaluated. It is assumed that the clinician has the acumen to discern the pathologic condition, a solid understanding of the relevant anatomy, and the technical expertise to undertake the appropriate treatment with the expectation of a reasonable outcome. One cannot assume that a patient has a definable disorder and is not, consciously or subconsciously, feigning the symptoms. In general terms, a patient's complaints can be subdivided into three groups: real, feigned, and exaggerated. No further discussion about real symptoms is warranted. If a physician determines that a patient is properly motivated and has real symptoms, then a search for the cause of the problem and its solution should be relatively straightforward. If the symptoms are deemed to be feigned or exaggerated, it is helpful for the physician to have at least a basic understanding of the implications so that a referral to a psychiatrist, psychologist, or other professional can be made swiftly.

Feigned symptoms can be broken down into two general subtypes: those with a conscious intent and those with an unconscious intention to deceive. The presentation of symptoms that do not actually exist is known as simulation, and concealing true symptoms is known as dissimulation [2]. Either type of presentation may be related to malingering or a factitious disorder [3]. Malingering is the feigning of symptoms motivated by external incentives, such as financial reward or avoidance of physical demands (eg, decreased work duties). A factitious disorder involves the feigning of symptoms motivated by internal rewards of playing the role of a patient [3]. Feigned symptoms that are presented on an unconscious level fall into three broad categories: dissociative disorders, somatoform disorders, and nonsomatoform medical disorders. These disorders usually can be sorted out by an experienced psychiatrist or other appropriate mental health professional [3].

The point of introducing these disorders into this discussion is that in some circumstances the physical findings do not explain the described symptom or symptom set. The evaluating physician should understand that some disorders are nonorganic in nature. If at any time the evaluating doctor is uncomfortable with making a diagnosis and treatment plan because of concern overfeigned symptoms, a referral to an appropriate mental health professional should be offered or recommended. Although this offer may not be well received by a prospective patient, it certainly is in his or her best interest. If the surgeon commits to an operation or procedure without objective physical findings or supportive diagnostic testing, he or she is doing the patient a disservice. If there is no anatomic basis for the symptoms, the surgeon runs the chance of iatrogenic injury for a procedure that was not indicated. For patients with underlying psychiatric disorders, they have surgical scars that validate their problem to themselves and to future physicians [2,4–6].

Sir William Osler once said, "It is more important to know what kind of a patient has a disease than what kind of a disease a patient has." He also added, "A good physician treats the disease, while a great physician treats the patient with a disease." No two points could better describe the constant evaluations a physician must make of patients and the care that he or she is rendering. A doctor not only must diagnose a patient accurately but also develop a sense of a patient's emotional or mental status beyond the anatomic diagnosis [7]. Although most patients have anatomically definable diseases or injuries, disturbed, impaired patients experience the most pain or loss of function [5]. For example, disfigured patients experience diminished self-image. In someone with a weak ego and poor work ethic, even a minor injury may be socially incapacitating. Thus begins the acting-out process.

The patient selection process should begin before a patient ever meets the physician. Office staff members, from the receptionist to the nurse or medical assistant, interact with the patient from the beginning. An attentive, alert staff can get a sense of a patient's demeanor. Rudeness, hostility, impatience, or a self-proclaimed importance should be scrutinized carefully. Any of these behaviors should be reported to the doctor and considered grounds to recommend that a patient seek care elsewhere.

At the first encounter, these same patients will put on their best face. A physician who does not have an open line of communication with staff may accept patients who have the potential to insinuate themselves between office staff members or between the doctor and staff. This situation ultimately can lead to a nonproductive conflict. Dismissal is a decision ultimately left to the physician but should be considered warranted when office staff inform the physician of unacceptable behavior.

On the initial evaluation, the doctor must begin to establish good patient rapport, which often begins with a brief discussion of how and why the patient was referred. The source may be from a regular referring physician or a satisfied former patient. Some patients may be referred by an attorney. We have found that the best lawyers call and speak personally with a physician before the referral. Be cautious about accepting patients if an attorney does not call. To the contrary, a few scenarios should raise the level of suspicion. The first situation involves that in which an angry or tearful patient begins describing how he or she was "butchered" by another doctor. A common variation of this scenario involves a potential patient simply wanting to make sure the previous doctor performed the surgery correctly. This scenario may represent a completely rational patient who felt that he or she could not communicate with the physician; it also could depict a situation in which the previous physician chose not to meet the needs of the patient. It also could represent a patient with an agenda looking for a reason to initiate a claim against the original physician. We feel it is safe to say that this type of patient should be avoided [8].

Another situation involves a patient who has undergone numerous operative procedures (the so-called "surgiholic"). Often these surgeries have been performed by several different surgeons. The fact that the patient is in your office should, at a minimum, raise an eyebrow. It is important to find the reason or reasons why this patient decided to change doctors. The truth may be that the other physician already dismissed the patient. If a patient is a perfectionist, his or her goals may not be realistically attainable [6]. Direct questions to evaluate their goals are appropriate. Be aware of the patient with SHAFT syndrome [6]. These patients are *s*ad, *h*ostile, *a*nxious, *f*rustrating, and *t*enacious. They can be disarming and clever. They want the surgeon to inflict the injuries.

Be cognizant of the patient who hits the door singing your praises. He or she may say that you are the "best," or the "only" doctor who can help them, or "I've even been to the Mayo Clinic." If an early decision not to accept the patient has been made, it may be prudent not to continue the consultation. The onus is on the doctor to establish an open dialogue such that a patient trusts the doctor and feels able to adequately vent feelings. During this initial encounter, the patient and the physician develop first impressions. If a patient dislikes a doctor, it is possible that he or she may go elsewhere for treatment.

If a doctor dislikes a patient for any reason, he or she should not agree to accept responsibility for the patient's care. Personality clashes are a natural part of human existence. Eventually every physician meets someone with whom he or she cannot establish rapport. A general ill will for a particular patient or a member of the family, regardless of whether it is deserved, may color future dialogue. This situation ultimately may compromise patient care because of a lack of adequate communication. There is no binding agreement from an initial consultation, and the doctor who is immediately suspicious for any reason may elect to render an opinion but not actually assume responsibility.

Moody, unpredictable behavior exhibited by a patient when giving the history should be viewed with caution. This fact especially holds true when a patient cries when giving the medical history. Pain itself does not incite tears, and this outburst should be a harbinger that a patient has nonanatomic factors involved. Emotional stability is paramount to a successful recovery and rehabilitation process. Consider the situation in which a postoperative complication arises. A properly prepared and mentally balanced patient can be coached through almost any unexpected setback. Patients who are emotionally labile may deteriorate, however, and never be able to cope with what is required to overcome the mental and physical hurdles of a complication.

Another important aspect of the patient history that should be assessed during the initial evaluation involves work, social, and family history. There seems to be a link between persons who pursue disability for work-related claims and persons with family members who are already on disability. In one study, the percentage of the working control group who have a disabled family member is 15%. Of persons seeking disability, 52% have disabled family members. The mechanism for this disparity is not completely clear but likely is multifaceted. There is obviously financial reward and secondary gain. Because there are no role models for hard work and success, disability may be looked at as socially acceptable [9].

The appearance of a patient should be noted, both on a physical and an emotional level. A patient who comes to a physician's office for a consultation and is unkempt and disheveled should have a more detailed psychosocial history obtained. The natural question that arises is "How can this patient take care of additional needs postoperatively when he or she cannot take care of *basic* hygiene?" A surgeon must remember that every patient becomes a living testament to his or her skill. If the result of an otherwise well thought out and executed procedure is hidden by layers of dirt, grime, and a broken cast, then a negative outcome may result, including a negative reflection for the doctor's reputation.

Be especially cautious of the patient who assumes a dysfunctional posture and has been labeled with reflex sympathetic dystrophy [10]. An extremity held in an awkward nonanatomic position should send up a red flag. The general affect or outward appearance of a patient's expression should be evaluated carefully. Clinically depressed patients should be referred for evaluation. A physician should look for disproportionate signs of verbalization of symptoms, facial grimacing, and pulling away from the examiner when there are no objective anatomic findings. Patients who are currently living through particularly stressful times, such as losing a job, going through a divorce, or coping with a death in the family, should be allowed a period of bereavement before considering elective surgery.

For the prospective patient, the degree of deformity or impairment versus the degree of concern must be assessed. A poor candidate is an individual who presents with a minimal (possibly imagined) deformity or functional impairment and who is focused and overly concerned. A rush to invasive treatment by the physician leads to disappointment on the part of the patient and perhaps results in hostility, violence, or litigation. Conversely, a patient who presents with an obvious deformity, seeks some improvement, and has a realistic goal most likely will be satisfied.

Dr. Mark Gorney has summed up this idea in a visual aid. The chart in Fig. 1 shows the degree of deformity along the horizontal axis. The patient concern is shown along the vertical axis or ordinate. The slanting line in the middle of the chart represents appropriate concern for a given degree of deformity. Any deviation toward the upper left-hand corner represents a patient whose concern outweighs the actual deformity [2]. The physician should be alert to this potential problem patient and avoid invasive treatment if at all possible. Any potential patient who falls into the lower right-hand corner represents a patient whose deformity outweighs the amount of concern. This patient is likely to be satisfied with any result and is considered safe. Most patients fall somewhere in between, along the slanted line.

The physician should select for management patients who he or she feels may be treated successfully. This goal sounds simple and painfully obvious; however, appearances can be deceiving. A patient may have psychological con-

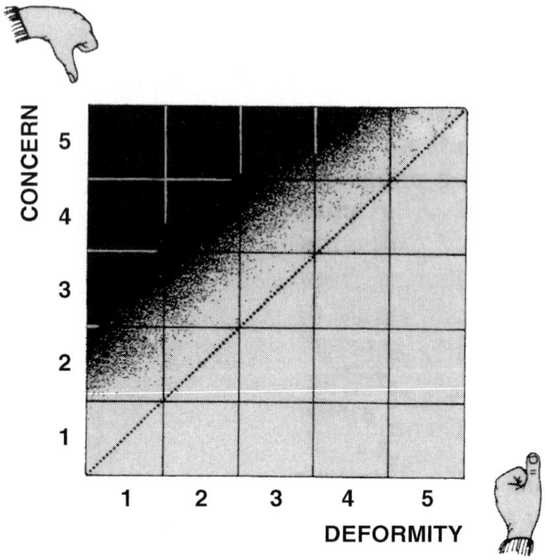

Fig. 1. A patient's objective deformity (as judged by the surgeon) is shown along the horizontal axis. The patient's degree of concern about the deformity (as perceived by the patient) is shown along the vertical axis. (*From* Gorney M, Martello J. Patient selection criteria. Clin Plast Surg 1999;26(1): 37–40; with permission.)

ditions, either conscious or subconscious, or an agenda that precludes a successful outcome. A patient may have comorbidities that may not necessarily preclude, but hinder, their successful postoperative care. One of the most common examples involves the alcoholic patient who smokes.

The goal as a doctor is to take a patient as efficiently and safely as possible through the process from initial evaluation to final follow-up care and discharge. By carefully selecting patients with no hidden agendas who come to treatment with a healthy attitude, anatomically defined disorders, good motivation, and cooperation, the physician can expect a successful outcome.

References

[1] Goldwyn RM. The patient and the plastic surgeon. 2nd edition. Boston: Little, Brown and Company; 1991.

[2] Gorney M, Martello J. Patient selection criteria. Clin Plast Surg 1999;26(1):37–40.

[3] LoPiccolo CJ, Goodkin K, Baldewicz TT. Current issues in the diagnosis and management of malingering. Ann Med 1999;31:166–74.

[4] Hentz VR. Surgical strategy: matching the patient with the procedure. Hand Clin 2002;18: 503–18.

[5] Louis DS, Lamp MK, Greene TL. The upper extremity and psychiatric illness. J Hand Surg Am 1985;10A:687–93.

[6] Kasdan ML, Soergel TM, Johnson AL, et al. Expanded profile of the SHAFT syndrome. J Hand Surg Am 1998;23A(1):26–31.

[7] Carillo JE, Green AR, Betancourt JR. Cross-cultural primary care: a patient-based approach. Ann Intern Med 1999;130:829.
[8] Kasdan ML, Vender MI, Lewis K, et al. Carpal tunnel syndrome: effects of litigation on the utilization of health care and physician workload. J Ky Med Assoc 1996;94:287–90.
[9] Stutts JT, Kasdan ML. Disability: a new psychosocial perspective. J Occup Med 1993; 35(8):825–7.
[10] Stutts JT, Kasdan ML, Hickey SE, et al. Reflex sympathetic dystrophy: misdiagnosis in patients with dysfunctional postures of the upper extremity. J Hand Surg Am 2000;25A(6): 1152–6.

ELSEVIER
SAUNDERS

Clin Occup Environ Med
5 (2) 225–234

CLINICS IN
OCCUPATIONAL AND
ENVIRONMENTAL
MEDICINE

Determining Causation of Work-Related Upper Extremity Disorders

Robert M. Szabo, MD, MPH

Department of Orthopaedic Surgery, University of California, Davis, School of Medicine, 4860 Y Street, Sacramento, CA 95817, USA

Causation

Before addressing the specific topic of this article, it is important to consider criteria used for establishing causality. Ultimately, causality of a disorder is established based on systematic reviews of the available evidence provided by epidemiologic studies supported by biomechanical and biologic laboratory experiments. There are several types of epidemiologic studies, and each type has strengths and weaknesses particularly worth noting when trying to establish causation. The principal designs used for observational epidemiologic studies include surveillance, cross-sectional survey, case control design, prospective cohort study, and randomized, controlled trial.

Surveillance involves a systematic collection of data on cases of disease (or exposures of interest), the purpose of which is to monitor a population for departures in the typical number of cases observed over time. Surveillance data can be analyzed for trends, and they have been used for analyses to generate and test hypotheses. The cross-sectional study or prevalence study is typically a single survey in which exposures and the outcome of interest are determined at the same time. It is important to note that the temporal association between exposure and outcome cannot be established in this study design. The case control study starts

E-mail address: rmszabo@ucdavis.edu

doi:10.1016/j.coem.2005.11.003 **occmed.theclinics.com**

with identification of individuals with disease (or the outcome of interest) and a sample of individuals without the disease (or outcome of interest). The two groups are then compared for history of exposures. The principal limitation of this study design is the potential for recall bias because cases (with the outcome of interest) are more likely than their controls to recall details of their exposures. The prospective (cohort) study involves the identification of a population in which individuals are characterized by the presence or absence of exposure and then followed over time for development of the disease or other outcome of interest. Although this design is stronger than the others because temporal association can be established, it cannot discriminate whether the association of the exposure to outcome is caused by self-selection into the exposure condition. The randomized, controlled trial is essentially a prospective study that has the added feature of random allocation of the exposure of interest. The advantages of the randomized, controlled study and the prospective study are similar, yet the trial has the advantage of having a procedure to remove the influence of direct or indirect self-selection into the exposure categories. The principal disadvantages of the trial design include the fact that it may be unethical to randomize persons to exposures that are estimated from previous work to be harmful, that randomization of exposure works well on average but sometimes can result in an uneven distribution of characteristics in the subgroups being compared, and that maturation and historical changes can occur during the course of the study (which change the exposure categories of the two initial groups). Each study design results in a summary measurement that estimates the risk of disease or (outcome of interest) in the exposed to the unexposed. This measurement quantifies the strength of association.

For epidemiologic studies, the original criteria for causality have been ascribed to Sir Bradford Hill [1]. In addition to strength of association, his criteria include temporality of association, consistency of association, specificity of association, dose-response association, and biologic plausibility. The strength of association refers to the magnitude of the measure of the association; the larger the measure, the more confident one can be that the association might be causal. There are no cast iron rules for the minimum size of the association. Temporality of association refers to the need in establishing causality that the exposure must precede the outcome in time. Consistency of association refers to the finding of similar findings within subgroups of a study or similarity of findings in other populations studied at different times even using different study designs. The greater the degree of consistency across studies, the more confident one can be that the association under study is likely to be causal. Specificity of association means if a factor is associated with one outcome but not others, then a causal inference is more likely. The dose-response relationship involves noting a positive and direct association between levels of the exposure and levels of the outcome, along with interventions in which reduction in levels of exposure is associated with reduction in levels of the outcome. Biologic plausibility refers to likelihood to which an association is compatible with existing knowledge of biologic mechanisms.

Although we treat the process of establishing causation as a science, we must be aware that the basic principles are founded in philosophy. Causal inference is "the logical development of a theory based on observations and a series of arguments that attributes the development of a disease to one or more risk factors" [2]. Different philosophical constructs underlie the process for making an inference. Reasoned arguments can proceed from either the general to the particular (deductive reasoning) or from the particular to the general (inductive reasoning). The traditional view of science is that induction, the formation of a hypothesis based on observation, is cardinal to the scientific method. Without using the term "induction," David Hume asserted that the generalization of a necessary connection between cause and effect cannot be obtained from experience but depends on "contiguity and succession," which rely on repeated observations [3]. The flaw of a hypothesis derived by induction is that it can be refuted by the first observation that proves an exception. For example, if by induction we believe that all hearts are on the left side of the chest, our belief can be destroyed by one patient with dextrocardia.

Sir Karl Popper, one of the most influential philosophers of science of the twentieth century, rejected induction by claiming that it is always possible to produce a theory to fit any set of observations [4]. He popularized a so-called hypothetico-deductive system, which advocates deductive reasoning to make predictions from the hypothesis and state what it prohibits. Knowledge is advanced by testing hypotheses and discarding those that fail. In this refutation or falsification perspective, the epidemiologist starts with a hypothesis and collects data about some disease, which are then used either to refute or accept the hypothesis. By alternating between generating hypotheses and collecting data, many hypotheses can be discarded without performing any experiment. Experiments are reserved for testing the hypothesis that has survived the deductive efforts to falsify it in observational studies [5]. Others argue that no scientific theory can be falsified with certainty because a theory always uses auxiliary hypotheses, and if some of the consequences of the theory turn out to be false, one of the auxiliary hypotheses rather than the theory may be false [6]. For instance, every study involves the auxiliary hypothesis that no unknown bias is occurring, and it may be this hypothesis that is falsified rather than the main theory. Any study can only falsify a theory to a degree. Judgments about causality in epidemiology depend on scientific revolutions argued that the evidence that scientists draw on is determined by an overriding contemporary paradigm that dictates the way in which a causal sequence is construed [7]. For example, tuberculosis was thought to be a social disease in the nineteenth century and malaria was thought to be caused by bad air. Once Robert Koch discovered the tubercle bacillus and developed the germ theory, a new paradigm was used to attribute specific diseases to specific agents [8]. As the causality hypotheses are tested and refuted, similar paradigm shifts are occurring with the way we think about so-called "repetitive stress injuries." One of the first steps to be made in an epidemiologic study is agreeing on a case definition.

Sorting out the relevant definitions

"Repetitive stress injury" is a term that represents a spectrum of musculoskeletal complaints that are attributed to occupations believed to be hazardous by involving repetitive physical motions. Nonmedical diagnoses of "cumulative trauma disorder," "repetitive stress (strain) injury," and "repetitive trauma injury" are used interchangeably for disorders of soft tissues that are believed to develop over periods of weeks, months, and years as a result of repeated action [9]. Close examination reveals that the terms used to describe those disorders are no more than umbrella terms used to describe any painful condition of the upper extremity in workers engaged in repetitive activities, however. The vague definition of these disorders indicates that scientific studies have failed to show that low-force repetitive motion causes injury, which is partly because of an increased promotion of ergonomics as a solution to the incidence of repetitive motion injury in the workplace. This finding has been accompanied by a proliferation of ergonomic literature in which conclusions are based on associations and suggestions [10,11]. Many proponents of ergonomics assert that the elimination of certain risk factors that relate to force, repetition, posture, and duration can prevent or even cure repetitive motion disorders. Scientific support for this position is scant, however [12,13]. Given the uncertainty about causation, "work-related musculoskeletal disorders" (WRMSDs) is the more readily accepted term used to describe these phenomena.

Although pain from repetitive stress injury is attributed to mechanical tissue overload secondary to repetitive, forceful movements and awkward postures, repetitive work is often associated with "low job control, skill discretion, and decision latitude" [14]. Before embarking on preventive measure interventions, it is critical to establish whether musculoskeletal pain related to repetitive work is caused by the physical characteristics of the work or the psychosocial factors. One must examine the hypothesis: "Primary and secondary prevention strategies can reduce the incidence of musculoskeletal injuries, illnesses and disorders in the workplace." Primary prevention is defined as the intervention undertaken before members of the population at risk have acquired a condition of concern (eg, educational programs before starting employment). Secondary prevention is defined as the intervention undertaken after individuals have experienced the condition of concern (eg, introduction of ergonomic measures in individuals with symptoms of upper extremity pain).

In 2004, Williams and colleagues [15] performed a rigorous analysis by a systematic review of the literature to evaluate the available evidence on workplace rehabilitation interventions for work-related upper extremity disorders. They stated that the effectiveness of the available studies to date was limited by small sample sizes, lack of standardized outcome measures, and inadequate reporting of interventions and results, and they concluded that the evidence for workplace interventions for work-related upper extremity disorders has not been established [15]. More importantly, reliance on ergonomics to the exclusion of medical and health risk factors can have adverse consequence for patients because an underlying disease is often left undiagnosed when the symptoms are so easily ascribed to repetitive motion in the workplace. Repetitive stress injury is not a diagnosis, and the failure to make a correct diagnosis by labeling a patient with repetitive stress injury is harmful, as was witnessed in numerous repetitive stress injury legal cases described in the literature [16].

The incidence of WRMSDs is significant. According to Bureau of Labor and Statistics data, in 1994, 92,576 repetitive motion cases of the upper extremity resulted in lost days of work, with 37,804 (40.8%) of them being from carpal tunnel syndrome [17]. Although a high prevalence of WRMSDs has been reported in professions that require high force wrist motions, such as assembly line workers, meat packers, and materials handlers, much of the recent focus has been on keyboard operators, whose activities, although repetitive, do not require high force. In an effort to capitalize on the prominence and publicity surrounding claims that typing on computer keyboards has caused an epidemic of repetitive stress injuries, several years ago, prominent, well-financed plaintiffs' lawyers began filing claims against computer manufacturers under the products' liability theories of defective design and failure to warn. Their efforts, however, have met with abject failure before juries and judges and they have abandoned the litigation. Few, if any, "mass torts" have met with similar failure [16].

Much of the confusion surrounding WRMSDs arises from a misunderstanding of the definitions of the relevant terms. An occupational disease is one in which there is a direct cause and effect between a hazard and the disease. Silicosis is a clear example of an occupational disease in which silica, the hazard, is essential to producing the occurrence of the disease. A disease is considered work related, however, when the work environment and the performance of work contribute significantly, but as one of several factors, to the causation of disease. Epidemiologists refer to risk factors as being associated with rather than causes of a particular disease because it is often not possible to establish a link between cause and effect. Causal inference is the logical development of a theory based on observation and a series of arguments that attributes the development of a disease to one or more risk factors. Inference depends on prior knowledge, intuition, insight, and uncertainty (probability) [2,18].

Evaluating the association

In examining the association between risk factors (exposures) and a disease (outcome variable), the risk factors and the disease should be well defined. For an acute traumatic injury (eg, a fall that results in a fractured wrist), the relationship between the trauma and the injury is clear. This is often not the case for WRMSDs. For some conditions such as carpal tunnel syndrome, the pathology can be defined and measured objectively with electrodiagnostic studies. Most WRMSDs of the upper extremity fall into a more amorphous category, such as hand pain, in which there is no objective way to define the condition or measure its severity, and there is no clear anatomic correlate for the symptoms. For these disorders, we rely on workers' self-reports or survey data, which tend to overestimate the prevalence of a disorder. Social, cultural, and medicolegal issues significantly affect the reporting of WRMSDs. In the National Health Interview Survey in 1988, 1.4% (1.87 million) of working US adults reported that they had a "condition affecting the wrist and hand called carpal tunnel syndrome." Only 0.53% (675,000) indicated that this diagnosis was made by a "health care provider" [19].

A worker's decision to report a symptom is influenced by personal, psychosocial, and economic factors. The progression from symptom to disability is influenced strongly by these same factors. Monotonous work, high perceived work load, time pressure, low control on the job, and lack of social support are related to musculoskeletal symptoms [20]. When a worker reports an upper extremity musculoskeletal symptom while at work, the "workplace paradigm" automatically labels the symptom as a work-related disorder, and the search begins for what workplace physical factor caused the worker's pain. Many risk factors have been implicated with repetitive stress disorders, such as force, repetition, posture, and vibration. A major criticism of the term "repetitive stress" is that it implies that the cause is repetition. Medically, "injury" implies damage to tissues. "Repetition and stress" imply that repetitive mechanical forces applied to tissues cause the injury, yet no information exists regarding the frequency, magnitude, duration, or rate that renders these forces harmful. The relationship between physical loads and musculoskeletal disease still has not been quantified, and contradictory evidence persists because of poor measurement of exposures and lack of specific diagnoses. Arguably, symptoms of aches and pains that precede the status of disease or injury are important to recognize, because many patients present with such symptoms. Progression to disease, however, is the exception rather than the rule or one would expect a greater prevalence in reports of disease states.

Despite the fact that the relative contribution of occupational and nonoccupational physical loads has not been addressed sufficiently in epidemiologic studies, ergonomists promote the concept that from the perspective of prevention and treatment, all work-related factors can be modified and should be modified [21]. There is little doubt that most ergonomic interventions increase comfort in the work environment, which is of great benefit to the worker; however, WRMSDs have led ergonomists to recommend legislation that requires expensive redesign of the workplace based on the unproven claim that WRMSDs are disabling physical conditions. Although ergonomists may create a more comfortable environment, they have not lowered the incidence of these disorders. One study from Australia reported an increase in the incidence of repetitive stress injuries even after ergonomic redesign of the workstation and instituting rest periods from keyboarding every hour [22]. A Cochrane review evaluated 15 randomized, controlled trials that studied conservative interventions (eg, exercises, relaxation, physical applications, biofeedback, myofeedback, and work place adjustments) for adults who suffered from upper extremity WRMSDs. The conclusions were "There is insufficient evidence about the effectiveness of conservative interventions for people with upper extremity work related disorders" [23]. Specifically, the authors stated that "The benefit of expensive ergonomic interventions in the workplace (such as new chairs, new desks, etc.) is not clearly demonstrated" [23]. They also found limited evidence for the effectiveness of keyboards with an alternative force displacement of the keys or an alternative geometry [23].

Carpal tunnel syndrome is one of the most well-recognized hand diseases attributed to repetitive stress. The syndrome's clinical picture of pain and paresthesias on the palmar-radial aspect of the hand, which is often worse at night, is readily recognized. Carpal tunnel syndrome is a condition of middle-aged people and is more common in women. In the first population-based study on carpal tunnel syndrome, the mean age at diagnosis was 50 years for men and 51 years for women; women accounted for 78.5% of the cases [24]. The rise in frequency and distribution change of carpal tunnel syndrome is blamed on forceful and repetitive hand motion associated with advance of automation and work specialization. Much faster work rates may require that production workers or data entry personnel repeat a single or limited number of tasks tens of thousands of times a day. Of the 37,804 cases of carpal tunnel syndrome reported in the 1994 Bureau of Labor and Statistics data, 7897 (8.5%) were attributed to repetitive typing or key entry, 5106 (5.5%) to repetitive use of tools, and 10,960 (12%) to repetitive grasping or moving objects except tools [17].

We currently know that in the general population, however, people involved with repetitive activities at work have an equal prevalence rate of carpal tunnel syndrome as do persons who are not [25]. More specifically, Atroshi and colleagues [25] found that the prevalence for carpal tunnel syndrome for repetitive hand or wrist motion was 2.4% compared with 2.7% for nonrepetitive motion (95% CI for the difference, −2%, −1.5%; $P=0.69$). To deliver rational preventive measures for workers with carpal tunnel syndrome, valid and scientifically sound information about the true association between repetitive exposures and median neuropathy must be established [26]. Primary prevention is aimed at reducing or controlling the workplace risk factors. Although keyboarding actually seems to have a protective effect from developing symptoms of median nerve compression compared with many other occupations [27], a tremendous amount of money has been spent on the design, promotion, and use of new keyboards. Many of these ergonomic designs, which claim to reduce symptoms, are based on changing the forearm rotation to less pronation. One study suggests that 45° pronation is the ideal position to reduce carpal tunnel pressures [28]. When adjusting for the usual shoulder position when seated in front of a computer terminal (20°–30° abduction), this is the exact position of forearm rotation used with the common, everyday keyboard design. Wrist splints have been used in the treatment of carpal tunnel syndrome but are currently marketed as protection for people in so-called high-risk occupations. Because wrist flexion/extension increases carpal tunnel pressure, which in turn inhibits median nerve function, it seems reasonable to use a splint that maintains the wrist in neutral position; however, one study demonstrated that carpal tunnel pressures were higher with splint use at baseline and during repetitive hand activity (typing), which perhaps suggests some external compression [29]. For a detailed discussion of occupational carpal tunnel syndrome see the article by Szabo [26].

Barsky and Borus [30] consider repetitive stress injury a functional somatic syndrome that is more characterized by symptoms, suffering, and disability than by demonstrable tissue abnormality. As such, repetitive stress injury is a product of somatization, the reporting of somatic symptoms that have no pathophysiological explanation, amplified by medicalization in which uncomfortable bodily states and isolated symptoms are reclassified as diseases for which medical treatment is sought [31]. Other functional somatic syndromes include multiple chemical sensitivity, sick building syndrome, chronic fatigue syndrome, Gulf War syndrome, and fibromyalgia. Patients with these syndromes experience exacerbation of suffering by a "self-perpetuating, self-validating cycle in which common, endemic, somatic symptoms are incorrectly attributed to serious abnormality, reinforcing the patient's belief that one has a serious disease" [30]. Because the condition is portrayed as catastrophic and disabling, the condition is likely to worsen and the person assumes the sick role [30]. Macfarlane and colleagues [32] found that workplace dissatisfaction had a higher relative risk associated with forearm pain than did repetitive activity and that "no increased risk was associated with typing for more than 30 minutes without a break." They concluded that "Psychological distress, aspects of illness behavior, and other somatic symptoms are important predictors of onset of forearm pain in addition to work related psychosocial and mechanical factors. Misleading terms such as 'cumulative trauma disorder' or 'repetitive strain injury,' implying a single etiology should be avoided" [32]. Clauw and Williams [33] put forth another causal hypothesis that may be a compromise between the psychological and physiologic mechanisms. They presented a model in which the chronic regional pain and other symptoms that an individual experiences (eg, with repetitive stress injury) are attributable to what they call "chronic multisymptom illness" rather than to tissue damage or a biomechanical dysfunction of the upper extremity. They further claim that evidence supports centrally mediated physiologic changes manifest as symptoms of pain and fatigue in some individuals who experience chronic stressors and draw the analogy as Barsky and Borus did—to fibromyalgia and chronic fatigue syndrome [33].

Despite the absence of proof that ergonomics has effects beyond comfort, the National Institute for Occupational Safety and Health promotes the following perspectives [34]: there is a higher incidence of pain to disability in occupations with high levels of exposure to physical factors, there is a strong biologic plausibility of the relationship between incidence and causative exposure factors in high exposure settings, research clearly demonstrates that special interventions can reduce the rate of musculoskeletal disorders for workers who perform high-risk tasks, although none is universally effective, and high levels of exposure, especially in combination with exposure to more than one physical factor, provide strong evidence of a causal relationship between physical factors and WRMSDs. This hypothesis has been refuted, although disagreement still thrives.

The physician's role

It is our job as good, caring physicians to be knowledgeable and understanding of the social and political issues relevant to our workers' compensation patients. The importance of determining work relatedness goes beyond who legally assumes responsibility for paying the medical bills in the workers' compensation system. A straightforward discussion early in the medical evaluation of a patient with carpal tunnel syndrome, for instance, should take place when the patient claims that the computer causes his or her disease. A frank discussion often spares the patient the dehumanizing medical-legal merry-go-round brought into existence by physicians with conflicting opinions and by ergonomists and lawyers [35]. A patient caught up in this morass often becomes bitter, recalcitrant, anxious, and neurotic [35]. Rehabilitation and return to work are prolonged, and proper treatment may never be rendered because no further consideration is given to other potential diagnoses once the patient is labeled with occupational carpal tunnel syndrome or repetitive stress injury. Most patients' intentions is not to defraud the workers' compensation system. They become victims of a system that inadvertently promotes incapacity in the workers whom it was designed to help. Many patients do not understand the concepts of causation, and often a short discussion to explain these concepts is warranted. Time and money can be saved on useless physical interventions. Future intervention research should not neglect the potential biobehavioral pathways that must be addressed if we are to help our patients [36,37].

References

[1] Hill A. The environment and disease: association or causation. Proc R Soc Med 1965;58: 295–300.
[2] Kleinbaum DG, Kupper LL, Morgenstern H. Epidemiologic research: principles and quantitative methods. New York: Van Nostrand Reinhold; 1982.
[3] Hendel C. Hume selections. New York: Charles Scribner's Sons; 1955.
[4] Susser M. The logic of Sir Karl Popper and the practice of epidemiology. Regul Toxicol Pharmacol 1986;124:711–8.
[5] Buck C. Popper's philosophy for epidemiologists. Int J Epidemiol 1975;4:159–68.
[6] Pearce N, Crawford-Brown D. Critical discussion in epidemiology: problems with the Popperian approach. J Clin Epidemiol 1989;42:177–84.
[7] Kuhn TS. The structure of scientific revolutions. 2nd edition. Chicago: University of Chicago Press; 1970.
[8] Susser M. Falsification, verification and causal inference in epidemiology: reconsiderations in the light of Sir Karl Popper's philosophy. In: Rothman KJ, editor. Causal inference. Chesnut Hill (MA): Epidemiology Resources Inc.; 1988. p. 32–57.
[9] Armstrong T. Ergonomics and cumulative trauma disorders. Hand Clin 1986;2(3):553–65.
[10] Rempel D, Tittiranonda P, Burastero S, et al. Effect of keyboard design on hand pain. J Occup Environ Med 1999;41:111–9.
[11] Tittiranonda P, Rempel D, Armstrong T, et al. Effect of four computer keyboards on computer users with upper extremity musculoskeletal disorders. Am J Ind Med 1999;35:647–61.
[12] Stanton NA, Young MS. What price ergonomics? Nature 1999;399:197–8.

[13] Vender MI, Kasdan ML, Truppa KL. Upper extremity disorders: a literature review to determine work-relatedness. J Hand Surg Am 1995;20A:534–41.
[14] Bonde JP, Mikkelsen S, Andersen JH, et al. Understanding work related musculoskeletal pain: does repetitive work cause stress symptoms. Occup Environ Med 2005;62(1):41–8.
[15] Williams R, Westmorland MG, Schmuck G, et al. Effectiveness of workplace rehabilitation interventions in the treatment of work-related upper extremity disorders: a systematic review. J Hand Ther 2004;17:267–73.
[16] Szabo RM, King KK. Repetitive stress injury: diagnosis or self-fulfilling prophecy? J Bone Joint Surg Am 2000;82A(9):1314–22.
[17] Mackinnon SE, Novak CB. Repetitive strain in the workplace. J Hand Surg Am 1997;22A(1): 2–18.
[18] Rothman K. Causes. Am J Epidemiol 1976;104:587–92.
[19] Tanaka S, Wild DK, Seligman PJ, et al. The US prevalence of self-reported carpal tunnel syndrome: 1988 national health survey data. Am J Public Health 1994;84:1846–8.
[20] Bongers PM, deWinter CR, Kompier MJ, et al. Psychosocial factors at work and musculoskeletal disease. Scand J Work Environ Health 1993;19:297–312.
[21] Viikari-Juntura E. Risk factors for upper limb disorders: implications for prevention and treatment. Clin Orthop 1998;351:39–43.
[22] Hocking B. Epidemiological aspects of repetition strain injury in Telecom, Australia. Med J Aust 1987;147:218–22.
[23] Verhagen AP, Bierma-Zeinstra SMA, Feleus A, et al. Ergonomic and physiotherapeutic interventions for treating upper extremity work related disorders in adults. Cochrane Database Syst Rev 2004;1:CD003471.
[24] Stevens JC, Sun S, Beard CM, et al. Carpal tunnel syndrome in Rochester, Minnesota, 1961 to 1980. Neurology 1988;38:134–8.
[25] Atroshi I, Gummesson C, Johnsson REO, et al. Prevalence of carpal tunnel syndrome in a general population. JAMA 1999;282(2):153–8.
[26] Szabo RM. Carpal tunnel syndrome as a repetitive motion disorder. Clin Orthop 1998;351: 78–89.
[27] Nathan PA, Takigawa K, Keniston RC, et al. Slowing of sensory conduction of the median nerve and carpal tunnel syndrome in Japanese and American industrial workers. J Hand Surg Br 1994;19B(1):30–4.
[28] Rempel D, Bach JM, Gordon L, et al. Effects of forearm pronation/supination on carpal tunnel pressure. J Hand Surg Am 1998;23A:38–42.
[29] Rempel D, Manojlovic R, Levinsohn DG, et al. The effects of wearing a flexible wrist splint on carpal tunnel pressure during repetitive hand activity. J Hand Surg Am 1994;19A:106–10.
[30] Barsky AJ, Borus JF. Functional somatic syndromes. Ann Intern Med 1999;130:910–21.
[31] Barsky AJ, Borus JF. Somatization and medicalization in the era of managed care. JAMA 1995;274:1931–4.
[32] Macfarlane G, Hunt I, Silman A. Role of mechanical and psychosocial factors in the onset of forearm pain: prospective populated base study. BMJ 2000;321:1–5.
[33] Clauw DJ, Williams DA. Relationship between stress and pain in work-related upper extremity disorders: the hidden role of chronic multisymptom illnesses. Am J Ind Med 2002;41(5): 370–82.
[34] Bernard BP, editor. Musculoskeletal disorders and workplace factors. Cincinnati (OH): US Department of Health and Human Services; 1997. p. 5a1–29.
[35] Ireland DCR. Repetition strain injury: the Australian experience—1992 update. J Hand Surg 1995;20A:553–6.
[36] Bongers PM, Kremer AM, ter Laak J. Are psychosocial factors risk factors for symptoms and signs of the shoulder, elbow, or hand/wrist? A review of the epidemiological literature. Am J Ind Med 2002;41(5):315–42.
[37] Feuerstein M. Biobehavioral mechanisms of work-related upper extremity disorders: a new agenda for research and practice. Am J Ind Med 2002;41(5):293–7.

ELSEVIER
SAUNDERS

Clin Occup Environ Med
5 (2) 235–247

CLINICS IN
OCCUPATIONAL AND
ENVIRONMENTAL
MEDICINE

Prevention of Delayed Recovery and Disability of Work-Related Upper Extremity Disorders

Jane Derebery, MD, FACOEM[a,*],
William H. Tullis, MD, FAPA[b]

[a]*Concentra Health Services, 10200 Broadway Boulevard, Suite 201, San Antonio, TX 78217, USA*
[b]*Neuropsychiatric Associates of Austin, 1600 West 38th Street, Austin, TX 78731, USA*

Work relatedness has been identified as a risk factor for delay in recovery and disability, which essentially means that an occupational medicine clinician can expect to face challenging, at-risk patients on a daily basis [1–4]. The workers' compensation system was developed to ensure that workers who were injured or made sick by their work would receive the needed medical care. The structure of the system that has gradually evolved, however, is unfortunately one that can promote disability in certain high-risk patients.

In most cultures it is the norm for some members of society to transform emotional or social distress into somatic complaints. Distressed persons tend to develop symptoms that are medically correct in a given society at a given period of time. Since 1986, when Occupational Safety and Health Administration (OSHA) first mandated that repetitive trauma cases were reportable, we have seen an exponential growth in claims being filed, based on the premise that routine repetitive activities in American workplaces can cause injury and disease of the upper extremity, despite considerable controversy in the scientific literature about the credibility of this premise [5–8].

Social and economic reinforcers of the idea that repetitive arm use causes repeated trauma have spawned entire heath care industries, and although this has most certainly provided economic benefit to health care providers, it is an unhealthy solution for high risk patients, and a costly one for industry.

A clinician's attitude about an illness/injury and its prognosis is a major influence on a patient's attitude about recovery and disability. Perhaps the great-

* Corresponding author.
E-mail address: Jane.derebery@concentra.com (J. Derebery).

doi:10.1016/j.coem.2005.11.013 **occmed.theclinics.com**

est obstacle to successful treatment of a patient with a work compensable disorder is the inability of a clinician to differentiate between a patient's pain and distress. Pain is not solely a sensory response but is influenced by many factors, including genetics, personal history, current health, and broader social, emotional, and cultural factors of each patient. Our Western culture's biologic model of disease focuses on the physical aspects of illness, and the nonphysical suffering associated with disease and injury is often ignored. With the disease model, a physician may be inclined to misinterpret a patient's distress or anxiety about a medical condition as indicating a more serious physical condition that requires more elaborate treatment or diagnostic testing rather than understanding the distress as an indication that a patient is having difficulty coping because of psychosocial or other extraneous stressors.

Treatment that focuses on physical fixes, such as carpal tunnel release for nonspecific hand pain and tingling, may appeal to the patient and physician, but it is invariably ineffectual in addressing the problem. The marked increase in disability from work-related upper extremity disorders in the United States this past decade attests to the dismal success rate of this model of management [9]. Since the mid-1980s, societal focus on repetitive work activities as the cause of hand and arm pain has motivated many people to seek treatment for upper extremity aches and pains, whereas previously they would not have done so [10]. Some workers present for assessment of even minor symptoms for fear of developing arthritis, carpal tunnel syndrome, or some other serious problem. This occurrence should come as no surprise considering the stories in newspapers and magazines about the dangers of repetitive use of our arms and hands.

Another fallacy of the workers' compensation system is that physicians are expected to treat each presumably work-related disorder as if the main or only cause were an activity, accident, or toxin at the workplace. This flies in the face of the widely accepted biopsychosocial model of disease causation as being generally multifactorial and complex in origin. When the causation of a given disorder is oversimplified and poorly understood, as it often may be when approached one dimensionally, the treatment may be inadequate or inappropriate, which results in poor and unsatisfactory outcomes.

Nontraumatic musculoskeletal pain is caused and influenced by multiple factors, as are many other medical conditions (eg, diabetes and heart disease), and identifiable disease need not be present. Musculoskeletal aches and pains are generally self-limiting and are viewed as normal occurrences that we all experience intermittently throughout our lives. Although certain industries have a predominantly higher incidence and prevalence of musculoskeletal or cumulative trauma complaints, there may be wide variation among similar and even identical companies within each industry, which illustrates that the problem is not caused simply by the repetitive or demanding physical activities of the workers but also by other factors, including poor management, job dissatisfaction, socioeconomic circumstances, and differences in the overall health status of individual workers [1,6,10].

Not uncommonly, evaluations of disabled patients with chronic pain syndromes reveal evidence of varying degrees of iatrogenicity caused by clinicians who treated patients when a problem was still acute or subacute. Perhaps having a better understanding of the more commonly associated factors that can lead to disability and using some practical cognitive behavioral therapy (CBT) early in the course of treatment enable a physician to reduce the likelihood that a patient will experience delayed recovery, disability, and chronicity.

There is a focus on incorporating CBT techniques and principles into the treatment of acute and subacute physical disorders in the office setting by a treating physician. Using CBT also may be an effective way for a clinician to interact with a worker whose condition is not progressing as anticipated. CBT has not been studied in the acute or subacute setting; however, the techniques of CBT can be applied in just a few minutes during the course of an office visit, which often saves a clinician time in the long run. Doing so also may reduce the recovery time and risk of recurrence. CBT initially was developed by a psychiatrist, Aaron Beck, in the 1980s and refers to an approach to treatment that recognizes the role of physical, psychological, and social factors in how pain and illness are experienced. More recently it has been combined with elements of the older discipline of behavioral therapy to make a technique called CBT, which has proved effective in treating various mental and physical disorders. It is based on the idea that a patient's thought and behavior patterns can affect the experience of illness and injury and may either impede or facilitate recovery [11,12].

CBT is being used in the treatment of chronic pain conditions, and in formalized chronic pain programs the technique has met with good success. CBT is also a widely accepted therapy for treatment of clinical depression, anxiety, addictions, eating disorders, stress, relationship problems, anger, and insomnia [11,12].

Evaluation of a patient who is experiencing a delayed recovery

Most patients who receive compensation recover uneventfully. If, at any point in the course of treatment, a patient is identified as having a delay in recovery or a disproportionate disability, the clinician must determine if the primary problem is physiologic or psychological. Patients at risk of developing chronic complaints generally can be identified early in the course, and outcome improves greatly when these patients are identified within the first few weeks after an injury. Although a physician must assess appropriately for physiologic explanations for a delay in recovery, psychosocial factors also must be assessed actively and thoroughly, because statistically it is more likely that psychosocial factors are causative rather than that the problem is a physiologic one. Either sociodemographic or psychosocial measures can provide accurate predictions of disability risk for patients with low back pain by the subacute period [13,14].

Because the workers' compensation system does not reward rapid recovery, some patients may use an injury maladaptively as a solution to some problem and do not necessarily have any significant degree of psychopathology, although there may be issues such as the personal integrity or maturity level of the patient. Such employees may use an injury as a means to escape responsibility, avoid noxious work, retaliate against a supervisor or company, or receive sympathy and attention. Frank malingering and conscious fraud are relatively uncommon and are discussed in the article by Dean S. Louis elsewhere in this issue.

Disability is a learned behavior that may have little correlation with the degree of actual impairment, and a patient's ability to recover is influenced by factors such as motivation, social support, attitudes about work, and family dynamics. In cases in which a patient is found to have significant psychogenic or nonorganic components to an injury, generally some true physical component exists that also must be addressed [15,16].

When negative beliefs delay recovery

There are two particularly common belief systems of patients with workers' compensation claims that can present primary obstacles to recovery. One is the belief of being exploited or mistreated by a boss or company. The other is a belief that a problem is not being taken seriously and that an underlying disorder is being missed. In communication we are ambivalent about what and how much we want to express ourselves. Part of us wants to make ourselves known and part of us wants to stay in hiding, so we code our messages. Decoding is always guesswork in which we can only infer what words and actions mean. Behaviors are easily observable; they are on the outside. Thoughts, however, are not directly observable; our only clues are a person's words and actions (behavior). Emotions are often concealed carefully. Our only clue to a person's feelings comes to us indirectly through behaviors.

The belief by a patient of being exploited or mistreated frequently manifests as hostility and rejection toward health care providers. The belief by a patient of being ignored and misdiagnosed often takes the form of distress and anxiety that do not respond to reassurances by the health care provider.

The hostile patient

Obstacle: Belief of being exploited and mistreated

A patient with this type of belief often manifests behavior that is accusatory, provocative, or even offensive. Such angry behavior may mask fear and frustration and is likely to elicit defensive or antagonistic responses by a physician if the physician does not recognize the process. Such responses reinforce a patient's belief that he or she is the victim of an uncaring or even hostile system.

The anxious/distressed patient

Obstacle: Belief that a serious disorder is being missed

The other major belief category that can be an obstacle to recovery involves the idea that a patient has a debilitating illness that could be overlooked by the physician. A patient's anxiety and distress, if not properly understood, can engender anxiety in a physician and often are misinterpreted as pain, which leads to misdirected care. The behaviors that such patients who are at high risk for chronicity may manifest include passivity, dependency, and helplessness. Behaviors of this kind often invoke responses of caretaking and enabling on the part of health care providers and others. Health care providers can find themselves colluding with patients by placing them on medical leave or restricted duty even when it does not seem warranted by the findings.

When psychiatric disorders contribute to disability

There is always a psychological component to any illness or injury, and unless appropriately addressed, such factors can complicate or delay recovery from illness or injury. When a patient's recovery is delayed and medically unexplained physical symptoms are associated with or caused by an underlying psychiatric disorder, the prompt recognition and proper management of the disorder can improve greatly a patient's prognosis. Box 1 lists psychiatric diagnoses that should be included in the differential diagnosis of medically unexplained physical symptoms in a patient with a work-related injury or illness [17,18]. All but depression and anxiety are included in the Diagnostic and Statistical Manual-IV classification of somatoform disorders. The common feature of somatoform disorders is the presence of physical symptoms that suggest a general medical condition but cannot be explained fully as the direct effects of a given medical condition or as an effect of a known substance [18].

Box 1. Psychiatric causes of medically unexplained physical symptoms

Anxiety
Depression
Delusional disorder: somatic type
Somatoform disorders
Conversion disorder
Hypochondriasis
Body dysmorphic disorder
Pain disorder

Most patients who have a psychiatric diagnosis that leads to medically unexplained physical symptoms are assessed and treated in medical settings, not psychiatric ones. Because the patients can be frustrating to a physician, they may have their care terminated early or shunted to a consultant and are at risk of undergoing excessive and inappropriate diagnostic evaluations and procedures [17].

Depression

Depression is the most common concomitant disorder associated with chronic pain disorders. When present, it must be identified and treated appropriately along with the painful condition if a good outcome is to be expected [19]. Some common treatments of depression have been found to be efficacious in treating patients with chronic pain [20,21]. Patients should be questioned regarding past history of depression, change in weight, attention, or appetite, tearfulness, trouble concentrating, low energy, difficulty sleeping, and suicidal ideation.

Anxiety

Anxiety disorders also can impede recovery and contribute to disability. A patient who is not progressing should be assessed for symptoms of distress, such as disproportionate symptoms, excessive anxiety, complaints of shortness of breath, and stocking glove arm or hand symptoms. There may be a clear element of anxiety with evidence of fearfulness, pressured speech, agitation, tearfulness, and emotional lability [18].

Somatization disorder

Historically this disorder was known as hysteria, and to fit Diagnostic and Statistical Manual-IV criteria for inclusion, a patient must have a pattern of recurring, multiple somatic complaints that start before age 30. The complaints cannot be explained fully by any known medical condition or be the direct effects of some substance. If they occur in the presence of a medical condition, such as a work-related injury, the physical complaint or disability cannot be in excess of what would be expected. A variant of this disorder is the undifferentiated somatoform disorder, which is a residual category for persistent somatoform disorders that do not meet the full criteria for somatization disorder or another somatoform disorder. The common feature of undifferentiated somatoform disorder is one or more physical complaints that persist for 6 months or longer, cannot be explained fully by any known medical condition, and are not produced intentionally or feigned by a patient (eg, malingering or factitious injury) [10,11,18].

Conversion disorder

This disorder refers to a patient's loss of function that cannot be explained solely by known medical processes. The deficits involve either motor or sensory dysfunction that suggests a neurologic or other medical condition. An example is that of a patient who presents with a paralyzed or weak hand that he or she attributes to typing. Disorders are usually monosymptomatic and time limited, with most patients experiencing symptom resolution within 1 month. Approximately 25% of patients may have a recurrence [18,22].

Hypochondriasis

This disorder has been described as stemming from inappropriate processing of somatic information, which causes a patient to believe that he or she has a serious disease [17]. The patient is hypervigilant, with attention paid to benign body sensations, and is convinced that a pathologic process is responsible. The hypochondriacal patient has obsessions and fears serious disease, despite negative medical evaluations and reassurance. It is estimated that hypochondriasis occurs in 5% to 10% of primary care patients [22]. Hypochondriacal tendencies also can indicate underlying depression [18].

Body dysmorphic disorder

This disorder refers to a condition in which a patient has a preoccupation with an imagined or exaggerated physical defect, which subsequently causes significant psychological and social disability [17,22]. An example is that of a woman whose second-degree burn on her hand dorsum from a work-related accident subsequently heals with a mild hyperpigmented discoloration. Despite having full hand function, she is adamant that the scar is disfiguring and insists that she receive further treatment.

Psychogenic pain disorder

Psychogenic pain, which is seen commonly in general practice, refers to the situation in which pain causes significant distress and disability and yet is inadequately explained pathophysiologically. A patient's pain is the predominant focus of clinical attention. Patients who have chronic pain seek medical attention at a rate almost five times that of the general population. This disorder is difficult to differentiate from other somatoform disorders, factitious disease, or malingering and is associated with a real potential for abuse of drugs in a minority of these patients [17]. Sleep disturbances are common in patients with persistent, chronic pain or depression and can be secondary to these conditions or can be the primary disorder that causes depression or chronic pain [23].

Taking a history

Patients with persistent pain and a delayed course of recovery must be asked about depression and sleep disturbance, because often they do not associate these conditions with their physical symptoms, may fear that if the pain is associated with depression it may not be taken as being real, or fear that it might adversely affect their workers' compensation status. If these comorbid conditions are not identified and treated, however, a patient is likely to experience misdirected treatment and a delayed recovery.

Other aspects of the history also may shed light on what an illness/injury may mean to a patient. Did the patient's job recently change? Did the patient feel that he or she did not receive adequate training for the job? Does the patient feel that he or she has been neglecting children? Did the symptoms occur after an argument with a supervisor? Did a friend or family member recently have a major health problem? Such information can give the health care provider a better idea of what the symptoms may be triggering in the patient's mind or what things in the patient's mind may have triggered the symptoms. Does the patient fear that this is a progressive condition that could cripple him or her? Is the illness a means to escape what feels like an overwhelming situation? Could the injury be symbolic of perceived neglect and maltreatment by employers?

Questions should be directed toward identifying what a patient's beliefs and thoughts are regarding the injury/illness. Knowing the beliefs and thoughts is key to understanding the feelings and behaviors that are likely to elicit responses that may reinforce the beliefs. For example, if a patient feels that a company does not care about his or her welfare, one can be sure that if a complete history and thorough examination are not performed, the patient is apt to see the physician as an extension of the uncaring company. If a clinician is too quick to reassure that nothing is seriously wrong, then the doctor is likely to be viewed as a company doctor speaking for the company, which is not concerned about the patient.

Management

Maladaptive beliefs or contributing psychosocial factors that are identified during the evaluation must be addressed or at least understood by the clinician. Using cognitive behavioral techniques may be helpful in dealing with maladaptive beliefs. Regardless of whether they are aware of this, most skilled and effective clinicians already use certain CBT techniques with their patients. Breaking down the individual CBT principles and clarifying how and why they work can help to use them more effectively. CBT is based on the following principles:

- Patients have an underlying belief (often erroneous) about an illness or injury
- The belief generates automatic thoughts when patients experience symptoms
- These thoughts generate feelings
- The feelings lead to behaviors

- The behaviors elicit responses
- The responses reinforce the underlying belief or conception

For example, a person with hand and arm pain may have a firm belief that activity and exercise will increase pain and worsen the condition, whereas regular activity and exercise actually hasten recovery. The patient avoids activity, which causes him or her to experience pain on the occasions of activity, which reinforces the belief that hinders recovery. Another person may have the belief that exercise is good for most problems and that "no pain means no gain." This person likely will have a shorter duration of hand pain and reinforce the belief that facilitates recovery.

If a clinician can alter an underlying maladaptive conception, automatic thoughts, or behaviors, the whole cycle can be changed for the better. The goal of CBT is to replace unhealthy ways of thinking and behaving with ways that are healthier. The fact that 50% of patients with carpal tunnel syndrome symptoms improve with placebo treatment illustrates how strong an influence the patient's belief system is [24].

Managing the hostile patient

With hostile patients it is important not to become defensive or antagonistic, which is easier said than done. It is helpful to keep in mind that a patient does not really know you and that it could not be personal. When the hostility is overt it can be helpful to comment to the patient that he or she seems angry and ask what that is about.

Hostility is usually a reaction to fear, which indicates that such a patient believes that he or she is at risk of being mistreated or neglected by an employer or a health care provider. Changing such a belief requires the physician to convince the patient that he or she is concerned about the patient's welfare and not just carrying out the policies of the "oppressive" employer. Convincing requires showing concern by active listening (periodically repeating or rephrasing a patient's comments to indicate hearing the concerns) and occasionally making empathic comments (ie, "that must have been terrifying" or "I can see how that was very frustrating for you"). A hostile patient is projecting a role onto the physician that fits with the patient's belief system. You can help to change the belief if you respond empathically and in a caring manner rather than in the way the patient expects. This does not mean that the physician, therapist, or staff should tolerate abusive behavior. If it occurs, appropriate limits should be set as calmly as possible, like a good parent with an out-of-control child.

A clinician must understand that in many cases a hostile patient has an unconscious fear of abandonment by the clinician and consequently must be given the message repeatedly that the physician is concerned about and committed to the patient's health and well-being.

Managing the anxious, distressed patient

Performing a thorough history and physical examination is important for changing the beliefs of anxious patients. It is also crucial to take their concerns seriously and explain that you are looking for the type of problem they fear that they may have. Active listening and empathic comments are also helpful. Clinical judgment and cost concerns should limit the number of diagnostic tests ordered, but the rationale for such decisions should be explained carefully to patients. Such patients can be helped to change this particular cycle by physicians actively involving them more in their assessment and treatment. Let them know how important their history is and demonstrate by your responses that you value their input. Approach their problem as if they were athletes eager to return to participation in their sport.

Giving such patients a way to conceptualize their illness helps to relieve some of their fear of the unknown. Involving them actively in their treatment gives them more of a sense of control and counters the feelings of helplessness. Giving them some sort of time schedule as to when they can expect certain improvements in their condition helps to neutralize their fears that the illness may be progressive or long-term. It is not so important that patients understand the pathophysiology of the illness, but it is helpful for them to learn that the clinician knows and cares enough to educate. In this way, patients can feel understood.

Treating distressed or anxious patients requires active listening. When patients have talked out the distress, offer feedback and suggestions for management. Providing a conceptual model of the condition to patients gives them a sense of control. When making suggestions, give choices. Provide reassurance, and when terminating treatment, do not say you are "discharging" a patient. Instead, tell patients that because they are doing well, no follow-up appointment is necessary, but they can return if needed.

A key aspect of a physician's duties regarding patient care is to provide reassurance to apprehensive patients. Waddell and colleagues [25] confirmed the importance of allaying fears and apprehensions that patients may have regarding their injury or condition. A key aspect of allaying fears is providing reassurance that a condition will resolve and not be disabling. Experts in interpersonal communication feel that reassurances frequently can have a negative impact on communication, particularly when one or more persons is interacting under stress [26]. Because as physicians we must advise and reassure regularly, we must understand the possible negative impact of doing so and develop the skill to advise and reassure in an effective manner. How could reassurance possibly act as a negative barrier? Reassuring is a way of seeming to comfort another person while actually doing the opposite. The word "comfort" comes from two Latin words and literally means "strengthened by being with." Reassuring does not allow the comforter to really be with the other. It can be a form of emotional withdrawal. If a physician reassures prematurely, patients are at risk of viewing the reassurance as a brush off.

Providing reassurance

Before offering reassurance, the following first six steps must be completed to have maximal probability of effectiveness. (1) Elicit a detailed description of the symptoms. (2) Elicit the affective meaning of the symptoms. (3) Examine the patient. (4) Make a diagnosis. (5) Explain the pathophysiology of the symptoms. (6) Permit the patient to have the symptom. (7) After all the above, provide reassurance. Making a diagnosis does not mean that a disease must be found. The diagnosis can be nonspecific, such as myalgia, arthralgia, backache, or headache. Understanding patients' concepts of an illness allows you to incorporate their fears in your explanation. "It is not arthritis." "It is not cancer." "It is not a blood clot." It may be important to include pertinent negatives in our reassurance.

Other management components

Treating underlying depression and anxiety may reduce physical symptoms significantly and reduce disability. Antidepressants may benefit medically unexplained physical symptoms [27], fibromyalgia [28], and chronic pain. The analgesic effect of antidepressants is independent of the antidepressant effect and seems strongest in the mixed receptor or predominantly noradrenergic activity (eg, bupropion, venlafaxine, and duloxetine) [29,30]. CBT has shown promise, even when used for brief periods when the focus is on beliefs about etiology, sick role behaviors, and symptom amplification [10–12]. Regular aerobic exercise is effective not only in treating mild depression but also in improving work endurance. Evidence suggests that regular aerobic programs can be beneficial to median nerve function and may reduce hand symptoms from carpal tunnel syndrome [31–33].

Return to work

Hand and arm pain occurs commonly in working and the nonworking populations and is seldom disabling. The pain is real; most patients are not faking. Lost time disability is rarely indicated, however, and if restrictions are needed they should be time contingent, not pain contingent. When objective evidence justifies lost time or prolonged restrictions, a physician has the responsibility to specify what the needed restrictions are. When patients have persistent pain that cannot be substantiated by objective means, they must decide if they are willing to tolerate their job duties. Patients, not the physician, should make the decision regarding whether to return to work or work under restrictions. Patients must understand that in such cases, the work is not considered disabling nor are patients considered to be disabled from work [33,34].

Summary

The mind clearly plays an important role in every patient's presenting symptoms and the course of their recovery. A patient's beliefs produce the thoughts that lead to the feelings that result in the behaviors that elicit the responses that reinforce the original beliefs. Sometimes the beliefs may be healthy ones or at least ones that are not an obstacle to recovery. With these patients, the path to recovery should be straightforward. When a patient's beliefs present an obstacle to successful treatment, however, the cycle must be broken with techniques such as the ones discussed previously if a prolonged, complicated, and costly course of illness and treatment is to be avoided. CBT can be a helpful adjunct in treating such patients.

There is always a psychological component to any illness or injury, and unless appropriately addressed, such factors can complicate or delay the recovery from illness or injury. When a worker experiences a delayed recovery and unexpected disability, psychosocial contributing factors must be assessed for and managed.

References

[1] Derebery VJ, Tullis WH. Delayed recovery in the patient with a work compensable injury. J Occup Med 1983;25:829–35.
[2] Hirschfeld A, Behan R. The accident process: etiological considerations of industrial injuries. JAMA 1963;186:193–9.
[3] Krusen E, Ford D. Compensation factor in low back injury. JAMA 1958;166:1128–33.
[4] Peterson M, Wilson J. Job satisfaction and perceptions of health. J Occup Environ Med 1996;38: 891–5.
[5] Nathan P, Meadows K, Istvan J. Predictors of carpal tunnel syndrome: an 11 year study of industrial workers. J Hand Surg [Am] 2002;27A:644–51.
[6] Hadler N. Arm pain in the workplace: a small area analysis. J Med 1992;34:113–9.
[7] Nathan P, Keniston R, Meadows K, et al. Longitudinal study of median nerve sensory conduction in industry: relationship to age, gender, hand dominance, occupational hand use, and clinical diagnosis. J Hand Surg [Am] 1992;17A:850–7.
[8] Vender M, Kasdan M, Truppa K. Upper extremity disorders: a literature review to determine work-relatedness. J Hand Surg [Am] 1995;20A:534–41.
[9] Bureau of Labor Statistics. Survey of occupational injuries and illnesses, nonfatal (OSHA recordable) injuries and illnesses: case and demographic characteristics. Available at: www.bls.gov/iif/oshcdnew.htm.
[10] Barsky A, Borus A. Somatization and medicalization in an era of managed care. JAMA 1995; 274:1949–54.
[11] Kreonke K, Swindle R. Cognitive-behavioral therapy for somatization and symptom syndromes: a critical review of controlled clinical trials. Psychother Psychosom 2005;69(4):205–15.
[12] Barsky A, Ahern D. Cognitive behavior therapy for hypochondriasis: a randomized controlled trial. JAMA 2004;291(12):1464–70.
[13] Burton AK, Waddell G, Bartys S, et al. Screening to identify people at risk of long-term incapacity: a conceptual and scientific review. Disability Med 2003;3(3):73–83.
[14] Pincus T, Burton AK, Vogel S, et al. A systematic review of psychological factors as predictors of chronicity/disability in prospective cohorts of low back pain. Spine 2002;27:E109–20.

[15] Ford CV. Illness as a lifestyle: the role of somatization in medical practice. Spine 1992;17: S338–40.
[16] Lucire Y. Constructing RSI: belief and desire. Sydney (Australia): UNSW Press; 2003.
[17] Neimark G, Caroff S, Stinnet J. Medically unexplained physical symptoms. Psychiatr Ann 2005;35(4):298–305.
[18] Somatoform disorders. In: First M, editor. Diagnostic and Statistical Manual. 4th edition. Washington, DC: American Psychiatric Association; 1994. p. 445–70.
[19] Blair M, Robinson R, Katon W, et al. Depression and pain comorbidity: a literature review. Arch Intern Med 2003;163(20):2433–45.
[20] Lin E, Katon W, VonKorff M, et al. Effect of improving depression care on pain and functional outcomes among older adults with arthritis: a randomized controlled trial. JAMA 2003;290(18): 2428–9.
[21] Sindrup B, Bach F, Madsen C. Venlafaxine versus imipramine in painful polyneuropathy: a randomized controlled trial. Neurology 2003;60(8):1284–9.
[22] DeMichele S, Stinnett J. Somatoform and related disorders. In: Gliatto MF, Caroff S, Kaiser R, editors. Psychiatry for primary care practioners. Washington, DC: American Psychiatric Publishers; 1999.
[23] Smith MT, Haythornthwaite J. How do sleep disturbance and chronic pain inter-relate? Insights from the longitudinal and cognitive-behavioral clinical trials literature. Sleep Med Rev 2004; 8(2):119–32.
[24] Goodyear-Smith F, Arroll B. What can family physicians offer patients with carpal tunnel syndrome other than surgery? A systematic review of nonsurgical management. Ann Fam Med 2004;2:267–73.
[25] Waddell G, Newton M, Henderson I, et al. A fear-avoidance beliefs questionnaire and the role of fear-avoidance. Pain 1993;52(2):157–68.
[26] Bolton R. Barriers to communication. In: People skills. New York: Simon & Schuster; 1979. p. 14–26.
[27] O'Malley P, Jackson J, Santro J, et al. Antidepressant therapy for unexplained symptoms and symptom syndromes. J Fam Pract 1999;48(12):980–90.
[28] O'Malley P, Balden E, Tomkins G, et al. Treatment of fibromyalgia with antidepressants: a meta-analysis. J Gen Intern Med 2000;15(9):659–66.
[29] Maizels M, McCarberg B. Antidepressants and antiepileptic drugs for chronic non-cancer pain. Am Fam Physician 2005;71(3):483–8.
[30] Songer D. Psychotherapeutic approaches in the treatment of pain. Psychiatry 2005;19–24.
[31] Dunn AL. Exercise treatment for depression: efficacy and dose response. Am J Prev Med 2005; 28:1–8.
[32] Nathan P, Wilcox A, Emerick P, et al. Effects of an aerobic exercise program on median nerve conduction and symptoms associated with carpal tunnel syndrome. J Occup Environ Med 2001; 43(10):840–3.
[33] Melhorn JM. Working with common upper extremity problems. In: Talmage J, Melhorn J, editors. A physician's guide to return to work. Washington, DC: American Medical Association Press; 2005. p. 181–213.
[34] Van der Windt D, Croft P, Penninx B. Neck and upper limb pain: more pain is associated with psychological distress and consultation rate in primary care. J Rheumatol 2002;29:564–9.

ELSEVIER
SAUNDERS

Clin Occup Environ Med
5 (2) 249–266

CLINICS IN
OCCUPATIONAL AND
ENVIRONMENTAL
MEDICINE

Ergonomic Considerations in Work-Related Upper Extremity Disorders

Brian Pearce, MSc

Humane Technology Ltd., 203 Swithland Lane, Rothley, Leicestershire LE7 7SJ, UK

It is customary, indeed it almost seems to be obligatory, in any commentary on ergonomic considerations in work-related upper extremity disorders (WRUEDs) to pay homage to Ramazzini and his observations on scribes in 1713. Although this is no bad thing, many commentators leave the impression that WRUEDs were first recognized in the eighteenth century, whereas Dembe [1] noted that the ancient Egyptian writer of the Sellier Papyrus observed that the arms of masons were often "worn out by work," and Hippocrates provided one of the earliest known accounts of chronic disorders caused by repetitive occupational hand movements, in 550 BC. Although anecdotal comments by long-dead doctors and their predecessors may suggest that they were ahead of their times, it is possible that their perceptions of the causes of the maladies they observed were not necessarily correct.

The other apparently obligatory observation in more recent commentaries on WRUEDs is the dramatic growth in reports of such disorders in the last few decades. The paradox from an ergonomics perspective, which few commentators seem to have addressed, is that this has occurred at a time when, compared with the conditions in the first half of the twentieth century, working hours have been reduced, work in general is physically less arduous, extensive health and safety legislation has been introduced, occupational health facilities have improved, and ergonomics knowledge has been disseminated widely.

It can be argued that it is precisely because of these societal developments that we have become more aware of and more concerned about such disorders. Employees have become less tolerant of experiencing aches and pains, let alone serious injuries, which in less enlightened days were considered part and parcel of

E-mail address: b.g.pearce@HumaneTechnology.co.uk

doi:10.1016/j.coem.2005.11.012 *occmed.theclinics.com*

a job, an inevitable consequence of labor. Although the workplace has become safer, expectations also have grown and what we are observing is perhaps an increase in reporting rather than an increase in incidence. A more controversial explanation is that expectations have grown to the extent that virtually any ache or pain in the neck, back, or upper limbs can be perceived as being caused by repetitive strain or cumulative trauma, and what we are observing, at least in part, is the redefinition of "the heartache and the thousand natural shocks that flesh is heir to" as work-induced injuries.

Another explanation is that the dramatic growth in reports of WRUEDs is at least in part and despite moves toward an evidence-based approach the result of an increase in the willingness of some medical practitioners to ascribe a diagnostic label to that which might previously have been put into the "do not know" category. Some disorders and dysfunctions of the upper extremities are more clearly defined than others. Some conditions present with clear, objective, clinical signs of abnormality, whereas others are diagnosed on the basis of a patient's response to examination or merely a patient's report of a certain pattern of symptoms. Although it would be nice to think that all medical practitioners used common diagnostic criteria, it is clear that they do not [2]. Differing sensitivity and specificity of diagnostic criteria can lead to discrepancies in diagnosis and prevalence estimates in different countries.

Denotations and connotations

The failure to distinguish the denotation from its connotations has been described by Cohen and colleagues [3] as the fundamental epistemologic error in the epidemic of upper extremity disorders that swept (parts of) Australia in the 1980s. The use of terms such as "cumulative trauma disorder" and "vibration white finger" as diagnostic labels presumes the mechanism that has caused the dis-ease or disease. The term "repetitive strain injury" (RSI) has the added disadvantage of implying that someone, usually the employer, is culpable.

Even terms such as "work-related upper extremity disorder" and "work-related upper limb disorder," the term preferred in the United Kingdom, can be misinterpreted. It is clear that common upper extremity disorders, such as carpal tunnel syndrome and lateral epicondylitis, can be constitutional in origin and inevitably arise in the workplace and are almost inevitably perceived by some individuals as work-related. A condition can be perceived as work related when work activities merely make the sufferer aware of some previously asymptomatic condition or influence an individual's ability to work. It does not necessarily follow that a condition that is perceived or referred to as work related has been caused, aggravated, exacerbated, or accelerated by work activities. Many people die in bed, but that does not mean that beds are a serious hazard. Just because an upper extremity disorder manifests in the workplace does not mean that the work is hazardous.

The social construction of injury

Anecdotal evidence suggests that some individuals who have naturally occurring sensations or symptoms of a constitutional disorder can develop what might be described as an iatrogenic injury. For example, "I'm afraid you will continue to have this arm problem so long as you keep your current job" might be accurate advice, but it can be interpreted as implying a causal relationship between the work and the disorder. Moreover, some practitioners in medical and related disciplines seem willing to make categorical statements concerning the occupational nature of often vague signs and symptoms without giving due consideration to other possible causes and without ever having seen the workplace.

An individual with an upper extremity sensation becomes a patient upon visiting the practitioner, can leave the consulting room with the perception of being an employee with a work-induced disorder, and becomes a claimant with an injury upon encountering the compensation system. This is part of what is termed the "social construction of injury," in which various factors, including the press coverage of compensation claims, induce in employees the perception that they have suffered work-induced injuries for which someone is liable. This is in no way intended to suggest that such individuals construct their own injuries. It merely suggests that how individuals, health and safety practitioners, doctors, lawyers, and ergonomists perceive musculoskeletal sensations can be influenced strongly by external factors and the circumstances in which we find ourselves placed [4,5].

Unraveling the complex relationships between work activities and upper extremity disorders and quantifying the true scale of the problem requires sophisticated epidemiologic studies. Existing studies seem to be open to widely different interpretations, however. For example, using admittedly rigorous criteria, Vender and colleagues [6] concluded that none of the 2054 studies reviewed established a causal relationship between distinct medical entities and work activities. In contrast, in reviewing much of the same literature and acknowledging that epidemiologic evidence is often based on studies with weak designs, Buckle [7] suggested that the consistency in the results strongly supported a relation with factors arising from work. Criticism [8] of more recent reviews by NIOSH [9] and the National Academy of Science [10] seems to confirm that when it comes to the interpretation of the evidence, belief can be stronger than the rigor of the scientific method, such that supportive evidence is preferentially recruited and the inconvenient is downplayed or suppressed.

Acknowledging that psychological factors and factors extrinsic to work can play an important role in the recognition and interpretation of symptoms does not deny the reality of the symptoms or the legitimacy of the concerns. A country's system of compensation can promote or inhibit the reporting, presentation, and rehabilitation of upper extremity disorders [11,12]. Recognizing that WRUEDs can be contagious in that they can arise from ideas and beliefs about work, spread by word of mouth rather than mouth to mouth, acknowledges that factors intrinsic to the workplace but not necessarily to the work itself can play an important role in the interpretation and attribution of symptoms. Recognizing that for some employees a splint is more a badge of injury than a therapeutic aid and that illness behavior may be a natural response to the prevailing circumstances does not imply malingering but suggests that psychological factors and factors extrinsic to work can play an important role in the treatment and rehabilitation of upper extremity disorders.

Much of the ergonomics literature gives the impression that virtually all upper extremity disorders are caused primarily by work and that by applying an ergonomics approach they will be eliminated. They will not. Correctly applied, an ergonomics approach can reduce the likelihood of work-induced disorders and assist in accommodating individuals who have work-related disorders, but it cannot eliminate disorders that have been (mistakenly) attributed to work by social processes.

The role of ergonomics

Ergonomists view systems of work as involving complex interactions among human, social, and technological components. Unfortunately, a simplistic view of ergonomics has grown up that focuses on the physical aspects of work: force, repetition rates, and posture. Although the ergonomics approach emphasizes that psychosocial factors are equally important, they are frequently misunderstood or ignored. It has to be acknowledged, however, that it is often far easier to tinker with the physical features of the workstation than tackle the root cause of the problem (eg, the design of the job). Tinkering with the physical features of the workstation might well produce a Hawthorne effect, which gives the illusion of a successful ergonomics intervention.

In an ideal world, all equipment, workstations, and working environments would be designed to meet optimum ergonomics criteria. In practice, the degree to which ergonomics principles are applied—or should be applied—is a function of the duration and intensity of the task being performed and the anticipated adverse consequences on persons performing the task. Inevitably, ergonomics criteria are not absolute. A cost-benefit equation must be considered. Ergonomics principles clearly are not inconsistent with the need to protect the health and safety of employees, but ergonomists seek to provide not only a safe but also a satisfying and efficient system of work. The corollary of this proposition is that to describe a system of work as not meeting optimum ergonomics criteria does not necessarily imply that it is unsafe or potentially injurious. Herein lies fertile ground for the seeds of misunderstanding to flourish.

Where does discomfort stop and a WRUED start? Work can be tiring, but what level of fatigue is unacceptable? Is stiffness or soreness after unaccustomed work a WRUED? Take, for example, an employee who has some sort of (previously undiagnosed) constitutional disorder, the symptoms of which are exacerbated by work, or at least the employee perceives they are. In the current climate in which virtually any manual activity is perceived as being capable of causing injury, the employee reports a WRUED. Recommending some sort of change in the workstation or work regimen with the intention of making the employee more comfortable is not a bad thing, but unless this change is explained carefully, the change can be interpreted as confirmation that something about the work caused or materially contributed to the employee's disorder, particularly if the change is perceived by the employee as making work more comfortable.

At around the same time, the employee may have been prescribed some sort of medication or provided with a splint or physiotherapy, any or all of which may have reduced the discomfort experienced at work. However, the change in the work—the ergonomics intervention—rather than the treatment can be perceived by the employee as reducing the discomfort, reinforcing the perception that the work itself was the cause of the employee's disorder. Interventions, medical or ergonomic, must be accompanied by carefully considered explanations that are not aimed solely at the individual concerned.

If an employee's fellow workers interpret the ergonomics intervention as suggesting that something about the work caused their colleague's symptoms, there may be calls for similar changes in their work, which is newly and inaccurately perceived as hazardous. Herein lies fertile ground for localized epidemics of WRUEDs to flourish. Experiences of dealing with such epidemics in several organizations in which there was no obvious hazardous activity suggested that failing to deal appropriately with the early cases, which were subsequently shown to be primarily constitutional in origin, permitted ideas and beliefs to flourish and the reporting of WRUEDs to increase for no obvious reason.

In one such epidemic, in which clusters of WRUEDs appeared in some premises but not others, despite there being an identical system of (boring) work in all the premises, significant increases in reporting of WRUEDs occurred shortly after the visits of ergonomics consultants who had been called to solve the problem. A subsequent analysis of sickness absence data showed that the proportion of sickness absence caused by WRUEDs had increased significantly in the 'infected' premises but that the overall level of sickness absence was fairly constant throughout the epidemic and much the same in all the premises.

Problems also seem to arise when well-intentioned but inexperienced practitioners attempt to incorporate ergonomics principles into risk management strategies. This approach has given rise to the bizarre notions of ergonomic risk factors and, worse, ergonomic injuries. Such oxymorons demonstrate a fundamental misunderstanding of ergonomics principles and of the differences between dis-ease and disease and of the differences between hazard and risk. Ergonomic recommendations that are intended to promote comfort and efficiency are (mis)interpreted as essential health and safety requirements. The dumbing down of ergonomics principles results in attention being focused solely on that which is easy to measure or change.

Nowhere is the misunderstanding of ergonomics principles more apparent than in the way upper extremity disorders among computer users have become associated with deficiencies in the physical features of the workstation or some aspect of the posture adopted to use the computer, which might, at most, have a trivial influence on comfort. For example, most diagrams show a seated computer user in a bolt upright posture with the forearms horizontal. Simple observation of any large group of computer users shows that many individuals do not sit in this way.

One of the founding fathers of ergonomics, Professor Etienne Grandjean, referred to the bolt upright posture depicted in so many guidelines as wishful thinking and suggested that such diagrams were a throwback to the early days of mechanical typewriters, which required key forces of several hundred grams and were more easily operated in such a posture [13]. Modern electronic keyboards, which require much less force and have less key travel than mechanical typewriters, are mainly operated by finger movements with hardly any assistance of the forearms. Computer users do not sit and do not need to sit in a bolt-upright posture. Diagrams that purport to show optimum postures for computer use are useful aids but should not be interpreted too rigorously. The more general point is that the body is built to move. Maintaining a static, constrained posture quickly can lead to discomfort. There is no one perfect posture for any particular task. Unless constrained by some feature of the tools used or the workstation, users usually adopt postures that they find comfortable.

Upper extremity disorders among computer users are worthy of note for several others reasons, not least because of the sheer number of people whose work involves the use of a screen, keyboard, and mouse. If we have got it wrong about what constitutes ergonomically sound computer usage, there is potentially a big problem. Some apostles of RSI would undoubtedly argue that we have got it wrong and that the dramatic increase in the reporting of WRUEDs in the last few decades has run more or less in parallel with the dramatic increase in the use of computers at home and at work. However, the most significant contribution to the debate about ergonomic considerations in WRUEDs arising from considering upper extremity disorders among computer users is the explanatory models of WRUEDs that they have generated. It is to such explanatory models that attention is turned.

Explanatory models of work-related upper extremity disorders

In attempting to explain the abnormal, many models seem to ignore the normal (ie, that most work does not give rise to upper extremity disorders) and seem to assume that the cause of any WRUED is work. Many explanatory models look much like sketches of space stations and seem to exist in a vacuum, whereas in reality WRUEDs exist in a sea of potential influences. Sauter and Swanson [14] provide one of the most sophisticated explanatory models of the possible linkages between upper extremity disorders and computer use found in the literature. They describe their ecological model as "an integration of the generic psychosocial stress process into the traditional biomechanical model of musculoskeletal disorders." Although at various points they allude to environmental forces and to the literature arising from the epidemic of RSI in Australia in the 1980s, their ecological model does not explain what happened in Australia.

Explanations of the Australian repetitive strain injury epidemic

What is clear from the literature is that the Australian RSI epidemic in the 1980s was not caused simply by the physical demands of work. It was not resolved by simplistic ergonomic interventions but by changing perceptions of the hazards and the likely harms arising from work activities that had become distorted by the well-intentioned but misguided activities of the medical profession and related disciplines and various other factors unrelated to work.

A series of articles in the *Medical Journal of Australia* in September 1987 amounted to a recantation of the RSI concept by the Australian medical establishment. Ferguson [15] began his leading article entitled "Putting the epidemic to rest" by stating "With hindsight, the gigantic and costly Australian epidemic called 'repetition strain injury' (RSI) can be seen as a complex psychosocial phenomenon with elements of mass hysteria, that were superimposed on a base of widespread discomfort, fatigue and morbidity, The epidemic, to which the medical and legal professions, managements, unions, governments and the media have all contributed, is now waning, but endemic work-related musculoskeletal syndromes remain. It is important to examine the epidemic in the hope that its recurrence in some other guise may be prevented."

In an article entitled "RSI: a model of social iatrogenesis," Cleland [16] argued that clinical observations suggested that the pain may be caused by a disturbance of sensory function rather than a chronic unhealed tissue injury and went on to suggest that "With the model of disturbed sensory perception, one can predict a number of the effects of environmental influences upon disease expression and severity." He noted that educational programs and treatments that promote the idea that work activities can cause injury would be likely to cause further concern, which, in turn, could further heighten regional sensory awareness and complete a vicious cycle. In criticizing the term RSI, Cleland [16] also referred to "iatrogenesis by nomenclature."

Wright [17] argued that not only the term but also the concept of RSI should be abandoned. Hocking's article [18], which reported an inverse relationship between keystroke rate and rates of reporting of RSI in Telecom Australia, clearly showed the inadequacy of the traditional biomechanical model. Hocking [19] later postulated an iceberg of disease, the iceberg representing a mass of ill-defined bodily sensations and subclinical disease, only the tip of which is perceived as pain or clinically presented illness. Many other symptoms are coped with and remain subclinical. The iceberg floats in a social sea, however. If the density of the surrounding sea (ie, the social environment) increases because of organizational change or medical, media, or legal influences, the iceberg rises, the tip enlarges, and more illness is presented.

Dembe [1] concluded his detailed account of how social factors have shaped physicians' recognition and conception of cumulative trauma disorders in the United States by referring to events in Australia: "A question raised by the Australian experience is whether history will repeat itself in the United States, with CTDs eventually being subsumed as varieties of 'occupational stress,' 'nervous fatigue,' or some other comparable concept that implies a fundamentally psychological origin."

Another explanation of the Australian epidemic that is rarely referred to explicitly in the politically correct literature but was strongly hinted at in the Australian popular press, particularly as the epidemic declined, is that RSI was a good excuse for a 'sickie' (Australian slang for a sickness absence) and an easy route to unwarranted compensation. The press strongly hinted that many RSI sufferers were malingering or at least exaggerating their symptoms. Cynics suggested that the acronym RSI stood for retrospective supplementary income.

The most detailed account of the Australian RSI epidemic published so far is in a book entitled "Constructing RSI belief and desire," by an Australian forensic psychiatrist. Like many other Australians who have commented on the epidemic, however, Lucire [20] was involved intimately in the debate and holds trenchant views. Although many might question Lucire's explanation of the epidemic, there seems no reason to doubt her detailed account of the chronology of events and the key role played by the medical practitioners and related disciplines in initially legitimating and subsequently denouncing RSI.

No explanatory model of WRUEDs can afford to ignore the experiences in Australia. No satisfactory explanatory model can afford to ignore the possibility that some WRUEDs are (directly) induced by the (physical) demands of work, the possibility that some WRUEDs are a function of domestic and leisure activities, the probability that some WRUEDs are intrinsic to the individual, and the clear evidence that WRUEDs are multifactorial in origin and that factors extrinsic to work can shape ideas and beliefs about WRUEDs.

Beyond psychosocial processes: a contextual model

The contextual model presented in Fig. 1 draws heavily on Sauter and Swanson's ecological model but attempts to place work-related disorders in a broader context by explicitly drawing attention to the range of factors that, it is suggested, can influence perceptions of upper extremity disorders. As is fitting for a model based on ergonomics principles, at its center is the individual. Individuals come in different shapes and sizes and vary in their capabilities and limitations. A significant minority have some sort of constitutional condition or at least a predisposition to some sort of disorder. Virtually all individuals experience ephemeral, naturally occurring aches and pains at some point.

The interaction of an individual with work and domestic and leisure activities, for the most part, contributes positively to mental and physical well-being.

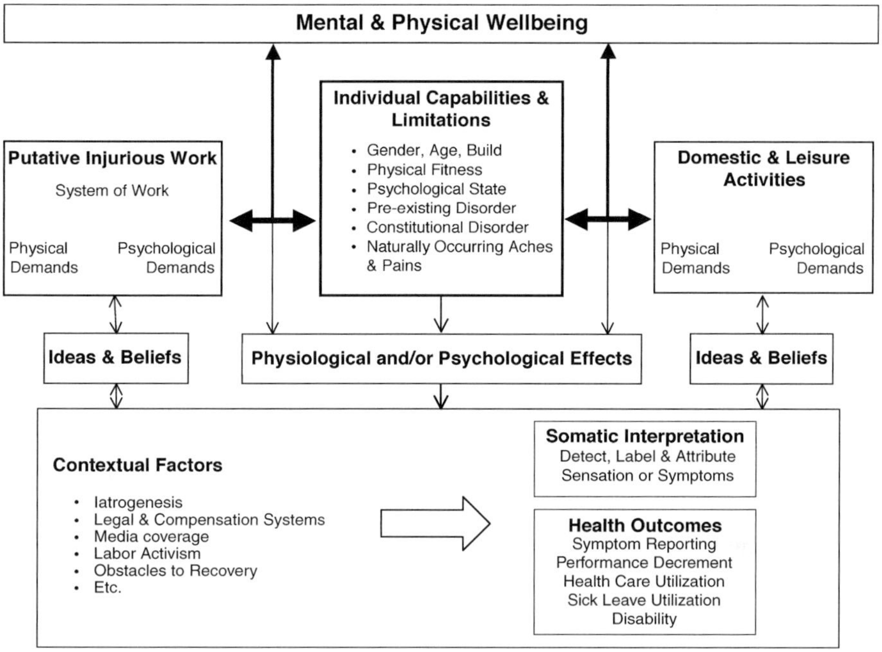

Fig. 1. A contextual model of work-related disorders.

However, if the physical or psychological demands exceed the capabilities of an individual, there is the potential for physiological and/or psychological effects. As in Sauter and Swanson's ecological model, physical damage or disease is not necessarily integral to the contextual model; however, the contextual model intentionally avoids using the terms "biomechanical strain" and "psychological strain." The other important point to note is that although physiological or psychological effects can arise from the interaction of an individual with work and domestic or leisure activities, there is also a direct path in which the etiologic focus is the individual.

As in Sauter and Swanson's ecological model, in the contextual model the psychological mediation of upper extremity disorders is considered in terms of normal psychological processes. While noting Sauter and Swanson's cautionary words about implicating psychological processes and psychiatric mechanisms in the cause of disease and possibly creating the impression that the disease is not real and of victim blaming and shifting the etiologic focus toward the worker and away from the job, an explanatory model must not prohibit an etiologic focus on the worker or ignore factors intrinsic to an individual. The contextual model implicitly acknowledges the possibility of malingering, somatization, and the exaggeration of symptoms as well as pre-existing conditions and constitutional disorders.

The contextual model explicitly acknowledges some of the factors extrinsic to work that can shape perceptions of upper extremity disorders and influence the process of somatic interpretation and the outcomes of experiencing physiological or psychological effects. Two pathways for the export and import of ideas and beliefs are shown to emphasize the sometimes starkly different and often distorted perceptions of the risks that arise from work and domestic and leisure activities. This approach is not intended to suggest that work activities are always perceived as hazardous, whereas domestic and leisure activities are not. It merely allows for the same actual level of risk or the same adverse health outcome to be perceived differently, depending on—among other things—whether the activity was indulged in voluntarily or was a requirement of work. To illustrate some of the contextual factors and pathways in this model, it is expedient to return to the issue of upper extremity disorders among computer users and focus attention on experiences in the United Kingdom.

Work-related upper extremity disorders in the United Kingdom

The first recorded epidemic of WRUEDs in the United Kingdom occurred in the civil service in the 1830s and was associated with the introduction of the steel nib to replace the quill pen [21]. The report of an enquiry into a subsequent epidemic in the early 1900s among telegraphists [22] was suggested by Lucire [23] to be the origin of the term "nervous breakdown." The rapid growth in the use of typewriters did not give rise to any reports of similar epidemics in the United Kingdom or, as Dembe [24] noted, in the United States.

Until the importation of the term RSI from Australia in the mid 1980s, a term popularly used in the United Kingdom for virtually any WRUEDs was "teno," which was short for tenosynovitis (eg, the trade union publication, *Tackling Teno*). Pheasant [25] suggested the connection between tenosynovitis and the repetitive, short-cycle tasks of the industrial assembly line had been recognized in the United Kingdom since the 1930s. The first guidance on WRUEDs issued by the Health and Safety Executive (HSE) in 1977 suggested that tenosynovitis can occur especially in industries in which rapid, repetitive twisting and gripping movements are common [26]. All the examples given were of blue-collar work that involved obvious force. It was with the introduction of the notion of RSI and its associations with computer use that the reporting of WRUEDs took off in the United Kingdom.

Upon visiting Australia in November 1986, Waugh [27] referred to RSI as a "great innovation" and "the disease England has been waiting for." His article concluded, "I prophesy a tremendous future for this wankers' disease in Britain, as soon as a few more people learn about it. It will go through the country like a dose of salts." Clearly a few more people did learn about it, if the results from a trailer questionnaire on the 1990 Labor Force Survey are to be believed [28]: "Self-reports of musculoskeletal conditions far exceeded those of any other disease category. The estimated number of prevalent cases caused by work is 593,000 of which 50,000 fall into the RSI category, the majority of the remainder (300,000) being related to back problems." Precisely what the individuals who self-reported RSI were suffering from and how they came by their diagnoses remain open to question.

The term WRULD came into use in the United Kingdom after 1990, following the publication by the HSE of a guidance document entitled "Work related upper limb disorders: a guide to prevention" [29]. This guidance document adopted an ergonomics approach but primarily focused on blue-collar work. The opening paragraphs of this guidance made clear that musculoskeletal problems that affect the upper limbs are "common in the general population" and that "they can arise spontaneously and without any link to work." It also suggested that "The musculoskeletal system is well suited to produce repeated motions at low force levels." It dismissed the term RSI in one sentence in a footnote: "Although in recent years the term 'Repetitive Strain Injury' (RSI) has been commonly used it is medically imprecise and not sufficiently accurate to cover the conditions observed." Nevertheless, the term RSI continued to be used by the media and in trade union publications.

Media coverage of work-related upper extremity disorders

A review of the UK national press over the 10 years from the beginning of 1985 until the end of 1994 revealed that reports of compensation claims dominated the coverage of WRUEDs [30]. The image often portrayed in the national press was that of a metaphorical David, a victim of RSI, but with hand in sling rather than sling in hand, fighting several Goliaths including negligent employers, ignorant doctors, and inadequate compensation systems, but usually winning a substantial award.

A comparison of the press reports of court judgments in the five daily broadsheets with the actual wording in the judgments showed that in every case the press reports referred to RSI despite the fact that most of the disorders for which damages were awarded involved one of the more well-defined clinical conditions, such as tenosynovitis. Two further themes emerged from this analysis: the portrayal of WRUEDs as predominantly associated with keyboard or computer use and, possibly linked to this, the preoccupation of journalists to write about RSI among journalists.

From 1989, there was a significant growth in the number and the proportion of press cuttings each year that primarily referred to keyboard users. In part, this growth merely reflected the increase in the number of awards—in and out of court—to keyboard users and the consequent increase in news reports of these awards. However, most features on WRUEDs also emphasized RSI among keyboard users. Examination of the database of court judgments in claims for WRUEDs in England and Wales [http://www.HumaneTechnology.co.uk/wruld/] suggests that there were four times more blue-collar WRUED claims than white-collar claims fought through the courts during the 10 years in question. Most of these blue-collar WRUED court judgments received no press coverage whatsoever.

It can be argued that the journalists' apparent preoccupation with writing about RSI among keyboard users merely reflected the fact that literally millions of people were using keyboards. However, the journalists were themselves keyboard users and possibly had a personal and professional interest in these matters. For example, one of the longest running stories found in the five daily broadsheets concerned an apparent epidemic of WRUEDs among journalists at the *Financial Times*. Although not disputing that such an event and its subsequent industrial relations and legal ramifications were newsworthy, it is questionable whether a similar situation in an organization not associated with the media would have been afforded such extensive coverage. It can be argued that if journalists perceived that they were exposed to the alleged hazard about which they were writing when composing their stories at a computer, it would not be surprising if their objectivity in reporting on WRUEDs was sometimes compromised.

From partway through 2000, the press coverage of court hearings and judgments in claims for WRUEDs associated with computer use effectively ceased, despite several cases that might be considered noteworthy. It is perhaps no coincidence that by 2000, all known claims by journalists for WRUEDs had been thrown out and union backing for such claims seemed to have ceased. Subsequent coverage of WRUEDs usually included a reference to RSI being associated with computer use, even when the story concerned a completely different type of work. By 2000, an element of tongue in cheek writing also had begun to creep into the coverage of WRUEDs. Perhaps journalists were learning to live with their computers. It seems clear that whatever the story, RSI and computer use were, still are, and may be for some time to come indelibly (l)inked in the minds of some.

At approximately the same time that press coverage of WRUEDs associated with computer use was reaching its crescendo, the United Kingdom was introducing the first health and safety regulations that explicitly endorsed ergonomic principles by implementing European Directive 90/270/EEC "on the minimum safety and health requirements for work with display screen equipment" [31]. The resulting fiasco is a sobering lesson in how well-intentioned but misguided regulation can lead to distorted perceptions of ergonomics principles and of the low risks to which individual computer users are exposed and to the diversion of health and safety resources from arguably much more hazardous activities.

The implementation of ergonomic regulations in the United Kingdom

Despite the UK government's and employers' clear lack of enthusiasm for specific legislation on the use of computers, lawmakers decided to implement the Directive in the United Kingdom under the Health and Safety at Work etc. Act 1974, which resulted in the Health and Safety (Display Screen Equipment) Regulations 1992 (DSE Regulations) coming into force on January 1, 1993.

The HSE published its first guidance on the DSE Regulations in November 1992, that is, only 2 months before the DSE regulations came into force [32]. At approximately the same time, the HSE issued a press release to warn employers about exploitation of the DSE regulations by unscrupulous suppliers of furniture, equipment, and services [33]: "Many of the claims being made about what the legislation says and what firms must do are bogus, aimed at getting businessmen to buy advice and then undertake unnecessary measures, usually involving further services or products." The DSE regulations require employers to undertake individual risk assessments of computer users. A user is defined as "an employee who habitually uses display screen equipment as a significant part of his normal work." This risk assessment must be "suitable and sufficient" and be reviewed when "there is reason to suspect it is no longer valid" or when there has been "a significant change." The HSE's guidance suggested that before the risk assessment, the user should be provided with training and information on a formidable list of issues.

Employers are also required to ensure that any workstation meets the requirements specified in the Schedule to the Regulations, which are very similar to the requirements in the Annex to the Directive. The validity and use of many of these so-called "minimum ergonomic requirements" are open to question. For example, the schedule suggests that in designing, selecting, commissioning, and modifying software and in designing tasks using display screen equipment, the employer shall take into account five principles, one of which is that "the principles of software ergonomics must be applied, in particular to human data processing."

A "Review of Health and Safety Regulation" published by the Health and Safety Commission (HSC) in May 1994 highlighted continuing dissatisfaction with the DSE regulations and estimated that the recurring costs of the DSE regulations were similar to the recurring benefits, whereas similar cost benefit analyses of other health and safety regulations typically show the benefits far outweighing the costs [34].

Adding insult to injury

The DSE Regulations were amended by the Health and Safety (Miscellaneous Amendments) Regulations in 2002. The latest guidance on "What is a workstation?" now suggests the regulations apply to the prolonged use of "mobile phones and personal organisers that can be used to compose and edit text, view images or connect to the Internet" [35]. The revised guidance states: "Any prolonged use of such devices for work purposes will be subject to the DSE Regulations and the circumstances of such cases will need to be individually assessed." How hazardous is a personal digital assistant? "Mobile phones that are in prolonged use only for spoken conversations are excluded. . .because their display screens are small."

The guidance acknowledges that "It is not always practicable for the employer to send someone else to conduct a risk assessment for homeworkers/teleworkers (particularly in the case of mobile workers)" and that "in the case of mobile teleworkers working for very short periods in hotel rooms and similar places, the full (risk assessment) procedure may not be necessary." How hazardous is using a laptop in a hotel room? Users of laptops are told that "risk assessments for, say, half an hour's work in a borrowed office can be quite informal and need not be written down" and not to carry "equipment or papers unless they are really likely to be needed."

At the same time that the HSE published revised guidance on the amended DSE regulations, the HSE launched a revision of a leaflet that was entitled "Upper limb disorders: assessing the risks" [36] and is currently called "Aching arms (or RSI) in small businesses" [37]. Both versions of this leaflet are a triumph of graphic design over technical content. The choice of wording for the new title is difficult to understand given that, on page 3, the revised leaflet says "HSE prefers to use the general term ULD because problems might not be due to strain and there may not be any sign of injury." The HSE's revised guidance on the DSE Regulations includes the observation that "Media reports often refer to some, or all, ULDs as RSI but this term is not a medical diagnosis and can be confusing."

Why bother?

Employers who do not comply fully with the DSE Regulations, whether because of ignorance, misunderstandings, or a lack of conviction that the DSE Regulations address important health and safety issues, potentially expose themselves to criminal prosecution by the authorities responsible for the enforcement of health and safety legislation. The overall impression that can be drawn from the admittedly limited evidence currently available is that for various reasons, the authorities responsible for enforcement have viewed the DSE regulations as a low priority.

The revised guidance on the DSE regulations claims to bring the guidance up to date with "improvements in knowledge of risks." However, nowhere in the revised guidance is there any sound evidence or even a reference to a study, however, that shows that there are any significant health and safety risks to individual computer users. There is no evidence that the DSE regulations have or will bring about a significant reduction in the incidence of upper extremity disorders and the number of working days lost by computer users. More than 10 years after the DSE Regulations came into force, the organizations that foot the bill for implementing them, indeed the authorities responsible for enforcing them, might justifiably ask, "Where is the evidence of harm arising from computer use?"

The simplistic answer is in the civil courts. However, contrary to the impression given in the national press and by individuals who have a vested interest in promoting the risks of computer use, however, only a handful of the many millions of computer users in the United Kingdom have been awarded damages by the courts for WRUEDs. One of the consequences of the incorporation of the Directive into UK legislation is that the DSE Regulations can be used to assist an employee who brings civil proceedings against an employer for an injury arising from computer use by pleading a breach of statutory duty, which is generally considered to be less difficult to prove than negligence. The admittedly unusual case of *Conaty v Barclays Bank plc*, which was heard in Central London County Court in April 2000, illustrates what can happen when lawyers get involved in such matters [38].

Fiona Conaty claimed that she had developed De Quervain's syndrome in November 1994 at the age of 22 as a result of numeric data entry. Her employer accepted that they had been in breach of the DSE Regulations by failing to conduct a suitable and sufficient risk assessment, by not planning her activities so that her work at the screen was periodically interrupted by breaks and changes in activities, and by failing to train and advise her about health and safety. She was described by the judge as habitually adopting "what is agreed to be a bad posture whereby her wrist was flexed and whilst using the numeric keys subject to ulnar deviation instead of being kept straight, as is recommended." It was also noted, however, that "She used only her right hand and made no use of her thumb in keyboarding, which accordingly she stuck out to the side of her right hand." In other words, this was a claim for De Quervain's syndrome allegedly caused by the non-use of the thumb in a poor posture!

Both medical experts agreed that she had suffered De Quervain's syndrome and that they had no direct experience and were not aware of any cases in the literature of De Quervain's syndrome in a 22-year-old person without either a traumatic or hormonal cause. After reviewing the medical and ergonomics evidence, the judge said, "Although therefore there is no identified case where [De Quervain's syndrome] has been shown to be the result of deviation of the wrist not involving use of the thumb, I am not able on the evidence which includes acknowledgement of the lack of full knowledge of such relationships to dismiss such relationship as impossible." The judge found that the work was a possible cause and that he could find no other cause to identify as the probable or more probable cause. He concluded that the disorder was work related and "As such I have no difficulty in holding that it arises from the poor posture adopted by the Claimant which itself was caused by the Defendant's breaches of statutory duty, both in the layout of the workstation and lack of training and concentration of keyboarding which I have identified." He awarded a total of £235,000 damages.

Although this county court decision set no legal precedent, it seems that the DSE Regulations assisted the claimant in this particular case, the admitted breaches of statutory duty effectively determining the outcome, but where is the evidence of the DSE Regulations being of benefit in a wider context? Where is the evidence that the DSE Regulations actually reduce the incidence of work-related ill health or the number of working days lost? Persons responsible for dealing with the fallout from the DSE Regulations could be forgiven for concluding that DSE stands for "despite sound evidence."

WRUEDs among computer users have received much attention. Although there are no reliable statistics, anecdotal evidence suggests that there are probably significantly more blue-collar than white-collar WRUEDs. Regrettably, it seems as if their numbers are likely to increase, given that the HSE's latest guidance on blue-collar WRUEDs leaves the impression that virtually all upper extremity disorders, including nonspecific pain syndromes, are primarily caused by work and that by applying an ergonomics approach they can be eliminated [39]. RSI is dead—long live nonspecific pain syndromes.

Summary

This commentary perhaps has cast some light on how upper extremity disorders might be related to work and perhaps cast some doubt on the popular perceptions of ergonomics. It would be wrong, however, to leave the impression that most WRUEDs are mostly unrelated to work activities or that ergonomics has little to contribute. If a disorder influences an employee's ability to work efficiently, regardless of any ergonomic or health and safety considerations, an employer must be aware of and manage the issue. A balance must be struck, however, between encouraging employers to recognize and deal sympathetically with disorders that probably originate outside of work but influence the ability to work and disorders that probably are caused or at least are significantly aggravated or accelerated by work. The former may only require localized changes to accommodate an individual; the latter may require significant changes to be made to the overall system of work. Correctly applied, ergonomic principles can contribute to both situations. If the analysis above is even partially correct, however, neither simplistic ergonomic interventions that focus on the physical aspects of work nor elaborate ergonomic regulations will reverse the growth in reports of WRUEDs—they are part of the problem not the solution.

In the current climate, in which virtually any manual activity is perceived as being capable of causing injury and in which there is a perceived epidemic of WRUEDs, it is understandable that there are calls for the introduction of ergonomic programs and a proactive response to search out WRUEDs. Just as critical as having appropriate systems in place to identify, treat, and manage upper extremity disorders when they do arise at work is communicating to workers in kind and carefully considered words, using words that avoid overmedicalizing or attributing to work "the heart-ache and the thousand natural shocks that flesh is heir to." Although patients desire a diagnostic label for their symptoms, they should not be given labels presuming to know the causative mechanism of their condition.

Correctly applied, ergonomic principles undoubtedly can play a role in controlling the currently perceived epidemic of WRUEDs by making "workplaces that are comfortable when we are well and accommodating when we are ill" [40]. From an ergonomics perspective, however, there seems to be an urgent need to examine the true scale of the problem and the range of factors that promote and inhibit accurate perceptions of the risk of experiencing upper extremity disorders at work. There are strong arguments for promoting evidence-based practice by all the stakeholders in this complex problem.

References

[1] Dembe AE. Occupation and disease. New Haven (CT): Yale University Press; 1996.
[2] Diwaker HN, Stothard J. What do doctors mean by tenosynovitis and repetitive strain injury? Occup Med 1995;45(2):97–104.
[3] Cohen ML, Arroyo JF, Champion GD, et al. In search of the pathogenesis of refractory cervicobrachial pain syndrome: a deconstruction of the RSI phenomenon. Med J Aust 1992;156: 432–6.
[4] Spurgeon A, Gompertz D, Harrington JM. Non-specific symptoms in response to hazard exposure in the workplace. J Psychosom Res 1997;43(1):43–9.
[5] Cioffi D. Somatic interpretation in cumulative trauma disorders: a social cognitive analysis. In: Moon SD, Sauter SL, editors. Beyond biomechanics: psychosocial aspects of musculoskeletal disorders in office work. London: Taylor & Francis; 1996. p. 43–63.
[6] Vender MI, Kasdan ML, Truppa KL. Upper extremity disorders: a literature review to determine work-relatedness. J Hand Surg [Am] 1995;20A(4):534–41.
[7] Buckle PW. Clinical review: work factors and upper limb disorders. BMJ 1997;315:1360–3.
[8] Hadler NM. Occupational musculoskeletal disorders. 3rd edition. Philadelphia: Lippincott Williams & Wilkins; 2005.
[9] NIOSH. Musculoskeletal disorders and workplace factors: a critical review of epidemiologic evidence for work-related musculoskeletal disorders of the neck, upper extremity, and low back. 2nd edition. Cincinnati (OH): National Institute for Occupational Safety and Health; 1997.
[10] National Research Council and the Institute of Medicine. Musculoskeletal disorders and the workplace: low back and upper extremities. Washington, DC: National Academy Press; 2001.
[11] Hopkins A. The social recognition of repetition strain injuries: an Australian/American comparison. Soc Sci Med 1990;30(3):365–72.
[12] Waddell G, Burton AK. Concepts of rehabilitation for the management of common health problems. London: The Stationery Office; 2005.
[13] Grandjean E. Ergonomics in computerized offices. London: Taylor & Francis; 1987.
[14] Sauter SL, Swanson NG. An ecological model of musculoskeletal disorders in office work. In: Sauter SDMSL, editor. Beyond biomechanics: psychosocial aspects of musculoskeletal disorders in office work. London: Taylor & Francis; 1996. p. 3–21.
[15] Ferguson DA. RSI: putting the epidemic to rest. Med J Aust 1987;147:213–4.
[16] Cleland LG. RSI: a model of social iatrogenesis. Med J Aust 1987;147:237–9.
[17] Wright GD. The failure of the RSI concept. Med J Aust 1987;147:233–6.
[18] Hocking B. Epidemiological aspects of repetition strain injury in Telecom Australia. Med J Aust 1987;147:218–22.
[19] Hocking B. Some social and cultural anthropologic aspects of musculoskeletal disorders as exemplified by the Telecom Australia RSI epidemic. In: Moon SDS, editor. Psychosocial aspects of musculoskeletal disorders in office work. London: Taylor & Francis; 1996. p. 145–58.
[20] Lucire Y. Constructing RSI. Sydney, Australia: University of New South Wales Press; 2003.
[21] Bell C. Partial paralysis of the muscles of the extremities: the nervous system of the human body. Washington, DC: Duff Green; 1833.
[22] Great Britain and Ireland Post Office. Report of the departmental committee on telegraphists' cramp. London: His Majesty's Stationery Office; 1911.
[23] Lucire Y. Neurosis in the workplace. Med J Aust 1986;145:323–7.
[24] Dembe AE. The changing nature of office work: effects on repetitive strain injuries. In: Cherniack M, editor. Office ergonomics. Philadelphia: Hanley & Belfus; 1999. p. 61–72.

[25] Pheasant S. Ergonomics, work and health. Basingstoke: Macmillan Academic and Professional, Ltd.; 1991.
[26] Health and Safety Executive. Guidance note MS 10: beat conditions, tenosynovitis. London: Her Majesty's Stationery Office; 1977.
[27] Waugh A. Introducing kangaroo's paw, a wonderful new disease from Australia. Spectator 1986;Nov:8.
[28] Hodgson JT, Jones JR, Elliott RC, et al. Self-reported work-related illness. Health Safety Executive Research Paper No. 3; 1993.
[29] HSE. Work-related upper limb disorders: a guide to prevention. London: Her Majesty's Stationery Office; 1990.
[30] Pearce B. RSI and the media. Occupational Health Review 1995;Nov/Dec:14–8.
[31] European Economic Community. Council directive of 29 May 1990 on the minimum safety and health requirements for work with display screen equipment (fifth individual directive within the meaning of article 16 (1) of directive 87/391/EEC). Official Journal of the European Communities 1990;33:14–8.
[32] Health and Safety Executive. Display screen equipment work: guidance on regulations. London: Her Majesty's Stationery Office; 1992.
[33] Health and Safety Executive. Bogus burdens on business. London: Health and Safety Executive; November 16, 1992.
[34] Health and Safety Commission. Review of health and safety regulation: main report. London: Health and Safety Executive; 1994.
[35] Health and Safety Executive. Work with display screen equipment. London: HSE Books; 2003.
[36] Health and Safety Executive. Upper limb disorders: assessing the risks. London: HSE; 2001.
[37] Health and Safety Executive. Aching arms (or RSI) in small businesses. London: HSE Books; 2003.
[38] Clark L. £240,000 payout for bank victim of RSI. Daily Mail; April 7, 2000. p. 15.
[39] Health and Safety Executive. Upper limb disorders in the workplace. London: HSE Books; 2002.
[40] Hadler NM. Back pain in the workplace. What you lift or how you lift matters far less than whether you lift or when. Spine 1997;22(9):935–40.

ELSEVIER
SAUNDERS

Clin Occup Environ Med
5 (2) 267–283

CLINICS IN
OCCUPATIONAL AND
ENVIRONMENTAL
MEDICINE

Epidemiology of Work-Related Upper Extremity Disorders: Understanding Prevalence and Outcomes to Impact Provider Performances Using a Practice Management Reporting Tool

Geneva M. Giang, MBA

Concentra Health Services, 5080 Spectrum Drive, West Tower, Suite 1200, Addison, TX 75001, USA

Although overall incident rate for occupational injuries has declined in the US workforce, the percentage of work-related upper extremity disorders (WRUEDs) since 1986 has increased from 1% to 4% of all occupational injury claims. Correspondingly, average total medical and indemnity costs for these injuries are 80% higher than the average for all other claims, which results in enormous workers' compensation and other costs to the community [1,2]. Currently, limited information exists on the demographics and distribution of WRUEDs, their associated health care and indemnity costs, and impact on disability [3]. It is apparent that the quality of research in this area is generally poor, but research studies are being used as the basis for acceptance of workers' compensation claims, expensive ergonomic changes in the workplace, and even workplace closures [4]. The fact that the incidence of WRUEDs has crept up steadily despite these latter measures suggests that a causal relationship is not proven and that there may be misunderstanding in WRUED prevention and treatment. This article sheds light on WRUEDs through empirically quantifying detailed administrative data captured on this disorder available through a large nationwide occupational medicine network that is composed of 301 medical clinics and approximately 680 affiliated primary care physicians. This occupa-

E-mail address: geneva_iang@concentra.com

doi:10.1016/j.coem.2005.12.002 ***occmed.theclinics.com***

tional provider group sees approximately 600,000 injuries annually, with approximately 7% (42,000) cases diagnosed as WRUEDs, which offers a significant and valid population for analyses. The premise of the discussion is to understand better the prevalence and pattern of WRUED diagnoses, their impact on outcomes as a function of demographics and geography on metrics such as utilization, duration, disability status, and costs. By having a clear understanding of the outcomes metrics and cost drivers, we can appreciate better how provider performances can be impacted to achieve lower cost outcomes for the workers' compensation community while ensuring better patient outcomes for injured workers.

Opportunities to assess outcomes in occupational medicine

Efforts to measure outcomes in occupational medicine have benefited greatly from the wealth of experience offered by the benefit medicine world augmented by the simple fact that regardless of presenting complaints, goals for the stakeholders within the occupational health system remain the same—maximizing patient recovery while minimizing work restrictions, lost time, case duration, visit frequency, and costs. This homogeneity of goals facilitates the identification of key outcome variables that are of interest to patients, providers, employers, and payers. Measurement is also simplified in the occupational medicine sector because short- and long-term outcomes (eg, lost time, restricted duty, disability status) are standard components of the patient record as required for Occupational Safety and Health Administration (OSHA) or state workers' compensation entities [5]. This homogeneity in utilization drivers and desired patient outcomes allows for identification and employment of highly applicable and actionable metrics as we profile the WRUED claims population.

Case study: the outcomes reporting and management system that makes it all possible

At Concentra Health Services Incorporated, a nationwide network of 294 occupational medical centers, the value of operational and outcomes measurement lead to the development and ongoing refinement of a proprietary information management system. The system is composed of transactional and summarized process management data stored in a data warehouse. The transactional subsystem is used at the medical centers to document the operational, utilization, diagnostic, and outcomes information. Data from the transactional system are imported into the data warehouse using business rules to accept and summarize the data at multiple levels and create dimensions, including the case, visit, procedure, client/employer, and geographic region. Reports generated from the data warehouse, stratified by geographic region/market, injury category, or entity as appropriate permit ongoing analysis of practice trends.

The specific elements tracked within this outcomes system are dictated in part by medical standards and government regulations regarding documentation of encounters and disability. Stakeholder input also has been sought to define, incorporate, and interpret key outcomes/metrics of interest for reports. Duty restrictions, lost time from work, and referrals to specialists are critical to employers and payers because of their implications for costs. Specialist services result in higher medical costs, but lost time increases nonmedical/indemnity costs, which generally account for as much as 60% of the total injury [1,6].

In addition to lost income, prolonged lost time from work has critical implications for patients because it has been associated with increased morbidity and mortality, the development of various psychosocial problems, and decreased likelihood of complete recovery from injury [7,8]. These outcomes metrics are critical to providers from the perspective that they must maximize the health and well-being of their patients while demonstrating their efficiency value to employers/payers to maintain business.

Regular reporting, solicitation of stakeholder feedback, and ongoing revision of these measures and associated reports has had several benefits: (1) the assurance that the resulting information will be interesting and actionable for stakeholders, (2) the capacity to assess normal variation within different segments of the network, patient populations, or diagnostic groups, and (3) the ability to provide and measure the impact of evidence-based improvement initiatives [9].

Work-related upper extremity disorders profiled

The evaluation presented is an analysis of WRUED claims within the Concentra Medical Centers closed during 2000 through 2004. During the 5-year evaluation period, a total of 187,030 cases were diagnosed with tendonitis, epicondylitis, muscle syndromes, ganglions, carpal tunnel syndrome (CTS), and nonspecific pain, all of which fall into the WRUED diagnostic considerations,

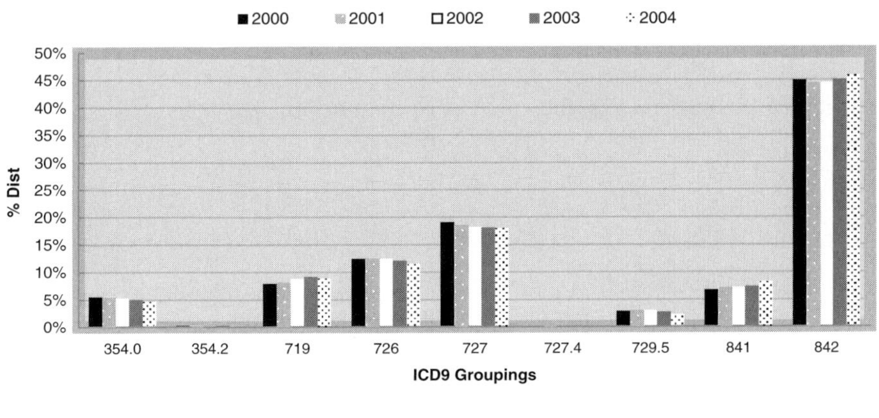

Fig. 1. Distribution of work-related upper extremity disorders.

Table 1
Case distribution for work-related upper extremity disorders[a]

Group	ICD-9	Description	% Distribution 2000	2001	2002	2003	2004	Total claims	% Distribution total
Mononeuritis (354)									
	354.0	Carpal tunnel syndrome	5.5	5.6	5.3	5.0	4.7	9758	5.2
	354.2	Lesion of ulnar nerve	0.2	0.3	0.2	0.2	0.3	483	0.3
Wrist/elbow pain (719)									
	719.40	Pain In joint	0.1	0.2	0.2	0.2	0.1	306	0.2
	719.42	Elbow pain	0.9	0.9	1.1	1.3	2.0	2395	1.3
	719.43	Wrist pain	6.9	7.1	7.4	7.7	6.8	13,427	7.2
Enthesopathies (726)									
	726.31	Medial epicodylitis	2.3	2.2	2.3	2.2	2.3	4195	2.2
	726.32	Lateral epicondylitis	10.2	10.4	10.2	9.9	9.3	18,655	10.0
Tendon disorders (727)									
	727.03	Trigger finger (acquired)	0.8	0.8	1.1	1.2	1.3	1947	1.0
	727.04	Radial styloid tenosynovitis	0.6	0.6	0.5	0.5	0.5	1002	0.5
	727.05	Wrist tenosynovitis	17.7	17.3	16.6	16.5	16.3	31,516	16.9
	727.4	Ganglion and cyst of synovium, tendon, and bursa	0.2	0.1	0.1	0.1	0.1	235	0.1

Soft tissues (729)								
729.5	Pain In limb	2.9	3.1	3.1	2.7	2.2	5195	2.8
Elbow/forearm pain (841)								
841	Sprains and strains of elbow and forearm	3.2	3.6	4.0	4.0	2.8	6593	3.5
841.0	Radial collateral ligament sprain	0.0	0.1	0.1	0.1	0.1	100	0.1
841.9	Elbow/forearm pain	3.6	3.5	3.1	3.3	5.4	7087	3.8
Wrist/hand pain (842)								
842	Sprains and strains of wrist and hand	1.7	1.6	1.3	1.4	1.2	2702	1.4
842.0	Wrist sprain	31.5	30.8	30.2	29.8	30.4	57,099	30.5
842.1	Hand sprain	7.9	7.8	7.7	8.1	8.5	14,975	8.0
842.11	Sprain of carpometacarpal (joint) of hand	0.1	0.1	0.1	0.1	0.1	154	0.1
842.12	Metacarpophalangeal joint sprain	1.4	1.7	2.5	2.8	2.8	4205	2.2
842.13	Interphalangeal joint sprain	2.3	2.3	2.7	2.8	2.7	4788	2.6
842.19	Other hand sprain	0.1	0.1	0.1	0.1	0.1	213	0.1
Total all WRUED ICD-9 codes		100.0	100.0	100.0	100.0	100.0	187,030	100.0

[a] For claims closed between 2000 and 2004.

according to the International Classification of Diseases, Clinical Modification (ICD-9-CM). These 187,030 injuries accounted for approximately 7% of Concentra's workers' compensation injury volume. The claims universe encompasses various types of employers and different jobs types and transverses 40 states and 90 different geographic markets, covered under one proprietary encounter data capturing system with uniform rules for outcomes metrics aggregation. This profile serves to provide descriptive data on WRUED cases, associated utilization, costs, and disability outcomes.

Prevalence and pattern of diagnoses

The broad spectrum of 187,030 disorders categorized as WRUEDs was segmented into nine categories (Fig. 1) for easier management: mononeuritis (CTS and lesion of ulnar nerve, 354), wrist/elbow pain (719), epicondylitis (726), tendon disorders (tenosynovitis and ganglion, 727), soft tissues (729), elbow/forearm pain (841), and wrist/hand pain (842). Based on the WRUED groupings identified, wrist/hand pain was the most prevalent class of disorder at 45%, whereas tenosynovitis and epicondylitis followed at 18% and 12%, respectively. The other six categories had distribution ranging from less than 1% to 9%. Of the mononeuritis diagnoses, CTS was the most common, accounting for 95% of the cases in this category. Lateral epicondylitis was the most prevalent enthesopathy, representing 82% of all enthesopathy-related diagnoses. For this provider group there is no significant change in case distribution from year to year for WRUED diagnoses. Table 1 details the claims distribution of WRUEDs by ICD-9 diagnoses for the five periods under evaluation.

Work-related upper extremity disorder utilization profiled

Based on the claim population of 187,030, 56% were male claimants and 44% were female claimants, with average age of 37 years. External referrals for diagnostic tests and specialists were 16%, whereas physical therapy referrals were 46% and averaged 5.4 visits per claim. Provider visits averaged 3.2, accounting for 1 initial visit and 2.2 recheck visits, at an average cost of $722 in primary care services per claim and average case duration of 28 days. Disability metrics show that 66% of the injuries were put on some form of restricted duty for a period of 23 days, and on average 2% were taken off duty and had lost time duration of 26 days.

Of greatest interest, although overall CTS accounted for only 5% or a little more than 1800 cases annually from the WRUEDs population, these claims have the highest referral rate, increased frequency of visits to providers and therapists, longer disability recovery, and corresponding highest claim costs. Fifty percent of CTS claims are referred on to a specialist, compared with 16% for the combined population; therapy referrals saw an increase of 9% from 46% for the total population to 55% for CTS. Provider visits increased by 1, whereas therapy visits increased by 3. Correspondingly, total primary care expenses for CTS are 75%

Table 2
Summary of outcomes statistics for work-related upper extremity disorder cases[a]

ICD-9 group	Description	No. of cases	% Ref to spec	% Ref to PT	Average PT visit/ PT case	Average PT chg/ case ($)	Average MD visits	Average MD chg/ case ($)	Average PC chg/ case ($)	Average case duration	% Limited	Limited days	% Lost	Lost days	Average paid/ claim ($)
354.0	Carpal tunnel syndrome	9758	49	55	8.45	1068	4.39	674	1261	76	60	61	6	54	20,902
354.2	Lesion of ulnar nerve	483	45	51	7.83	1046	3.92	594	1129	74	55	57	8	34	19,944
719	Wrist/elbow pain	16,128	20	46	5.32	674	3.10	398	705	34	56	29	2	22	11,425
726	Epicondylitis	22,850	24	73	6.68	858	4.46	521	1144	50	75	34	2	32	8519
727	Trigger finger/ tenosynovitis	34,465	25	68	5.95	730	3.99	488	985	43	76	31	2	30	7176
727.4	Ganglion and cyst of synovium, tendon, and bursa	235	34	20	5.45	623	2.58	328	452	40	37	24	2	15	6721
729.5	Pain in limb	5195	19	32	5.45	669	2.69	348	562	29	39	28	3	14	15,151
841	Elbow/forearm pain	13,780	14	56	4.99	656	3.24	390	757	23	72	19	2	25	3518
842	Wrist/hand pain	84,136	13	51	4.51	583	3.12	389	684	22	72	19	2	20	2748
Total All WRUED ICD9 Codes		187,030	16	46	5.37	683	3.23	408	722	28	66	23	2	26	10,935

Abbreviations: chg/case, charge per case; PT, physical therapist and/or occupational therapist; MD, medical doctor; Ref to spec; referred to specialist.

[a] For claims closed between 2000 to 2004.

higher ($1261 versus $722), whereas total claim costs (medical and indemnity expenses) are 91% more expensive at $20,902 compared with $10,935 for all WRUEDs. Total claim costs of $10,935 for WRUEDs already are 92% more expensive than the average for all injuries recorded at $5693 per claim. Case duration for CTS is 76 days compared with 28 days for the total WRUED population. Table 2 delineates the various outcomes metrics by ICD-9 groupings.

Clinicians long have hypothesized that gender may serve as a risk factor in treatment outcomes of patient who have chronic disability associated with musculoskeletal disorders [10]. It is appropriate to examine the impact of gender on utilization and cost outcomes. A review of this claims population showed that the male to female split is 56% to 44% (contrary to the scientific literature, which showed higher prevalence of repetitive motion injuries in women) [10], with male claimants averaging 36 years old—2 years younger than their female counterpart. There is a significant increase in treatment utilization for women who have WRUEDS directly correlated to the older population. Female claimants have significantly higher rate of referrals of 19% compared with 14% from their male counterparts. Higher rate to specialists potentially speaks to complications and severity inherent in the older population. WRUED female patients are referred to physical therapists at a 12% higher rate then their male partners (53%) and for an average of 6 visits as compared with 41% and 4.8 visits for men. Along with higher physical therapy utilization, provider visits also have increased in the female population by one (four visits versus three visits for men). More utilization translates to 30% higher cost per claim ($830 versus $638) and results in longer duration (37 days versus 22 days). In terms of disability, female claimants had 3% more claims with restricted duty; however, the rate of off-duty is comparable for both genders. Of significant variance is duration of disability. Restricted duty lasted 29 days for female claimants compared with 19 days for male claimants. Lost days lasted 31 days versus 21 days represented in the male population. Higher utilization and longer claim duration speak to longer recovery time for female patients with a WRUED diagnosis.

Tables 3 and 4 provide comparative distribution and outcomes metrics by age bands and gender. The age distribution of claimants with WRUED diagnosis indicated that most were between 21 and 50 years of age, with the highest volume of claims between 31 and 40 years of age. This pattern is true individually for female and male populations. Results from this study group seem younger than a prior study conducted by Feuerstein and colleagues [11], which found prevalence in claimants between ages 41 and 50. This result is understandable considering that the claims sample was for the federal workforce as compared with private industry, which dominates in this provider network.

For this provider network, their top ten states account for 72% of all WRUED claims. Table 5, which profiles utilization metrics by geography, shows great variations in outcomes and points to differences in practice patterns beyond age and gender influences of patients. Colorado is the only state in which the ratio of male/female is inverse; there are more female claimants with WRUED than male claimants by 2%. Because Colorado is a concurrent care state, utilization and

Table 3
Summary of work-related upper extremity disorder outcomes metrics by male age groups[a]

Age group	% Distribution	Average age	% Ref to spec	% Ref to PT	Average PT visit/PT case	Average MD visits	Average PC chg/case ($)	Average duration	% Limited duty	Limited duty days	% Lost	Lost days
20 & under	6	19	6	28	3.4	2.3	436	11	64.5	11	0.8	7
21–30	28	26	9	37	4.0	2.7	543	16	66.3	15	1.2	13
31–40	30	35	15	43	4.9	3.0	667	23	66.4	19	1.7	23
41–50	23	45	19	45	5.5	3.2	746	28	65.4	22	2.1	24
51 +	13	56	21	42	5.6	3.3	743	29	63.7	23	2.1	22
Total male	100	36	14	41	4.8	3.0	638	22	65.0	19	2.0	21

[a] For claims closed between 2000 and 2004.

Table 4
Summary of work-related upper extremity disorder outcomes metrics by female age groups[a]

Age group	% Distribution	Average age	% Ref to spec	% Ref to PT	Average PT visit/PT case	Average MD visits	Average PC chg/case ($)	Average duration	% Limited duty	Limited duty days	% Lost	Lost days
20 & under	4	19	8	41	4.1	2.8	537	18	69.0	17	1.2	14
21–30	23	26	13	51	5.1	3.2	711	29	68.3	23	1.5	23
31–40	23	36	19	54	5.8	3.6	842	36	69.0	29	2.0	34
41–50	27	45	24	54	6.5	3.9	933	44	68.4	33	2.4	35
51 +	17	56	27	53	6.7	3.9	952	45	67.1	33	2.8	32
Total female	100	38	19	53	6.0	4.0	830	37	68.0	29	2.0	31

[a] For claims closed between 2000 and 2004.

Table 5
Summary of work-related upper extremity disorder outcomes metrics by top ten volume states[a]

State	No. of cases	M/F ratio (%)	Average age	% Ref to spec	% Ref to PT	Average PT visit/PT case	Average MD visits	Average PC chg/case ($)	Average duration	% Limited duty	Limited duty days	% Lost	Lost days
TX	39,303	56/44	37	14	48	5.4	2.9	661	29	60.3	23	1.2	45
MI	27,537	58/42	37	14	36	4.9	2.9	594	18	71.0	17	1.6	17
CA	20,332	51/49	37	19	45	7.4	4.2	834	45	64.2	34	4.9	36
AZ	16,862	55/45	37	20	44	6.0	3.4	754	31	72.6	25	2.3	25
CO	13,933	49/51	37	27	56	7.4	4.6	937	63	78.2	50	1.3	19
GA	13,791	53/47	38	15	51	5.1	3.2	692	25	69.9	21	0.6	24
MD	12,600	62/38	37	10	48	3.9	3.1	441	20	67.9	17	2.1	21
IL	10,997	63/37	38	17	46	5.0	3.2	1085	20	66.8	19	2.0	20
PA	10,985	53/47	38	17	55	4.4	3.1	592	18	64.2	15	1.0	20
NV	8279	52/48	38	17	36	5.9	3.4	714	35	78.1	26	0.5	7

[a] For claims closed between 2000 and 2004.

outcomes metrics do not seem as favorable as the other nine states. Specialist referrals are at 27% compared with 16%, physical therapy referrals are 56% for 7.4 visits versus 46% with 5.4 visits; average provider visits are 4.6 versus 3.2; restricted duty claims account for 78% with duration of 50 days, whereas the total claim duration is 63 days compared with the WRUED universe of only 28 days.

How the information can be used to improve provider performances

Within this provider organization the data are used to describe the vital signs of provider practices, identify trends and explain outlier activities, discover opportunity for improvement, and identify best practices. Outcomes reports that depict the metrics describe aggregate levels of performance for an entire population or subpopulation. This report offers broad perspective on performance achieved at the global rather than individual level, which permits performance evaluation without revisiting each treatment decision.

How are the data evaluated?

The data are examined for trends to identify outcome patterns that are inconsistent with benchmarks. Potential outliers are defined as values that are inconsistent with the average (defined model/ benchmark) or unexpected values, assuming that the benchmark sets and appropriate expectations are identified. Trends are evaluated to differentiate practice changes from system changes. For example, is the higher specialist referral rate for women with WRUEDs observed consistently throughout the evaluation period, or are the results more a function of operational/system changes? Values that differ dramatically from the average, from benchmarks, or from other extremes are reviewed in detail.

What is being measured? With rate, the influence of a single case on the average or benchmark depends on the size of the comparison group. With duration statistics there is more potential to be meaningfully influenced by outliers than rate statistics, however. What is the intended response to outliers? Percentages above and below a benchmark are tracked to identify improvement opportunities that have maximum impact. The decision must be made as to whether it is reasonable to expect that value to hit the same benchmark as other values. Potential outliers are identified by looking for extremes, which offers an objective approach and determines whether the expectation for the value is appropriate allows for the subjective balance. One must decide on an appropriate action plan. Often the requests to exclude outliers are frequently unidirectional or one dimensional. In some cases, the "majority" statistics reflect things that actually happened. Excluding unusual occurrences can give a false-positive depiction of performance. Opportunities to improve performance are more evident when one considers the whole, and sometimes ugly, truth. Finally, the descriptive and quantitative outcomes metrics obtained through monitoring outcomes data facilitate the organization's goals to continually improve performance. In the final analysis, outcomes data help an entity to quantify successes and demonstrate their effectiveness.

A successful intervention to promote demedicalization and early activation of patients who have upper extremity complaints

Review of the literature shows that in medical arenas, such as with cardiac patients, postsurgical patients, and patients with back pain, there has been a successful move toward more aggressive activity recommendations during recovery. This has not been the case for work-related upper extremity nontraumatic pain complaints, however. It is common practice to restrict most patients who present with cumulative trauma upper extremity disorders [12–14]. Motivated by these studies and variations observed in her region's practice patterns, a regional medical director performed an intervention plan aimed at reducing restriction and lost time while advising against splinting and immobilization of the injuries to improve outcomes for the patient and provider within her management region [15]. The intervention included a communication of a change strategy in treatment based on the premise that although physical factors of the workplace might contribute to pain, with WRUEDs the physical factors of the job are generally not the primary contributing problem. Medical providers from two occupational medicine clinics were educated regarding this treatment approach. They were encouraged to keep patients at their regular jobs unless there had been a recent significant job change for which a patient was not properly conditioned or a patient had a systemic health condition that made it temporarily necessary to restrict certain activities. The providers were also advised against splinting or immobilizing a joint unless there was frank edema and clear evidence that it was indicated [16].

Because the primary goal of managing a work-related condition is to restore and maximize function, it was emphasized that avoiding unnecessary, excessive, or prolonged restrictions should be a main focus of the provider. The treatment includes keeping patients at their regular jobs and giving them a program to increase strength, flexibility, and stamina. Stress reduction techniques, such as regular aerobic exercise and relaxation, also are advised. Patients with arm and hand complaints are treated with strengthening, stretching, ice, and aerobic conditioning. When appropriate, nonsteroidal anti-inflammatory drugs are also prescribed. Problem solving and appropriate ergonomic suggestions are also made [17–19]. The medical director stressed the importance of developing expertise in the practice of aggressive nonrestriction of WRUEDs. Specific suggestions were provided on how to reduce the amount and duration of restricted duty and lost time for patients being treated.

Measuring change: improved performance

The success of this intervention was measured by comparing change scores for outcome statistics collected before and subsequent to the intervention.

Table 6
Change scores on outcomes metrics of educational intervention[a]

	Intervention group			
Treatment outcomes	Pre-training (%)	Post-training (%)	±	P-values
Specialist referral rate	20.5	11.8	2.46	<0.05
Splinting rate	40.2	14.3	5.91	<0.05
Restricted duty rate	68.8	30.4	8.10	<0.001
Restricted duty duration	27.4	21.7	2.35	<0.01
Off-duty rate	3.4	1.0	2.67	<0.01
Case duration	37.0	29.4	4.12	<0.05

[a] Shares positive results from an educational intervention to promote "demedicalization" and early activation of patients with upper extremity complaints.

Providers who were part of the same network but outside of the intervention region served as a control group. Differences in demographic, diagnostic, and severity characteristics of patients were controlled to better establish a meaningful comparison. The observed changes in the intervention group corresponding to the treatment time and differential changes between the intervention group (reduction in duty restrictions before and after intervention) and the no-intervention group (no change over the same time period) are consistent with a positive treatment effect. Table 6 summarizes these positive intervention results.

A key factor in the success of this intervention was the ability to identify objectively an improvement opportunity. Certainly not all practice variation is negative. Duty restrictions are necessary for some cases, and failure to restrict duty in patients with more serious injuries (eg, more pronounced functional limitations or injuries that require surgical interventions) would be impractical and unsafe. The medical director was able to perceive and convince her colleagues, via regular monitoring of practice trends and published results, that changes in treatment strategies were possible for some portion of patients. These findings elaborate on the premise that some variations in patient outcomes are within the providers' control.

Discussion

The current findings indicate that the most prevalent diagnostic grouping, classified under WRUEDs, seen by this large provider network is wrist/hand pain. Profile of utilization outcomes for this injury category revealed that it aligns well within the median range in terms of referral rates and utilization of services and total cost per claim of $2748, which is favorable compared with overall average cost per claim of $5693 for all injuries. The second most prevalent diagnoses group is tenosynovitis. For these disorders average claim costs rise to $7176, which accounts for increases in referrals and utilization. Epicondylitis, third in queue, account for 12% of WRUED claims at a cost of $8519 per claimant. Most significant, however, continue to be costs associated with CTS; although CTS cases only account for 5% of the WRUED population they account for 24% of total WRUED expenses. An average claim costs approximately $20,909. CTS continues to be a focused concern because of its relative low prevalence yet high cost implications. It is the execution of the 80/20 rule in health care cost containment.

Within this population 12% more men were diagnosed with WRUEDs compared with their female counterparts. Although women have lower volume of WRUED claims, they are associated with higher utilization, longer disability duration, and higher total cost per claim partly because the female population is 2 years older than the comparative male population. Most claimants are between the ages of 21 and 50, with heaviest volume seen between 31 and 40 years old. Most revealing in terms of work disability is that although the percentage of cases with restrictions are high and duration is long, only a relatively small group of claimants is taken off work for any substantial length of time. The ability to achieve fewer lost time claims is facilitated by this provider organization's focus on reducing lost time claims by understanding provider practices through active measurement and intervention to change/mold provider behavior to ensure best outcomes.

The infrastructure that makes this all possible is the outcomes tracking system, which demonstrate the feasibility and positive impact of ongoing practice pattern evaluations. The success of this system may be attributed to several factors:

- Capitalizing on opportunity. The homogeneity of treatment goals in occupational medicine facilitates the measurement of outcomes and assessments of utilization and cost. As a result, it is possible to identify operational opportunities to impact outcomes in a quantifiable fashion.
- Organizational commitment. The development and maintenance of a system capable of collecting, summarizing, and tracking utilization, costs, and outcomes require substantial financial and time investments. Without management support at the highest levels of the organization, earned by tireless efforts to demonstrate the validity and value of the system, results like the ones presented in this article would not be measurable.
- Ongoing revision and evaluation. The occupational outcomes captured in this system and the ways in which they are calculated have evolved over time. Data are evaluated constantly to ascertain whether the metrics reflect the intended constructs or operational anomalies in the data.
- Stakeholder input and communication. Solicitation of ongoing feedback from stakeholders (especially providers and payers) provides valuable insight on the appropriate interpretations of metrics, assists in the identification of new measurement needs, and helps assure that reports provide useful information.
- Focusing on the big picture. The focus of this effort is on practice trends and outcomes within particular regions or diagnostic groups rather than on individual treatment decisions. Attention to aggregate statistics rather than individual providers/patients is advantageous because it does not duplicate the functions of other areas (eg, utilization review), it is less intrusive in the

day-to-day operations of providers, and it offers greater statistical reliability by using more data points. Interventions made at this level are likely to have higher return on investment because the observed trends are not likely driven by idiosyncrasies (eg, outliers) in the data.

Summary

Ongoing efforts to measure and report patient outcomes are critical to demonstrating system performance, justifying expenses, establishing the need for change, and understanding the benefits of specific operational processes [10]. To assess outcome measurements, a good reporting and management system must be in place to allow ongoing evaluation and data analysis. Measuring and understanding outcome data can be used to develop intervention programs to improve provider performances and, ultimately, patient outcomes.

References

[1] National Safety Council. Injury facts. Itasca (IL): National Safety Council; 2004.
[2] Mayer TG, Gatchel RJ, Polatin PB, et al. Outcomes comparison of treatment for chronic disabling work-related upper-extremity disorders and spinal disorders. J Occup Environ Med 1999;41(9):761–70.
[3] Proctor TJ, Mayer TG, Gatchel RJ, et al. Unremitting health-care-utilization outcomes of tertiary rehabilitation of patient with chronic musculoskeletal disorders. J Bone Joint Surg Am 2004;86-A(1):62–9.
[4] Lincoln AE, Feuerstein M, Shaw WS, et al. Impact of case manager training on worksite accommodations in workers' compensation claimants with upper extremity disorders. J Occup Environ Med 2002;44(3):237–45.
[5] Office of the Federal Register, National Archives and Records Administration, US Department of Labor. Recording and reporting occupational injuries and illnesses: code of federal regulations [Revised as of July 1, 2002]. 29 CFR 1904. Available at: http://www.access.gpo.gov/nara/cfr/waisidx_02/29cfr1904_02.html. Accessed August 30, 2005.
[6] Hashemi L. Length of disability and cost of workers' compensation low back pain claims. J Occup Environ Med 1997;39(10):937–45.
[7] Panzarella J. The nature of work, job loss, and the diagnostic complexities of the psychologically injured worker. Psychiatr Ann 1991;21(1):10–5.
[8] Ross JF. Where do real dangers lie? Smithsonian 1995;Nov:42–53.
[9] Novotny-Devenport J, Giang G, Derebery VJ, et al. Using provider profiles to monitor outcomes and improve performance. Journal of Workers Compensation 2003;12(4):26–37.
[10] McGeary DD, Mayer TG, Gatchel RJ, et al. Gender-related differences in treatment outcomes for patients with musculoskeletal disorders. Spine J 2003;3(3):197–203.
[11] Feuerstein M, Miller VL, Burrell LM, et al. Occupational upper extremity disorders in the federal workforce: prevalence, health care expenditures, and patterns of work disability. J Occup Environ Med 1998;40(6):546–55.
[12] Carragee EJ, Han MY, Yang B, et al. Activity restrictions after posterior lumbar discectomy: a prospective study of outcomes in 152 cases with no postoperative restrictions. Spine 1999;24(22):2346–51.
[13] Carragee EJ, Helms E, O'Sullivan GS. Are postoperative activity restrictions necessary after posterior lumbar discectomy? A prospective study of outcomes in 50 consecutive cases. Spine 1996;21(16):1893–7.

[14] Hall H, McIntosh G, Melles T, et al. Effect of discharge recommendations on outcome. Spine 1994;19(18):2033–7.

[15] Goodman CS, Ahn R, Rubin RJ. Outcomes and effectiveness research in the private sector. Health Aff 1998;17(5):75–90.

[16] Wuori JL, Overend TJ, Kramer JF, et al. Strength and pain measures associated with lateral epicondylitis bracing. Arch Phys Med Rehabil 1998;79:832–7.

[17] Hay E, Paterson S, Lewis M, et al. Pragmatic randomized controlled trial of local corticosteroid injection and naproxen for treatment of lateral epicondylitis of the elbow in primary care. BMJ 1999;319:964–8.

[18] Smidt N, van der Windt D, Assendelft W. Corticosteroid injections, physiotherapy, or a wait-and-see policy for lateral epicondylitis: a randomized controlled trial. Lancet 2002;359:657–62.

[19] King JC, Kelleher WJ, Stedwill JE, et al. Physical limitations are not required for chronic pain rehabilitation success. Am J Phys Med Rehabil 1994;73(5):331–7.

ELSEVIER
SAUNDERS

Clin Occup Environ Med
5 (2) 285–298

CLINICS IN
OCCUPATIONAL AND
ENVIRONMENTAL
MEDICINE

The Role of Imaging of Work-Related Upper Extremity Disorders

Robert G. Hassett, DO, MPH

Concentra Health Services, 15800 Midway Road, Addison, TX 75001, USA

The colder the X-ray table, the more of our body is required to come in contact with it.

Anonymous

Work-related upper extremity disorders can pose a diagnostic and management challenge because the nontraumatic disorders that are often believed to be caused by repetitive work activities can and do occur without any apparent provoking activity and can be caused or associated with many systemic medical conditions. One mainstay in the assessment of hand and arm disorders remains imaging. In fact, William Conrad Roentgen's first human radiograph was of his wife's hand in 1895. Over the decades since that first x-ray, imaging capabilities have made incredible advances with the advent of MRI, CT, ultrasound, bone scan, and numerous technologies that enable clinicians to view fine details of anatomy and pathology. This article reviews the potential imaging choices and clinical indications for work-related injuries of the elbow, hand, and wrist.

Regarding imaging, it is best to remember that just because one can image something does not mean that one should. Clinicians should avoid unnecessary radiologic examinations for various reasons, including cost control, avoidance of unnecessary radiation exposure, wasting resources, and the need to avoid medicalizing patient condition. Unnecessary studies indicate that a provider is not following a logical thought process in the diagnostic evaluation [1]. Imaging studies should not provide the diagnosis but confirm it.

E-mail address: bob_hassett@concentra.com

doi:10.1016/j.coem.2005.11.015 ***occmed.theclinics.com***

Imaging of the elbow

Plain radiography remains the mainstay of imaging when evaluating elbow trauma [2]. Injuries result mainly from direct trauma or force that is transmitted axially from the wrist and forearm.

Specific elbow pathology

Epicondylitis

Lateral and medial epicondylitis are common diagnoses in the occupational medicine arena. Imaging is not routinely necessary for either lateral or medial epicondylitis, although plain radiography remains the mainstay of evaluating refractory cases of epicondylitis. Plain film radiography of the elbow may demonstrate faint calcification along the lateral epicondyle. MRI and CT play no role in the clinical evaluation of lateral epicondylitis [3].

Radial head fracture

Radial head fracture tends to be a subtle radiologic finding that should be given a high index of suspicion based on the clinical examination and history. A visible posterior fat pad should be considered a radial head fracture until proven otherwise. Missed radial head fractures may result in permanent impairment of the elbow with concomitant medicolegal implications. Fractures that produce an effusion also may displace the anterior fat pad outward from the humerus, which produces the "sail" sign. Often in the instance of a visible posterior fat pad, the fracture itself may not be visualized. In that case it is not necessary to obtain special views, CT, or even MRI scans, because the pathologic condition will be treated the same regardless of whether the pathology is radiologically documented [1].

Olecranon fracture

Olecranon fracture is usually straightforward and easily seen on plain film radiographs. Mechanism of injury is primarily direct trauma.

Osteochondral and other fracture patterns

Impaction injuries to the elbow may produce subtle chondral flaps and loose bodies that result in mechanical symptoms. More severe injuries should be visible on plain radiographs; however, more subtle cases require cartilage pulse sequencing on MRI [2].

Lateral collateral ligament

The ulnar band of the lateral collateral ligament is one of the primary stabilizers of the elbow [2]. Tears of this ligament allow the radial head to subluxate inferiorly when the forearm is supinated. This injury typically occurs after falling on an outstretched hand with axial compression, valgus load, and forearm supination [2]. Suspected tears require thin slice MRI to observe the ligamentous elements.

Medial collateral ligament

The medial collateral ligament is composed of anterior, posterior, and transverse bundles, with the anterior bundle being composed of anterior and posterior bands [2]. Primary restraint of valgus rotation falls to the anterior band of the anterior bundle, which may suffer injury to valgus overload while in extension [2]. The posterior band may be affected when the elbow is flexed [2]. It is important to image the ligament with MRI in flexion and extension as a result. One particular subset of pathology that is primarily encountered in athletes is "handball elbow," which results from repetitive hyperextension trauma, either with a hyperextension mechanism (usually seen while blocking a shot) or overhead throwing, which produces medial sided elbow pain [4]. Any occupation that mimics these activities puts an individual at risk for developing this condition. Plain film radiographs may demonstrate bony hypertrophy, and stress films may reveal medial elbow laxity. Imaging may demonstrate thickening of the ligament along with a hypertrophic spur off the coronoid of the ulna [2]. MRI is the modality of choice for evaluating cartilage injury [4].

Imaging of the forearm

A Colle's fracture is one of the most common arm fractures and involves the distal radius and ulna after a fall on the outstretched arm [1]. When the same fracture angulates in the volar direction, it is known as a Smith's fracture [1]. The forearm consists of two bones, the radius and ulna, which act as a bony ring [1]. There is not a break in only one location. If the second fracture is not evident, a dislocation of the nonfractured bone usually occurs. An example of this is a fracture of the ulna with a dislocation of the proximal radius, known as a Monteggia's fracture. A fracture of the radius with dislocation of the distal ulna is known as a Galeazzi's fracture [1]. A nightstick fracture occurs with trauma to the mid ulna, exemplified by being struck by a blunt object while holding the arm up in a flexed defensive position [5].

Typically, imaging of the forearm is limited to plain film radiography, with anteroposterior and lateral projections. If one suspects trauma to either the wrist or elbow, forearm views are not sufficient. Forearm views should be ordered when there is suspicion of abnormality to the midportion of the radius or ulna [5].

Imaging of the wrist

Injuries to the wrist and hand can arise as the result of direct trauma that causes crushes, contusions, and strains. When significant trauma is present, the decision to obtain radiographic imaging is generally straightforward. Some nontraumatic conditions of the wrist historically have been deemed as work related from repeated trauma, although a consistent dose response relationship between upper extremity use and upper extremity disorders has not been found. The wrist has been called the low back of the hand, and like the low back, the painful, nontraumatized wrist is at risk for overuse of radiographic imaging, particularly as imaging technology advances.

Many conditions can produce wrist pain—some work related, some not—and some conditions may predispose an individual to an exacerbation or aggravation from a work activity. In general, work-related wrist disorders that call for radiographic assessment require no more than plain film radiographs. Anatomy of the wrist is complex, with the distal radius and ulna articulating with the proximal row of four carpals: the scaphoid (navicular), lunate, triquetrum, and pisiform going from radial to ulnar side. These carpals in turn articulate with the second row of four carpals: the trapezium, trapezoid, capitate, and hamate. This second, distal row of carpals then articulates with the five metacarpals. The anterolateral margins of the scaphoid and trapezium protrude anteriorly to form the attachment for the flexor retinaculum. Various ligamentous and cartilaginous structures are also present in the wrist, along with nerves, vascular elements, muscles, and tendons.

When evaluating the wrist, a clinician should follow a logical thought process when making the determination as to whether imaging is indicated and what type of imaging is most appropriate. Obtaining a thorough history is essential. Comparing the mechanism of injury with the physical examination assists in the interpretation of imaging studies. Should abnormalities be found that do not correlate with the examination or history, another cause should be sought [6]. Age and sex should be considered, particularly when evaluating chronic wrist pain, because there is a direct relationship between age and cartilage and ligamentous attrition [6].

Posteroanterior, lateral, and oblique views should be a starting point when evaluating the wrist, with additional views (ie, radial and ulnar deviation views or clenched fist views) reserved for assessment of more subtle problems [6]. In assessing radiographs of the wrist, it is important to remember that radiographs project three dimensions onto two. An examiner can determine the medial/lateral position of an object identified on a posteroanterior view of the wrist but can tell nothing of whether it is located more anteriorly or posteriorly. One common mistake in ordering films of the wrist is requesting wrong or insufficient views [7]. At least two projections are required to evaluate any structure. Another common error involves ordering one set of films to evaluate the wrist and the hand, which proves to be a false economy, because the standard views of the hand differ from the wrist [7]. A dedicated set of films for the area being evaluated frequently provides a better diagnosis [7].

Because the wrist has a complicated anatomy with many structures overlying each other (particularly on the lateral view), it is prudent to have radiographs of patients with traumatic wrist injuries overread by a qualified radiologist to confirm that a pathologic condition has not been missed. It is important to assess each radiograph for pathologic condition, technical quality, and proper positioning [7]. On the lateral view, the scaphoid on the radial side of the wrist and the pisiform on the ulnar side of the wrist serve as landmarks for forming what is, in essence, a line of sight along the lateral projection of the wrist. In an optimally positioned lateral view, the palmar margin of the pisiform should project midway between the palmar margins of the distal pose of the scaphoid and the capitate head, forming what has been referred to as the S-P-C lateral (Fig. 1). Positioning for lateral view of the hand differs from the wrist, because a foam step wedge is used to spread and obtain lateral views of the digits [7].

Specific wrist pathology

Triangular fibrocartilage complex

The triangular fibrocartilage complex (TFCC) provides stability to the distal radioulnar joint and is composed of the articular disc (TFC proper), the meniscus homolog (ulnar carpal meniscus), dorsal and volar radioulnar ligaments, ulnar collateral ligaments, and the sheath of the extensor carpi ulnaris tendon [8,9]. This complex helps absorb stresses directed longitudinally along the wrist and distribute them, and it acts as a buttress to support the proximal carpal row [8,10]. Normally, 80% of the mechanical force is transmitted across the radius, and the remaining 20% is transmitted through the ulna [11]. A mere 1 mm change in ulnar variance can increase the ulnar load by 25% [11]. Lesions of the TFCC can be traumatic or degenerative, with the incidence of degenerative lesions increasing with age [12]. Typically, lesions of the TFCC produce ulnar-sided wrist pain, which may become chronic and associated with a clicking or popping

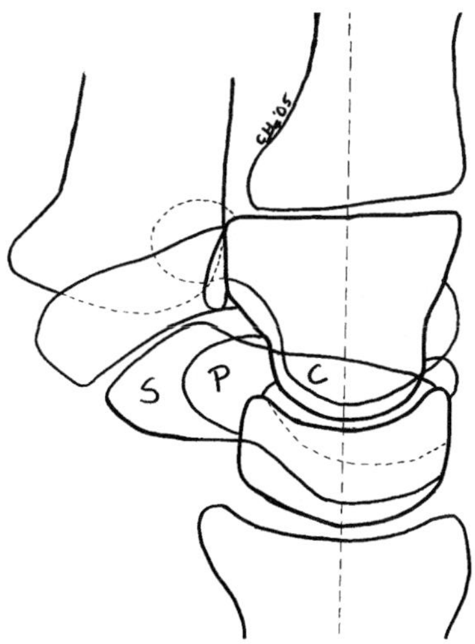

Fig. 1. Schematic of the lateral wrist demonstrates the relative positions of the scaphoid (S), pisiform (P), and capitate (C).

sound with certain movements. If TFCC injury is suspected, plain film radiography is indicated with posteroanterior and lateral views. The radiographs should be examined for ulnar variance, degenerative joint disease of the distal radioulnar joint, instability of the lunate-triquetrum or scapholunate areas, chondromalacia of the lunate or ulnar head, and either dorsiflexed intercalated segment instability or volar flexed intercalated segment instability. Assessment for ulnar variance may be accomplished by several techniques [7], each of which has proved to be accurate. One method is shown in Fig. 2. Negative ulnar variance occurs when the distal cortex of the ulna projects proximal to the adjacent radial sigmoid notch, whereas positive ulnar variance exists when the ulna extends distal to the sigmoid notch The amount of ulnar variance that is clinically significant is as yet undetermined, because investigators have reported a 13-mm swing in normal individuals (−6 mm–7 mm); however, the mean variance in asymptomatic individuals is approximately 1 mm [7].

Other than plain radiography, there is no clear consensus on which modality is best to evaluate potential TFCC lesions [8,11–19]. For years, three-compartment wrist arthrography was the gold standard for evaluating wrist instability and TFCC lesions [17,18]. The sensitivity and specificity have been demonstrated to be low, however, so arthrography is seldom recommended since the advent of arthroscopy [6,18].

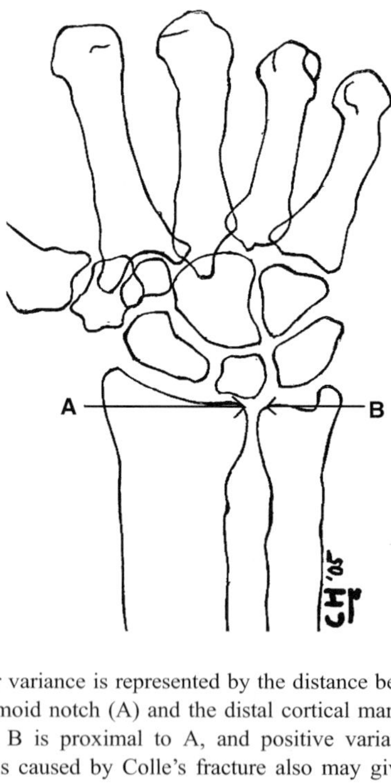

Fig. 2. Measurement of ulnar variance is represented by the distance between the transverse line that passes through the distal sigmoid notch (A) and the distal cortical margin of the ulna (B). Negative ulnar variance occurs when B is proximal to A, and positive variance occurs when B is distal to A. Impaction of the radius caused by Colle's fracture also may give the appearance of positive ulnar variance.

Use of MRI of the wrist has had a slower development than for other joints [1]. Several authors have reported that MRI gives satisfactory results in the evaluation of TFCC lesions [1,8,16]. Other investigators have found that MRI was not helpful in investigating instability of the wrist, however [6,20]. In two separate reports, Haims [13,14] noted that MRI is inadequate in visualizing peripheral attachment tears of the TFCC and that indirect arthrography does not improve diagnostic accuracy for lesions of the central disc of the TFCC.

Cineradiography has been used in the past for evaluating chronic wrist pain, which involves moving the wrist through full range of motion in an attempt to recreate the stresses and positions known to cause clicks or pops [21]. Along with assessing TFCC lesions, it can demonstrate scapholunate, lunatotriquetral, midcarpal, capitolunate, and distal radioulnar joint instability [6]. Numerous studies have demonstrated ligament perforations in asymptomatic individuals, which casts further confusion on the significance of these findings as they relate to ulnar wrist pain [1,6]. In a young patient with wrist pain that has failed conservative care, however, most hand surgeons intervene surgically if a lesion is found [1]. For this reason, imaging may play a role.

Carpal instability

Excessive forces applied to the wrist may produce various pathologic conditions. Directing focus solely toward identifying a TFCC lesion may cause a clinician to miss another cause of wrist pain, such as carpal instability. Carpal instability may be either static or dynamic [7]. Static instability is demonstrated by misalignment of the carpals on posteroanterior and lateral radiographs, whereas dynamic instability may appear normal on neutral films and require stress views for identification [7]. Carpal instability results from tears of the extrinsic and intrinsic carpal ligaments and presents as varying patterns of instability [8].

Perilunate instability. This condition may result from a fall on the outstretched arm. Mayfield described a progression of instability centered around the lunate [7]. Stage I involves the scapholunate joint. Stage II results as loading increases and involves the capitate, which allows the capitate to dislocate from its articulation with the lunate and rotate posteriorly (Fig. 3). In Stage III instability, the triquetrum is involved, dislodging all ligamentous attachments of the lunate and the carpals [7]. In this instance, the capitate pushes the lunate volarly and is termed lunate dislocation [1]. At stage IV there is disruption of the dorsal radiocarpal ligaments, which allows the lunate to rotate into the carpal tunnel. Lunate or perilunate dislocation can be seen on the anteroposterior view of the wrist, with the lunate appearing as triangular instead of the normal rhomboid shape. One always should look at the alignment of the lunate and capitate on every lateral film. Failure to diagnose this condition could result in impingement of the median nerve by the lunate with permanent impairment [1].

Dorsal intercalated segmental instability. The lunate has been referred to as the intercalated segment [7], which means "between two others," and is subject

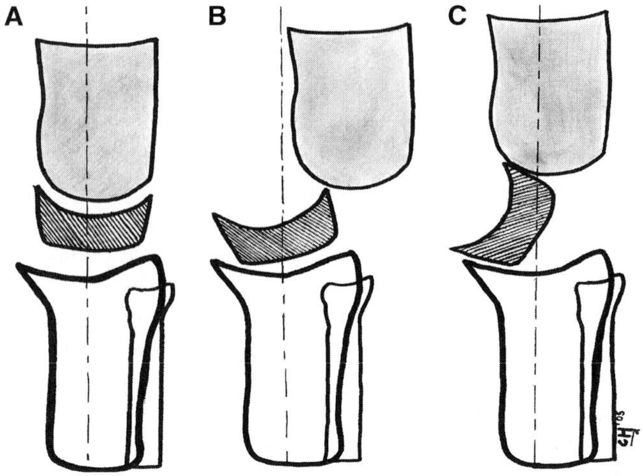

Fig. 3. The illustration portrays the lunate (*crosshatched bone*) and capitate (*shaded bone*). Note the normal lateral wrist with ventral to the left (*A*), perilunate dislocation (*B*), and lunate dislocation (*C*).

to various patterns of instability. Intercalated segment instability is evaluated by looking at the alignment of the lunate relative to the scaphoid and capitate, primarily in lateral radiographs [7]. Dorsiflexed intercalated segment instability is the most frequently encountered form of intercalated instability and is represented by a lunate dorsiflexed relative to the radius and subluxed in a palmar direction [7,8]. Often dorsiflexed intercalated segment instability is associated with disruption of the scapholunate ligament or the volar extrinsic ligaments [8].

Volar intercalated segmental instability. This condition occurs uncommonly [8].

Scapholunate advanced collapse. This condition is noted to be the most common pattern of degenerative arthritis in the wrist [22]. It is seen more commonly in men than women, has an association with performing manual labor, and tends to affect the dominant hand [22]. Plain films may demonstrate joint narrowing, sclerosis, osteophytes, cysts, scapholunate dislocation, and carpal collapse. If there is a question of avascularity, MRI is the modality of choice [8,12].

Scapholunate dissociation. Injuries to the scapholunate ligament have been referenced previously but may be seen as an isolated injury after a fall on the outstretched hand [1]. When seen radiographically, there is a gap between the scaphoid and the lunate on the anteroposterior view, which was known previously as the Terry Thomas sign, named after a famous British actor with a gap between his front teeth [1]. Current generations of radiologists have taken to renaming it the David Letterman sign [1]. In suspected scapholunate dissociation that is not radiographically obvious, indirect arthrography demonstrates improved sensitivity over unenhanced MRI [20].

Ulnar translocation of the wrist. This condition is normally seen in cases of rheumatoid arthritis or other wrist arthritides but rarely is noted in cases of post-traumatic carpal instability [7]. Two types have been noted, with type I involving translocation of the entire carpus and type II demonstrating a scapholunate gap as the scaphoid remains in anatomic position [7]. Ulnar translocation is determined by measuring the amount of lunate overhang on the posteroanterior wrist [7].

Carpal fracture

Fractures of the carpal bones are most common in the scaphoid, lunate, and hamate [8]. Scaphoid fractures are encountered most frequently and usually are the result of a fall on the outstretched hand [8], with pain in the anatomic snuffbox a clinical indicator [21]. Scaphoid fractures may be difficult to identify on standard views. Obtaining an ulnar deviated posteroanterior view elongates the scaphoid and may provide better visualization (a scaphoid view) [7]. Hamate fractures result from direct trauma to the hypothenar eminence from falls or from sports impact via racquet, bat, or golf club, and they usually involve levering off the hook portion. Lunate fractures are usually caused by avascular necrosis (AVN) and fragmentation. Carpal fractures often are radiographically occult and not visualized on initial radiographs and may take up to 6 weeks to become visible [8,23]. AVN is a potential serious consequence to carpal fracture, particularly of the scaphoid [1,8]. Because the blood supply to the scaphoid originates distally, the proximal segment tends to develop AVN [1]. Several authors have recommended obtaining MRI scans on patients suspected of having radiographically occult scaphoid fracture [1,23]. In lieu of casting for 4 to 6 weeks with repeat radiographs, MRI or CT can identify the problem with earlier treatment and potentially decrease lost productivity [1,23].

Fractures of the hook of the hamate can be difficult to diagnose and may require the carpal tunnel view, which is accomplished by placing the wrist palm down on the cassette and pulling the fingers and the palm dorsally [1]. The x-ray beam is angled 45° parallel to the palm. The hook of the hamate is seen as a bony protuberance on the ulnar aspect of the carpal tunnel. This fracture also may be visualized on a lateral radiograph. CT scanning may be indicated if this fracture is clinically suspected but not radiographically evident [1]. One other uncommon fracture seen is a triquetral fracture, which is best seen as a small chip of bone on the dorsum of the wrist [1,5].

Ulnolunate abutment syndrome

Also known as ulnar impaction syndrome or ulnar impingement syndrome, ulnolunate abutment syndrome involves changes related to chronic repetitive ulnar loading [8]. This syndrome also has been associated with distal radius fracture [11]. A long ulna may predispose to this condition with recurrent impaction on the lunate and triquetrum [8]. There is subsequent degeneration of the TFCC with chondromalacia of the ulnar head and lunate. MRI can depict the abnormalities, including subchondral cystic changes, subchondral sclerosis of the lunate, lunate-triquetral tears, and central perforation of the TFCC. Many of the abnormalities coexist and do not present as discrete entities because of the complex and interactive nature of the wrist anatomy. Familiarity with the potential lesions, how they may occur concomitantly, and presentation on history and physical examination allows an examiner to decide logically on which imaging modality to use along with necessary views and imaging findings.

Avascular necrosis

AVN previously was mentioned in relation to carpal fracture. Kienbock's disease is AVN with associated deformity of the lunate bone [1,12]. Bone scanning has high sensitivity but low specificity for AVN [1,6,8]. Late effects of AVN may be seen on plain film radiography with increased density [1]. CT is another option and is less expensive than MRI [6,8]. MRI also can demonstrate AVN early by noting marrow changes, which enhances early diagnosis [8,12].

Carpal tunnel syndrome

Many studies have been conducted recently on the use of imaging for carpal tunnel syndrome. Advances in imaging have allowed more detailed anatomic examination of the wrist and the structures in the carpal tunnel, primarily through MRI [24,25]. MRI findings in patients with carpal tunnel syndrome include median nerve enlargement proximal to the transverse carpal ligament, flattening of the nerve in the carpal tunnel, and bowing of the flexor retinaculum [8,12,26–29]. These anatomic findings have not been demonstrated to add significantly to the diagnostic armamentarium, however. To date, clinical examination and electrodiagnostic studies have been the gold standard for diagnosis of carpal tunnel syndrome. Even with the improved ability to visualize anatomy, several authors have stated that imaging does not add to diagnostic accuracy [1,8,26,30–32] MRI or other imaging should be reserved for patients with equivocal presentation or for patients who have diabetes and diffuse peripheral neuropathy that confounds electrodiagnostic studies [29].

Ulnar hammer syndrome

This condition is a vascular abnormality that involves lesions of the ulnar artery caused by repetitive compression to the hypothenar eminence, typically caused by vibrating tools. Patients exhibit pain, stiffness, and whitening of the affected fingers. Magnetic resonance angiography establishes the diagnosis.

Ganglion cysts

Ganglion cysts occur 70% of the time on the dorsum of the wrist and can occur on the volar region in the area of the trapeziotrapezoid joint [12]. Imaging is generally not helpful or necessary.

Osteomyelitis

Osteomyelitis can be evaluated by bone scanning or MRI.

Other disorders

Two other conditions that should be mentioned are DeQuervain's tenosynovitis and disorders of the flexor or extensor tendons of the forearm and wrist. DeQuervain's tenosynovitis remains a clinical diagnosis with no indication for routine imaging. Similarly, tendinous structures are well visualized on MRI, but no indication for this modality is documented for flexor and extensor disorders of the wrist and forearm. With regards to DeQuervain's tenosynovitis, some recent studies have explored the use of high-resolution ultrasound or MRI in this condition, but further studies are needed to validate these techniques [33–35].

Imaging of the hand

Traumatic injuries to the hand can be evaluated routinely by plain film radiography. The hand consists of the five metacarpals and five digits, with the thumb having two phalanges and the remaining fingers having three. Erkonen [36] proposed that proper nomenclature of the hand should refer to the digits as thumb, index, long, ring, and short. This naming removes potential confusion of numbering systems, particularly in a patient who has had previous amputation.

A significant portion of injuries to the hand that require imaging involves fractures, which may be simple, compound, spiral, transverse, oblique, nondisplaced, overriding, distracted, offset, or comminuted. Common fractures encountered in the hand include the following:

- Bennet's fracture, which is a fracture at the base of the thumb into the carpometacarpal joint that poses the risk of the metacarpal sliding out of alignment [1].
- Rolando's fracture, which is a comminuted fracture at the base of the thumb that extends into the joint [1].
- Pseudo-Bennet's fracture, which is a fracture at the base of the thumb that does not involve the joint [1].
- Gamekeeper's thumb, which occurs when there is an avulsion on the ulnar aspect of the MCP joint of the thumb at the insertion of the ulnar collateral ligament [1].
- Mallet finger, which occurs with an avulsion at the dorsal base of the distal phalanx at the insertion of the extensor digitorum tendon [1].
- Phalangeal fractures, which may involve proximal, middle, or distal phalanges and may be seen occasionally on one view [7]. Normally on the lateral view, the condyles of the phalanges overlap. If there is a fracture with a rotational component, a bicondylar sign is seen because the condyles are offset, with both being visible [7]. Fractures frequently may involve the tuft, in which case the nail plate must be evaluated, whereas fractures of the shaft of the proximal and middle phalanges may be either transverse or longitudinal.

- Flexor digitorum profundus avulsion, which may demonstrate an avulsion from the anterior base of the distal phalanx.

Dislocations of the metacarpal phalangeal, proximal interphalangeal, interphalangeal, or distal interphalangeal joints may be noted on radiographs. Other defects, such as Swan- neck deformity or Boutonniere deformity, may be seen, particularly in patients who have rheumatoid arthritis. Boutonniere deformity is a condition in which the middle finger joint is bent in a fixed position volarly and the distal joint is bent excessively posterior away from the palm. This condition also may be the result of an extensor tendon injury. Plain film radiography may be useful in identifying foreign bodies in the hand. Metallic foreign bodies are most easily seen, but wood and glass may be visualized if of a large enough size.

Summary

In choosing an imaging modality for the upper extremity, it is important to understand the indications and limitations of each modality and follow a proper decision logic with imaging directed by history and physical examination. Plain film radiography remains the mainstay of imaging, and other imaging studies should be ordered properly and judiciously.

In summarizing imaging choices for the wrist and hand, it is necessary to remember the following points:

- Plain film radiography should be the study of choice and can identify many areas of pathology.
- MRI may have some use in diagnosing TFCC lesions, carpal ligamentous injuries, and fractures. MRI also can demonstrate soft tissue abnormalities. MRI evaluation of the intrinsic carpal ligaments is specific, however, but suffers from low sensitivity and cannot exclude an injury to these areas [16]. MRI also has been shown to lack sensitivity or accuracy for diagnosing cartilage defects in the distal radius, scaphoid, lunate, or triquetrum [14].
- CT scanning can be used to evaluate osseous and articular morphology, healing, cysts, and tumors.
- Bone scanning may be useful in assessing aseptic AVN or other conditions that produce rapid bone turnover, such as neoplasm.
- Imaging of the wrist in carpal tunnel syndrome is generally not necessary.

Acknowledgments

The author would like to give special thanks to Carolyn Hassett for providing illustrations.

References

[1] Helms C. Fundamentals of skeletal Radiology. 3rd edition. Philadelphia: Elsevier; 2005.
[2] Potter H. Imaging of posttraumatic and soft tissue dysfunction of the elbow. Clin Orthop Relat Res 2000;370:9–18.
[3] Pomerance J. Radiographic analysis of lateral epicondylitis. J Shoulder Elbow Surg 2002;11(2): 156–7.
[4] Popovic N, Ferrara MA, Daenen B, et al. Imaging overuse injury of the elbow in professional team handball players: a bilateral comparison using plain films, stress radiography, ultrasound, and magnetic resonance imaging. Int J Sports Med 2001;22:60–7.
[5] Mettler F. Essentials of radiology. Philadelphia: WB Saunders; 1996.
[6] Nagle D. Evaluation of chronic wrist pain. J Am Acad Orthop Surg 2000;8(1):45–55.
[7] Shreibman K, Freeland A, Gilula L, et al. Imaging of the hand and wrist. Orthop Clin North Am 1997;28(4):537–82.
[8] Girgis W, Epstein R. Magnetic resonance imaging of the hand and wrist. Semin Roentgenol 2000;35:286–96.
[9] Palmer AK. Triangular fibrocartilge complex lesions: a classification. J Hand Surg [Am] 1989; 14:594–606.
[10] Ishii S. An anatomic study of the ligamentous structure of the triangular fibrocartilage complex. J Hand Surg 1998;23-A:977–85.
[11] Steinborn M, Schürmann M, Staebler A, et al. MR imaging of ulnocarpal impaction after fracture of the distal radius. AJR Am J Roentgenol 2003;181:195–8.
[12] DiMarcangelo M, Smith P. Use of magnetic resonance imaging to diagnose common wrist disorders. J Am Osteopath Assoc 2000;100(4):228–31.
[13] Haims A, Schweitzer M, Morrison W, et al. Limitations of MR imaging in the diagnosis of peripheral tears of the triangular fibrocartilage of the wrist. AJR Am J Roentgenol 2002;178: 419–22.
[14] Haims A, Moore A, Schweitzer M, et al. MRI in the diagnosis of cartilage injury in the wrist. Am J Radiol 2004;182:1267–71.
[15] Keogh C, Wong A, Wells N, et al. High-resolution sonography of the triangular fibrocartilage: initial experience and correlation with MRI and arthroscopic findings. AJR Am J Roentgenol 2004;182:333–6.
[16] Hobby J, Tom B, Bearcroft P, et al. Magnetic resonance imaging of the wrist: diagnostic performance statistics. Clin Radiol 2000;56:50–7.
[17] Chung, Lektrakul, Gigena, et al. Magnetic resonance imaging of the upper extremity: advances in technique and application. Clin Orthop Relat Res 2001;383:162–74.
[18] Haims A, Schweitzer M, Morrison W, et al. Internal derangement of the wrist: indirect MR arthrography versus unenhanced MR imaging. Radiology 2003;227:701–7.
[19] Vander Eynde S, De Smet L, Fabry G. Diagnostic value of arthrography and arthroscopy of the radiocarpal joint. Arthroscopy 1994;10:50–3.
[20] Johnstone DJ, Thorogood S, Smith WH, et al. A comparison of magnetic resonance imaging and arthroscopy in the investigation of chronic wrist pain. J Hand Surg [Br] 1997;22: 714–8.
[21] van Vugt R, Gijlsma J, van Vugt A. Chronic wrist pain: diagnosis and management. Development and use of a new algorithm. Ann Rheum Dis 1999;58:665–74.
[22] Watson HK, Brenner LH. Degenerative disorders of the wrist. J Hand Surg [Am] 1985;10: 1002–6.
[23] Nikken J, Uei E, Ginai A, et al. Acute wrist trauma: value of a short dedicated extremity MR imaging examination in prediction of need for treatment. Radiology 2005;234:116–24.
[24] Kocharian A, Adkins M, Amrami K, et al. Wrist: improved MR imaging with optimized transmit-receive coil design. Radiology 2002;223:870–6.
[25] Saupe N, Prussmann K, Luechinger R, et al. MR imaging of the wrist: comparison between 1.5 and 3-T MR imaging. Preliminary experience. Radiology 2005;234:256–64.

[26] Jarvik JG, Yuen E, Haynor DR, et al. MR nerve imaging in a prospective cohort of patients with suspected carpal tunnel syndrome. Neurology 2002;58:1597–602.

[27] Bonel H, Howe F, Clifton A, et al. Carpal tunnel syndrome: assessment by turbo spin echo, spin echo, and magnetization transfer imaging applied in a low-field MR system. J Comput Assist Tomogr 2001;25(1):137–45.

[28] Jarvik J, Kliot M, Maravilla K. MR nerve imaging of the wrist and hand. Hand Clin 2000;16(1): 13–24.

[29] Jarvik J, Yuen E. Diagnosis of carpal tunnel syndrome. Neurosurg Clin North Am 2001;12: 241–53.

[30] Lee C, Kem T, Yoon E, et al. Correlation of high-resolution ultrasonographic findings with the clinical symptoms and electrodiagnostic data in carpal tunnel syndrome. Ann Plast Surg 2005;54:20–3.

[31] Cudlip S, Howe F, Clifton A, et al. Magnetic resonance neurography studies of the median nerve before and after carpal tunnel decompression. J Neurosurg 2002;96:1046–51.

[32] Wu H-T, Schweitzer M, Culp R. Potential MR signs of recurrent carpal tunnel syndrome: initial experience. J Comput Assist Tomogr 2004;28:860–4.

[33] Giovagnorio F, Andreoli C, De Cicco ML. Ultrasonographic evaluation of de Quervain disease. J Ultrasound Med 1997;16(10):685–9.

[34] Glajchen N, Schweitzer M. MRI features in de Quervain's tenosynovitis of the wrist. Skeletal Radiol 1996;25(1):63–5.

[35] Pilagian G, Herbert R, Hearns M, et al. Evaluation and management of chronic work-related musculoskeletal disorders of the distal upper extremity. Am J Ind Med 2000;37(1):75–93.

[36] Erkonen W. Radiology 101: the basics and fundamentals of imaging. Philadelphia: Lippincott-Raven; 1998.

ELSEVIER
SAUNDERS

Clin Occup Environ Med
5 (2) 299–322

CLINICS IN
OCCUPATIONAL AND
ENVIRONMENTAL
MEDICINE

Tendinitis and Tendinosis of the Elbow, Wrist, and Hands

Jeffrey L. Wainstein, MD*, Tracy E. Nailor, MD

Concentra Medical Centers, 5730 Glenridge Drive, Suite 308, Atlanta, GA 30328, USA

Tendinopathy in the upper extremity is a common occupational illness and a frequent cause of disability in the working population. Tendinopathy is found in working and nonworking populations and can have a significant impact on work and quality of life. Often, tendinopathy can result in lost time from work and can even result in permanent disability [1].

Tendinopathy is the preferred clinical term for tendon disorders. The term tendinitis historically has been used because inflammation of the tendon was assumed to be the underlying pathophysiologic process. Inflammation of the tendon, or tendinitis, rarely occurs, however [2]. The term "tendinitis" is still in common use among clinicians and lay people and may be used interchangeably with the term tendinopathy in this article.

Anatomically located at the intersection of muscle and bone, tendons transmit force to enable movement and function. Gross inspection of a normal tendon shows a white glistening structure. Microscopically, tendons are composed of three main elements: collagen bundles, cells, and ground substance [3]. The histologic appearance of a normal tendon shows tightly packed bundles of collagen with little ground substance or cellular material. A double layered synovial sheath encases a tendon in areas of increased mechanical stress in the wrist and the hand. The synovial sheath aids in the smooth movement of the tendon. The flexor digital tendon sheaths have an additional retinacular, or ligamentous, component found intermittently along the tendon and are commonly referred to as pulleys.

Two types of tendinopathy—tendinosis and paratendonitis—are responsible for most clinical disorders of tendons in the upper extremity (Table 1). Tendinosis

* Corresponding author.
E-mail address: Jeffrey_Wainstein@concentra.com (J.L. Wainstein).

1526-0046/06/$ – see front matter
doi:10.1016/j.coem.2006.01.001 *occmed.theclinics.com*

Table 1
Histopathologic classification of tendon disorders

Pathologic diagnosis	Macroscopic pathology	Histopathologic findings
Tendinosis	Intratendinous degeneration (commonly caused by ageing, microtrauma, vascular compromise)	Collagen disorientation, disorganization, and fiber separation by an increase in mucoid ground substance, increased preponderance of cells and vascular spaces with or without neovascularization, and focal necrosis or calcification
Tendinitis	Symptomatic degeneration of the tendon with vascular disruption and inflammatory repair response	Degenerative changes (as noted previously) with superimposed evidence of tear, including fibroblastic and myofibroblastic proliferation, hemorrhage, and organizing granulation tissue
Paratenonitis	Inflammation of the outer layer of the tendon (paratenon) alone, regardless of whether the paratenon is lined by synovium	Mucoid degeneration if the areolar tissue is seen; scattered mild mononuclear infiltrate with or without focal fibrin deposition and fibrinous exudate
Paratenonitis with tendinosis	Paratenonitis associated with intratendinous degeneration	Degenerative changes as noted in tendinosis with mucoid degeneration with or without fibrous and scattered inflammatory cells in the paratenon alveolar tissue

From Khan KM, Cook JL, Bonar F, et al. Histopathology of common tendinopathies: update and implications for clinical management. Sports Med 1999;27(6):393–408; with permission.

is thought to be caused by mechanical overload with microtrauma, vascular compromise, and aging [4] and presents as tendon degeneration without signs of inflammation. Tendons affected with tendinosis grossly appear dull, gray, friable, and amorphous [3]. Microscopically they show disorganized collagen fibrils, an increase in the amount of ground substance, an increase in cellular material (primarily fibroblasts) and neovascularization, with a proliferation of disorganized capillaries and arterioles [4].

Paratendonitis, or stenosing tenosynovitis, is an inflammation of the tissues that surround the tendon and occurs where a tendon rubs over a bony prominence [4]. Acute edema of the paratendon with infiltration of inflammatory cells is seen. A fibrinous exudate may fill the synovial sheath and can result in the clinical finding of crepitus. Paratendonitis may be associated with degenerative changes in the tendon (tendinosis) but is rarely associated with inflammation of the tendon itself (tendinitis).

Epidemiology and work relatedness

Tendinopathy has been recognized as a common work-related condition, although it is difficult to estimate the exact prevalence of this disorder in the working population, because few epidemiologic studies differentiate between tendinopathy of the upper extremity and other work-related upper extremity disorders. The prevalence of tendinopathy in the working population is likely underestimated because of underreporting by employees and employers.

According to the Bureau of Labor Statistics, 7730 cases of tendinitis that resulted in lost time were reported in the United States in 2003. This figure represented 0.6% of all lost time cases with a median of 11 days away from work [5]. In a study of workers in an automobile plant, the prevalence of pain in the forearm and hand among high-risk workers was 36% in men and 50% in women, whereas it was 17% and 28%, respectively, in a control group. The most prevalent clinical diagnoses were de Quervain's tendinitis in 9.8% of men and carpal tunnel syndrome (CTS) in 10.7% of women [6]. In a study of 749 workers who performed tasks not at risk for work-related upper extremity disorders, the incidence of lateral epicondylitis was only 0.2% to 0.3% and the incidence of wrist/hand tendinitis was 0.9% [7].

Most cases of tendinopathy in the United States are not work related. In a study by Tanaka and colleagues [8] in 1998, they estimated approximately 395,000 cases tendinitis of the distal upper extremity among US workers, with only 37% of cases identified in the study population determined to be work-related by medical personnel. In this study, 31% of these work-related cases were diagnosed as tendinitis and related disorders, with 69% of the cases being diagnosed as CTS.

Risk factors

The occurrence of tendinopathy seems to be related to certain types of work. A causal relationship between distinct medical entities and work activities has not been established, however [9]. Epidemiologic data show that the risk of tendinopathy of the hand and wrist in people who perform highly repetitive and forceful jobs is 29 times greater than in people who perform jobs that are low in repetitiveness and force [10]. In a group of textile workers, there was a statistically higher prevalence of tendinopathy in physically demanding job categories with no establishment of direct causation [11]. In a study of workers in a meat processing plant, the incidence of tendinopathy was 25.3% for female packers, 16.8% for female sausage makers, and 12.5% for male meat cutters, whereas the incidence was less than 1% in employees with nonstrenuous jobs. In the same plant, the incidence of epicondylitis was 7% for female packers, 11.3% for female sausage makers, and 6.4% for male meat cutters, compared with an incidence of 1% for employees in nonstrenuous jobs [12]. Many studies have confirmed this correlation with strenuous job tasks [10,13–20].

Specific mechanical risk factors for tendinopathy in the upper extremity include bending and twisting of the hand and wrist, high hand force, or forceful gripping and awkward wrist positions [21]. Vibration has been shown to be a risk factor for CTS, but it has not been shown to be a risk factor for tendinitis. Job types found to have a high incidence of tendinopathy include the textile, leather, and food industries, construction, manufacturing, assembly line work, wallboard installation, and wood products manufacturing [14].

Non–work-related risk factors, including personal and psychosocial factors, have been implicated in the development of some types of tendinopathy [22]. Gender, age, obesity, and poor general overall muscular conditioning have been found to be related to the development of tendinopathy [23]. Psychosocial risk factors, such as monotonous work, perceived high work load, time pressure, and low control and social support, play a role in the development and reporting of tendinopathy [24]. These psychosocial effects may be mediated indirectly through three mechanisms: (1) alterations of muscle tension or other physiologic processes [25], (2) altered perception of pain and its cause [24], and (3) increased willingness to report symptoms [24].

The risk factors found to have the highest predictive value for identifying a person who is likely to develop upper extremity tendinitis include age over 40, body mass index >30, a complaint of baseline shoulder or neck discomfort, a history of CTS, and a job with a higher shoulder posture rating [26].

Systemic risk factors for tendinitis include pregnancy, diabetes, rheumatoid diseases, gout, collagen vascular disease, Dupuytren's disease, thyroid disease, amyloidosis, and chronic renal disease [27]. The presence of rheumatoid factor has been found to be more common in people with recurrent wrist tenosynovitis, and HLA B27 has been found to be more prevalent in workers diagnosed with epicondylitis [28].

Causation

Work relatedness commonly goes unquestioned, although more than 60% of all cases of tendinopathy are not work related [8]. The symptoms of tendinitis can be exacerbated by manual work and are more commonly reported by employees who perform manual work compared with employees in nonmanual jobs [29]. Because of this, tendinitis may be assumed to be caused by work.

In an occupational setting, determination of causation or work relatedness should be performed using standard means of assessment. Clinicians should obtain the following information: specific job tasks, length of time at these tasks, exacerbation of symptoms with job duties, the presence of similar symptoms among co-workers, and a history of changing or increasing job demands, including higher productivity quotas and overtime work. The presence of any non–work-related physical risk factors also should be determined.

Clinical diagnosis

The diagnosis of tendinopathy is clinical and is based primarily on the history and physical examination. Ancillary testing is rarely helpful or necessary to confirm the diagnosis. Pain and tenderness over a specific tendon or tendon group are the hallmarks of this condition. Tendinosis, however, can be asymptomatic. Other clinical findings include localized swelling, impaired function, crepitus, pain with passive stretching of the tendon, and positive provocative testing. A clinician should be cautious when assigning someone a diagnosis of tendinopathy who has nonspecific upper extremity pain. Too often, vague pain with a lack of objective physical findings is attributed to tendinopathy. Accurate diagnosis of tendinopathy is essential. A complete examination of the upper extremity, including the neck, is recommended because coexisting clinical conditions are found frequently in patients who have work-related upper extremity pain.

Specific clinical conditions

Elbow

Elbow pain accounts for 2% to 3% of total lost workdays and 5% to 6% of workers' compensation claims [30]. The two important diagnoses to consider in a patient who presents with elbow pain are lateral and medial epicondylitis. Lateral epicondylitis results in an average of 12 weeks of absenteeism in as many as 30% of persons afflicted [31].

Lateral epicondylitis (tennis elbow)

Lateral epicondylitis was first described by Runge in 1873 [32]. Originally thought to be an inflammatory process, the precise pathology is uncertain, and as many as 30 different causes have been proposed [33]. The pathophysiologic mechanism responsible for the development of lateral epicondylitis is currently thought to be increased and excessive tensile loading on the tendon insertions of the proximal wrist extensors at the elbow, primarily the extensor carpi radialis brevis tendon [34]. This results in small tears, or microinjury, of the tendon structure. With repetitive injury, this microinjury overwhelms the tendons capacity for repair and incomplete healing occurs. Incomplete healing eventually leads to tendon degeneration. Surgical specimens show hyaline degeneration with neovascularization, which has been labeled angiofibroblastic tendinosis [35]. No histologic evidence of acute inflammation has been found in lateral epicondylitis [35,36]. Epicondylalgia and lateral tendinosis of the elbow are more appropriate clinical terms.

Clinical presentation. Lateral epicondylitis presents with pain at the lateral epicondyle in the elbow and localized tenderness just distal to the lateral epicondyle. The pain may radiate into the forearm and is exacerbated by active and resisted wrist extension and forearm supination, by grasping objects forcefully, and by lifting objects with the forearm pronated. Although persons affected may report muscular weakness, range of motion is typically unaffected. Symptoms are precipitated by overuse or acute trauma.

On clinical examination, Cozen's test is considered positive when, with the patient's forearm pronated and wrist radially deviated, the examiner elicits pain at the lateral aspect of the elbow upon resisted extension [37]. Because pain in other areas of the upper extremity is frequently found in association with lateral epicondylitis, a detailed examination of the neck and upper extremity is warranted to rule out comorbid conditions.

Differential diagnosis for lateral elbow pain includes lateral collateral ligament tear, radiocapitellar joint instability, bursitis, synovitis, arthritis, chondromalacia, osseochondritis dessicans, stenosis of the orbicular ligament, anconeus compartment syndrome, posterior interosseus nerve or radial nerve entrapment, lateral antebrachial nerve entrapment, triceps tendinitis, and cervical radiculopathy [38]. Radial tunnel syndrome may coexist in up to 5% of patients who have lateral epicondylitis and should be included in the differential diagnosis [33].

Epidemiology and work relatedness. The incidence of lateral epicondylitis is approximately 1% to 3% in the general population [39]. The prevalence of lateral epicondylitis among high-risk groups is as high as 15% [31], with women over 40 years of age commonly affected [40]. Lateral epicondylitis is five to nine times more common than medial epicondylitis [41].

Work relatedness of this disorder has been debated [42]. Use of the elbow has not been shown to cause lateral epicondylitis [29], although there is strong evidence for an association between exposure to a combination of risk factors, including high hand force, repetition, and awkward posture, and the presence of lateral epicondylitis [20,43]. Neither the performance of unaccustomed work nor work with a visual display unit or a computer mouse has been shown to be associated with the development of lateral epicondylitis [20]. High-risk occupations for lateral epicondylitis include construction, wall board installation, mechanics, carpentry, plumbing, wood products manufacturing, meat processing, and food handling [21,44].

Diagnosis and treatment. Specific diagnostic tests play no active role in the diagnosis and treatment of lateral epicondylitis. Elbow radiographs are generally unremarkable in lateral epicondylitis; however, in 20% of cases a small calcific deposit is noted in the region of the lateral epicondyle [35]. MRI and CT have no role in the clinical evaluation of lateral epicondylitis.

Little is known about the natural history of lateral epicondylitis, and there is a lack of consensus on its appropriate management. Limited research-based evidence exists regarding the efficacy of common treatment modalities. Poor prognosis at 1-year follow-up has been found to be related only to high baseline pain and manual work [45].

Conservative treatment is effective in up to 90% of cases of lateral epicondylitis, yet more than 40% of patients can experience prolonged minor discomfort [46]. Conservative treatment includes nonsteroidal anti-inflammatory drugs (NSAIDs), application of ice, and rest. NSAIDs are generally recommended acutely to provide symptomatic pain relief despite some controversy regarding their benefit [47]. Modified work duties with biomechanical correction of activity and reduction of excessive loads may be necessary. Workplace changes to consider include using lighter weight tools to help reduce forces needed to accomplish tasks and using modified hand tools to help avoid awkward hand positions. Loads should be lifted with the arm in a flexed position, because lifting with the arm fully extended tends to increase symptoms. No evidence shows that persistent use of the elbow with tolerant symptoms significantly alters the natural history of epicondylitis [29].

Tennis elbow bands or counterforce braces decrease the force transmitted to the tendon insertion to prevent further injury and allow for the healing process to proceed. Wrist splints that maintain the wrist at 30° to 45° extension also may help reduce continued trauma to the tendon by preventing forced wrist extension [48]. Wrist splints have not been shown to be superior to tennis elbow bands in the treatment of lateral epicondylitis [49]. There is some evidence that use of splints and bands in treatment actually may increase case duration [50].

Physical therapy and rehabilitation have been used in the treatment of lateral epicondylitis and are recommended as the first line of treatment in patients with symptoms of short duration. [51] Exercises aimed at stretching and strengthening are recommended along with modalities such as iontophoresis, e-stim, ultrasound, manipulation, soft tissue mobilization, and deep transverse friction massage. In a recent meta-analysis of clinical trials on treatments of lateral epicondylitis, however, a lack of evidence for the long-term benefit of physical interventions in general was found. A favorable effect of exercise on pain relief and some evidence of a positive effect of elbow manipulation suggested the need for further research. Some evidence supported the efficacy of acupuncture, ultrasound, and ionization in short-term outcomes, but this effect disappeared in long-term follow-up [31]. Deep tissue friction massage has not proved to be of benefit [52].

Corticosteroid injection around the lateral epicondyle is safe and effective in the short-term and is indicated if conservative treatment fails to relieve symptoms [53]. Corticosteroid injection has been found to be more effective than physiotherapy at 6 weeks of treatment, with success rates of up to 92% [54]. Recurrence rate is high in patients who receive steroid injection, however, and no long-term benefit (>6 months) has been found [55]. Minor complications, such as local skin depigmentation and skin atrophy, can occur with local corticosteroid injection. In rare instances, tendon rupture can occur [56]. The risk of tendon rupture increases with multiple injections.

Other treatments, such as acupuncture, manipulation, orthoses, low energy laser, glycosaminoglycan polysulfate injection, botulinum toxin injection, and topical nitric oxide application, have been used to treat lateral epicondylitis, although insufficient evidence exists to support or refute their use [57]. Extracorporeal shock wave treatment also has been used, but a recent study failed to prove any clinical benefit of this modality with lateral epicondylitis [58].

Surgical intervention is indicated for patients who fail conservative medical management after 6 to 12 months [33]. Surgical outcomes are generally excellent, with up to 90% success rates [33,59], although outcomes are less successful in work-related cases [29]. Failure to return to regular work occurs in up to 50% of patients in a workers' compensation population [38].

Medial epicondylitis (golfers' elbow)

Medial epicondylitis affects the proximal wrist flexors and pronators at the elbow, primarily at the interface between the pronator teres and the flexor carpi radialis. The histology and pathophysiology are similar to that of lateral epicondylitis [35,60].

Clinical presentation. Medial epicondylitis presents clinically as elbow pain and tenderness at or just distal to the medial epicondyle over the pronator teres and the flexor carpi radialis. Persons affected may report radiation of pain distally to the forearm. Typically, the pain is of gradual onset but may be precipitated by direct trauma or a single acute event. Compared with lateral epicondylitis, there is less impairment of overall arm function [61]. On examination, symptoms are exacerbated by resisted forearm pronation with wrist in flexion.

Other work-related upper extremity disorders are commonly associated with medial epicondylitis, including CTS, lateral epicondylitis, and shoulder tendinitis [62]. Ulnar neuropathy is found in up to 60% of patients who have medial epicondylitis [63]. The differential diagnosis includes medial collateral ligament instability or tear, ulnar trochlear synovitis, chondromalacia, arthritis, and cervical radiculopathy [38].

Epidemiology and work relatedness. Few studies are available regarding the epidemiology of medial epicondylitis, and most do not differentiate medial epicondylitis from lateral epicondylitis or other work-related upper extremity disorders. The prevalence of medial epicondylitis in a work population ranges from 4% to 5%% with an annual incidence estimate of 1.5% [64]. Medial epicondylitis accounts for 10% to 20% of all epicondylitis diagnoses [62]. Risk factors include forceful work but not repetitive work [64].

Diagnosis and treatment. The diagnosis is made clinically, and radiographs are typically normal, although up to 25% of patients can have soft tissue calcification in the area of the medial epicondyle [62]. Treatment considerations are similar to lateral epicondylitis. Initial treatment consists of ice, NSAIDs, and physical therapy with an emphasis on stretching and strengthening. Soft elbow pads may be useful to avoid direct trauma. Patient education, activity modification, and ergonomic workplace changes may be required. Corticosteroid injection around the tendon is used for cases unresponsive to medical management and provides short-term benefit similar to that seen with lateral epicondylitis [65]. Operative treatment is reserved for cases resistant to conservative management, and surgical outcomes are generally good [62].

Wrist

The wrist is an anatomically complex structure and a common site of tendinopathy. De Quervain's disease is the most frequent condition seen in the wrist.

Anatomy

The wrist and hand extensors originate at the lateral epicondyle of the distal humerus at the elbow and run on the dorsal surface of the forearm. They pass under the extensor retinaculum at the wrist. Six distinct compartments, or osseofibrous canals, are present deep to the extensor retinaculum at the wrist through which these tendons travel. The first extensor compartment contains the abductor pollucis longus and extensor pollucis brevis and is the site of involvement in de Quervain's syndrome. The second compartment contains the extensor carpi radialis longus and the extensor carpi radialis brevis, and involvement of this area is seen in intersection syndrome (Fig. 1). The wrist and hand flexors originate at the medial epicondyle of the humerus in the elbow and run on the volar surface of the forearm. They course under the flexor retinaculum at the wrist through the carpal tunnel.

Tendinopathy of the wrist extensors

De Quervain's disease

The most common tendinopathy in the wrist was first described by Swiss physician Fritz de Quervain in 1895 [66]. De Quervain's disease is classified as a stenosing tenosynovitis or tenovaginitis. The pathophysiologic changes include a thickening of the extensor retinaculum over the first extensor compartment [67] with a thickening of the tendon sheaths in the first extensor compartment and a proliferation of fibrous tissue. [68] Impaired gliding that leads to mechanical impingement of the abductor pollucis longus and extensor pollucis brevis tendons results from the narrowing of the fibro-osseous canal through which they travel [67]. Intrinsic degenerative mechanisms have been postulated as the cause of these changes. No signs of acute inflammation in the tendon itself are seen histologically [69].

Clinical presentation. The clinical hallmark of de Quervain's disease is pain located on the radial side of the wrist in the area overlying the first extensor compartment at the radial styloid. The pain may radiate proximally or distally and is exacerbated by flexion and abduction of the thumb and ulnar deviation of the wrist. Associated symptoms include swelling, warmth, and crepitus. Acute trauma may precipitate de Quervain's disease, although it most commonly has no specific antecedent. In 1930, Finklestein [70] described the provocative test for de Quervain's disease, which bears his name and is pathognomonic for the disorder. As he originally described the maneuver, "on grasping the patient's thumb and quickly abducting the hand ulnarward, the pain over the radial styloid

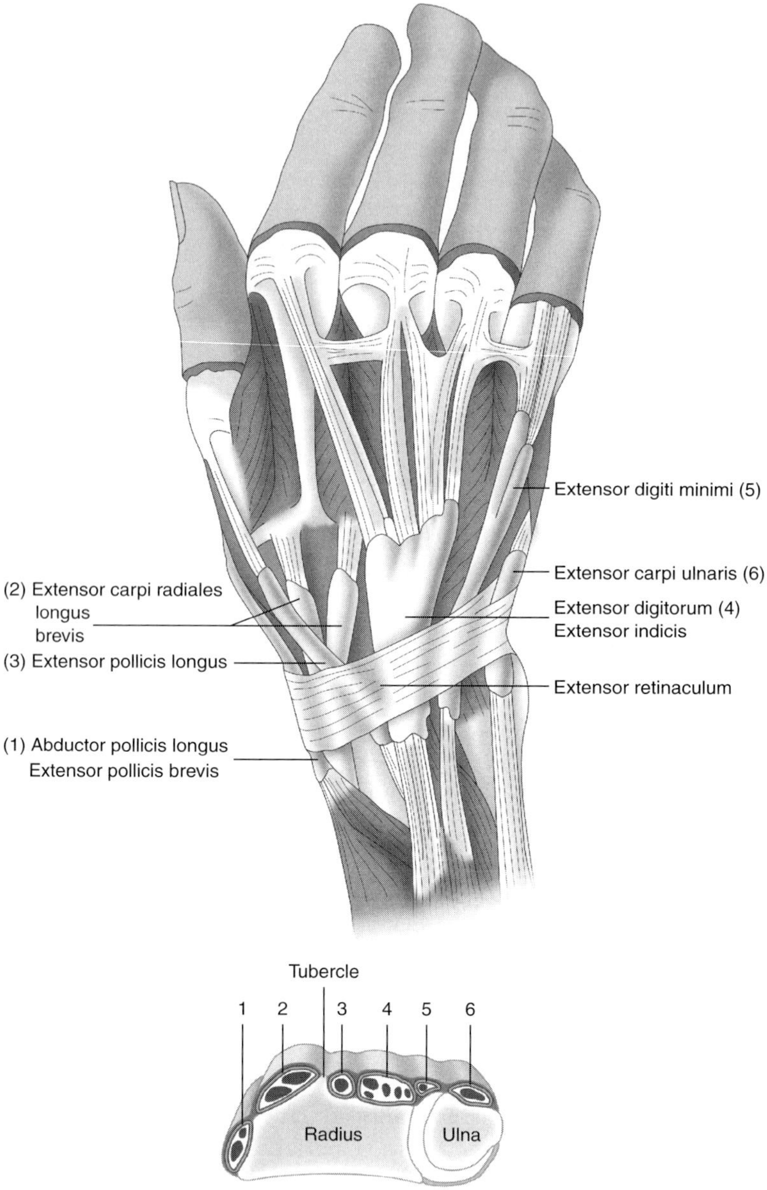

Fig. 1. A drawing of the synovial sheaths on the dorsum of the wrist.

is excruciating." Finklestein's test is more commonly performed by having a patient grasp the thumb with the fingers and forcibly deviate the wrist in an ulnar direction. Intense pain of the radial side of the wrist is considered a positive sign.

Epidemiology and work relatedness. De Quervain's tenosynovitis is most commonly seen in adults aged 30 to 50. Women are affected ten times more frequently than men [71]. De Quervain's occurs with equal frequency in the dominant and nondominant hands [72]. Repetitive, forceful, radial deviation of the wrist with abduction and extension of the thumb [73] and rapid rotational movements of the forearm with repetitive movements and forceful ulnar deviation at the wrist [74] have been identified as risk factors for de Quervain's disease. Pain symptoms can be aggravated by the use of the affected hand at work, which can be misinterpreted as being caused by work. There is, however, no validated evidence for causation by work [68].

Associated activities and occupations for de Quervain's tenosynovitis include prolonged piano playing, working at a typewriter or adding machine, excessive writing, washing, or wringing out clothes, chopping wood, carrying heavy objects, farm labor, sewing, knitting, weaving, and cutting cloth, working on a grinding or buffing machine, and repeated unaccustomed movement [21,67]. Nonoccupational risk factors, including rheumatoid arthritis and hormonal changes associated with pregnancy and menopause, have been shown to be associated with de Quervain's disease [68].

Diagnosis and treatment. Diagnostic testing has limited value in the evaluation of de Quervain's disease because the diagnosis is primarily a clinical one. As with other work-related upper extremity disorders, a thorough evaluation of the neck and upper extremity is mandatory to detect the presence of coexisting conditions. Approximately one third of patients who have de Quervain's disease may have associated conditions, such as cervical spondylosis, CTS, ganglions, trigger fingers, lateral epicondylitis, and rheumatoid arthritis [68]. Differential diagnosis includes osteoarthritis of the first carpometacarpal joint, Wartenberg's syndrome, Kienbock's disease, triscaphoid arthritis, and intersection syndrome [75,76].

Initial treatment is nonoperative and includes relative rest with consideration to modified work activity. Worksite modification may be necessary for long-term treatment and prevention of recurrence. Short-term splinting for acute painful cases may be used, although immobilization has not been shown to offer any long-term therapeutic advantage [77]. Immobilization is best accomplished with a thumb spica splint. NSAIDs and ice can be helpful for pain control. Physical therapy, with emphasis on stretching and strengthening, should be considered with judicious use of modalities such as cold, heat, ultrasound, and iontophoresis. Continuous low-level heat wrap therapy has been shown to be effective for pain control [78].

Injection of the tendon sheath of the first extensor compartment with a corticosteroid preparation is the preferred initial treatment for de Quervain's tenosynovitis [79,80]. Results of a recent meta-analysis showed that there is an 83% cure rate with injection alone, compared with 61% for injection and splinting, 14% for splinting alone, and 0% for rest and NSAIDs [81]. Corticosteroid injection can be repeated up to three times, although repeat injections increase the risk of complications, including tendon rupture. Treatment failure is more likely with chronic cases, which have a higher incidence of significant fibrosis of the tendon sheath. Anatomic anomalies, such as a septated first extensor compartment and duplicated or absent tendons, are common and can result in treatment failures.

Surgery is necessary for patients who fail conservative medical management. Results of surgery are excellent, with up to 96% of patients having total relief of symptoms [82]. The need for meticulous exploration to identify anatomic anomalies and avoid the superficial branch of the radial nerve is necessary for good surgical results.

Intersection syndrome

Intersection syndrome, first described by Velpeau in 1841 [83], affects the second dorsal compartment of the wrist. Other descriptive names for this condition include peritendinitis crepitans, crossover syndrome, squeakers, bugaboo forearm, Oarsman's wrist, adventitial bursitis, subcutaneous perimyositis, and abductor pollicus longus syndrome [83,84]. The pathophysiology of this condition was once postulated to be caused by friction between the abductor pollicus longus and extensor pollicus brevis where they cross over the tendon sheath that contains the extensor carpi radialis longus and extensor carpi radialis brevis. The cause is now thought to be stenosis of the second dorsal compartment, similar to the cause of de Quervain's disease (Fig. 2) [85].

Clinical presentation. Clinical findings include forearm pain and swelling 4 to 8 cm proximal to the radial styloid. Crepitus is a common associated finding that results from fluid accumulation in the synovium. Pain is provoked by pulling or twisting hand motions with radial deviation.

Epidemiology and work relatedness. The condition is found in approximately 0.37% of patients with arm or hand pain and is frequently misdiagnosed as de

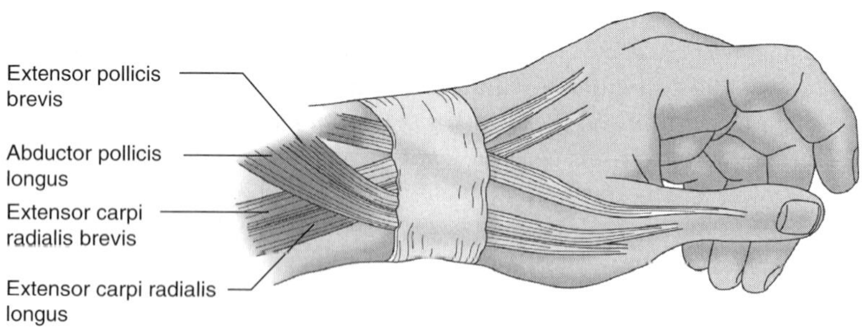

Fig. 2. Representation of the anatomy of the wrist. (*From* Hanlon DP, Luellen JR. Intersection syndrome: a case report and review of the literature. J Emerg Med 1999;17(6):970; with permission.)

Quervain's [84]. Work-related risk factors include repetition, awkward joint posture, and prolonged constrained posture, although causation has not been proved [84].

Diagnosis and treatment. Management of intersection syndrome consists primarily of conservative treatment, including modified work activity, ice pack, splint, and NSAIDs. Unlike with de Quervain's disease, corticosteroid injection is recommended only after 2 to 3 weeks of persistent symptoms [84]. Forty percent of patients do not respond to these nonoperative measures and require surgical release [85].

Extensor carpi ulnaris tendinopathy

The extensor carpi ulnaris tendon is contained in the sixth extensor compartment. Extensor carpi ulnaris tendinopathy is a stenosing tenosynovitis similar to that of de Quervain's. It is the second most common sports-related overuse injury of the wrist and presents with pain at the head of the ulna [86]. Extensor carpi ulnaris tendinopathy is related to excessive ulnar deviation of the wrist and can be associated with a subluxation of the extensor carpi ulnaris tendon over the head of the ulna. On clinical examination this subluxation can be elicited by active ulnar deviation with the wrist in supination. Corticosteroid injection may be useful in the treatment of extensor carpi ulnaris tendinopathy. Injury to the dorsal sensory branch of the ulnar nerve is a potential complication. Surgical decompression of the compartment may be warranted if conservative treatment fails, with surgical correction of the tendon subluxation if present.

Other

Tendinopathy that affects the third through fifth compartments presents similarly with pain and tenderness over the affected tendons. These tendinopathies generally respond to conservative medical management that consists of ice, relative rest, NSAIDs, and physical therapy. Surgery is rarely necessary.

Tendinopathy of the wrist flexors

Flexor carpi radialis tendinopathy

Flexor carpi radialis tendinopathy is an uncommon cause of radiovolar pain in the wrist [87]. The proximity of the flexor carpi radialis tendon to the carpal bones causes vulnerability of the tendon to primary stenosing tenosynovitis in an overuse syndrome or as a secondary process associated with soft tissue injury or osteoarthritis of the adjacent carpal structures [88]. Degenerative arthritis of the carpometacarpal joint of the thumb commonly is associated. Diagnosis of this disorder is difficult because of other more common conditions in the region and because it may be missed if a concomitant local lesion is present [88].

Clinical presentation consists of pain at the volar wrist near the scaphoid tubercle associated with crepitus. Diagnosis is confirmed clinically when resisted palmar flexion or radial deviation elicits pain and tenderness over the flexor carpi radialis tendon in its location at the wrist flexion crease [88]. The typical patient with flexor carpi radialis tendonitis is a woman older than age 50 with onset of radial wrist pain who also performs repetitive wrist motion during her daily tasks [4].

Conservative management includes immobilization, administration of NSAIDs, and physical therapy for up to 6 weeks [89]. Surgical decompression of the flexor carpi radialis tendon is warranted if conservative treatment fails.

Flexor carpi ulnaris tendinopathy

Flexor carpi ulnaris (FCU) tendinopathy is an uncommon entity but should be included in the differential diagnosis of ulnar wrist pain. In contrast to the flexor carpi radialis tendon, the FCU tendon does not have a sheath. The pathology related to the FCU tendon is not classified as a stenosing tenosynovitis but rather as a tendinosis, although calcific tendonitis of the FCU has been well described [90].

Diagnosis is made clinically by tenderness at the FCU tendon or pain elicited with resisted wrist flexion [91]. Plain lateral radiographs of wrist taken in slight supination and extension may show calcification at the FCU tendon [91].

Knowledge of the important anatomic distinction in FCU tendinopathy should guide therapeutic intervention more toward strengthening and stretching exercises after a period of rest and immobilization rather than anti-inflammatory medications and corticosteroid injections reserved for treatment of tenosynovitis. Surgical excision of the degenerative portion of the FCU tendon is warranted if conservative treatment fails.

Tendinopathy of the finger flexors

It is important to understand the anatomy of the hand to diagnose trigger finger (TF) and less common varieties of flexor tendinopathy appropriately in a patient who presents with hand or finger pain. Originating in the forearm, the extrinsic flexor tendons of the hand represent the terminal functional units of the deep forearm muscles, namely the flexor digitorum profundus, flexor digitorum superficialis, and the flexor pollicis longus tendons [92]. These tendons traverse the carpal tunnel entering the palmar surface of the hand enclosed in synovial sheaths, which are useful in delineating the five significant zones of the hand [92]. Zone 1, the most distal, includes the flexor digitorum profundus tendon. Zone 2, located just proximal to zone 1 and extending to the end of the fibrous digital sheath, includes the flexor digitorum profundus and flexor digitorum superficialis. The important pulley system of the finger is specific to this zone. Zone 3 extends from the proximal end of the digital sheath to the distal transverse carpal ligament. This zone is devoid of pulleys. Zone 4 is the carpal tunnel, and zone 5 is the start of the distal forearm (Fig. 3).

The finger pulley system housed in zone 2 of the hand is of particular interest when discussing TF. There are five segments of transverse (annular) or oblique (cruciate) thickenings situated in the synovial sheath on the flexor side of the

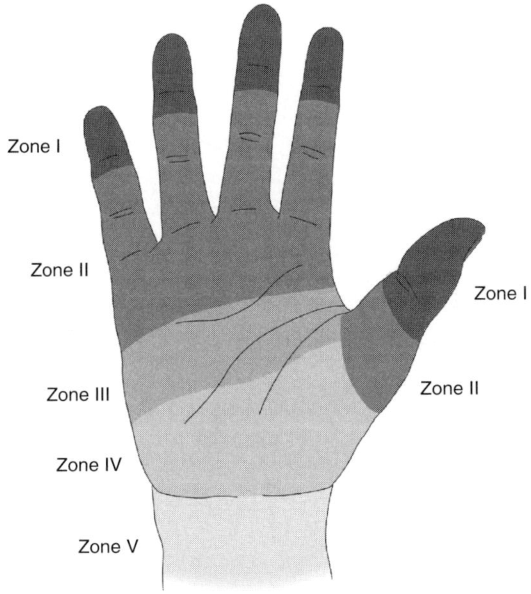

Fig. 3. Flexor tendon zones. (*From* Allan CH. Flexor tendons: anatomy and surgical approaches. Hand Clinics 2005;21:152; with permission.)

digits, referred to as pulleys. The annular pulleys begin proximal to the metacarpophalangeal (MP) joint and end at the distal phalanx (Fig. 4). Between the annular pulleys are the cruciate pulleys that are located typically over the interphalangeal joint. The thumb has just two annular pulleys with a cruciate ligament in between (Fig. 5). The purpose of the pulley system is to hold the flexor tendons

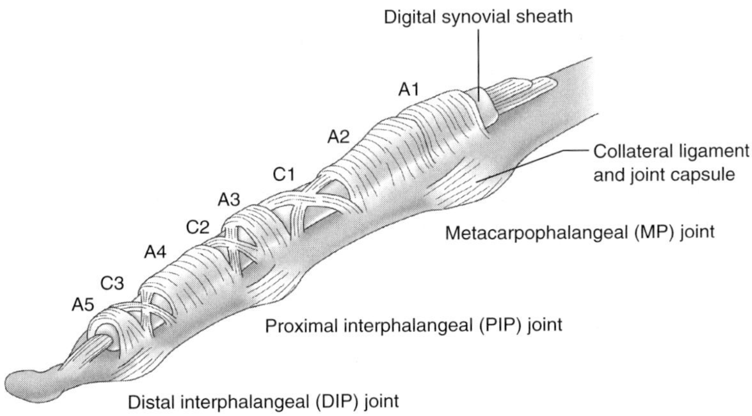

Fig. 4. Digital flexor sheath: annular and cruciate pulleys. (*From* Allan CH. Flexor tendons: anatomy and surgical approaches. Hand Clinics 2005;21:153; with permission.)

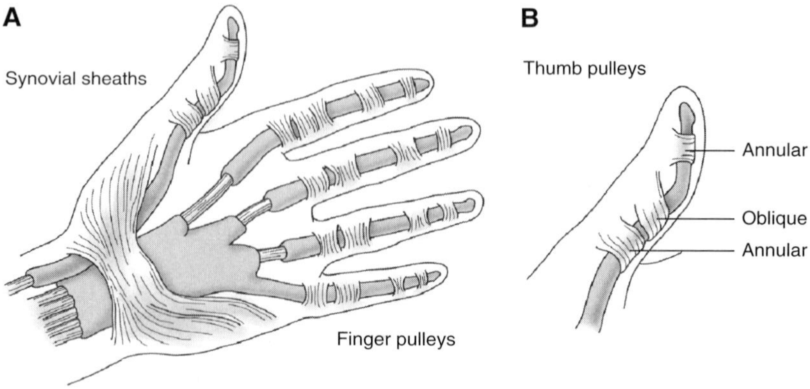

Fig. 5. (*A*) Synovial and retinacular pulleys at the wrist and digit levels. (*B*) The thumb pulley. (*From* Chase RA. Atlas of hand surgery. Philadelphia: WB Saunders; 1984. p. 32; with permission.)

close to the phalanges throughout range of motion and prevent bowstringing of the tendons across the joints when in flexion.

Trigger finger

TF was first described in the late eighteenth century by two French surgeons, Nelaton and Notta, who characterized "rebounding" or "springing" fingers as "doigt a resort" based on four case reports and cadaveric dissections [93–95]. Notta is credited as first describing the flexor sheath currently known as the pulley system, which is an important anatomic landmark in the discussion of TF [95]. Known also as stenosing tenovaginitis or tenosynovitis in the literature, TF is defined as a snapping or catching of the thumb or finger flexors because of inflammation of the tendon sheath [96]. In a recent literature review on TF, this disorder is redefined as a flexor tendon entrapment caused by stenosis of the digit's tendon sheath [97]. Whether viewed primarily as an inflammatory or stenotic process, TF ultimately results because of interference in normal gliding of the flexor tendon within the synovial lining of its sheath [97]. The thumb and ring and long fingers are the digits most commonly affected (Table 2) [96].

Clinical presentation. Patients who have TF typically present with pain and snapping, clicking, locking, or stiffness in the affected digit [97,98]. Onset of symptoms is usually insidious with more frequent occurrence in the morning [98]. Patients often note a gradual resolution in symptoms as the day progresses [98]. The triggering may range from barely perceptible to painful if the affected digit is forcefully extended [92]. Pain may be localized to the proximal interphalangeal joint of the finger, the interphalangeal joint of the thumb, or the palmar aspect of the MP joint sometimes associated with a painful nodule near the distal palmar crease [92,97]. Radiation of pain has not been reported [92].

Table 2
Digital distribution of the results of corticosteroid injection in the treatment of trigger finger and thumb

Digit	No.	Type	No.	Successful
Thumb	47	Nodular	35	32
		Diffuse	12	4
Fingers	54	Nodular	33	31
		Diffuse	21	6
TOTAL	101			

From Freiberg A, Mulholland RS, Levine R. Nonoperative treatment of trigger fingers and thumbs. J Hand Surg [Am] 1989;19A:554; ©1989, with permission from the American Society for Surgery of the Hand.

Physical examination may or may not reveal active triggering [99]. A painful nodule may be palpable at the distal palmar crease synonymous with the anatomic location of the A1 pulley. As a patient actively flexes and extends the affected digit, the nodule may move or the digit may become locked in a flexed position [97]. The lateral pinch test of Savill, a palpable thickening of soft tissue over the flexor tendons, has been mentioned historically in the literature as a method of detecting TF on physical examination [100].

Epidemiology and work relatedness. TF is more common in women in their fifties and sixties. This disorder also affects children, especially younger than 6 years of age. Although TF typically involves one digit, with the thumb affected most often followed by the long finger and ring finger, multiple digits may be affected, particularly in systemic illnesses, such as diabetes mellitus. The dominant extremity is affected more often than the nondominant one. In addition to diabetes, other systemic diseases associated with TF include rheumatoid arthritis, Dupuytren's disease, hypothyroidism, alcoholism, amyloidosis, and mucopolysaccharidoses. Comorbid conditions seen with TF include CTS, de Quervain's tenosynovitis, carpal and metacarpal fractures, and epicondylitis.

Early experiments by Sperling in the 1950s, in which he used himself as a test subject, confirmed that repetitive movement of the thumb and fingers could lead to symptoms consistent with TF [101]. Armstrong and colleagues [10] observed a statistically significant increased odds ratio for prevalence of hand and wrist tendonitis, including TF and trigger thumb, among workers who performed jobs characterized as high forcefulness and high repetitiveness. Moore and Garg's study [19] that compared incidence of distal upper extremity disorders in a pork processing plant found 15 cases of flexor tendon entrapment among 104 observed conditions. In this study, cases of TF were observed in hazardous jobs that involved one or more of the following tasks: repetitive grasping of pinch type, high speed, and nonneutral wrist position or hand-arm vibration. Gorsche and colleagues [102] conducted the first study to determine specifically the development of TF in the workplace. These investigators found a relative risk of 4.7 (95% CI 1.5–23.9; $P<0.02$) in hand tool users compared with non–tool users.

Diagnosis and treatment. Diagnosis of TF is essentially a clinical one. Radiographs are unnecessary. Although spontaneous recovery may occur in 20% of persons affected with TF, the natural history of the condition is characterized by progression from pain, snapping, and intermittent locking to continued triggering and potentially a digit locked in flexion [92,103].

The mainstays of treatment in TF have been splinting with or without concurrent physiotherapy, surgery, or corticosteroid injection. Until the advent of corticosteroids, the treatment of choice for TF was surgery if conservative management failed [96,103]. Patel and Bassini [104] devised a staging system for TF based on the grade of mechanical involvement noted on clinical examination (Table 3). Based on the stage at clinical presentation, a protocol was recommended for conservative versus surgical treatment. Essentially, only digits locked in flexion (stage 6 stenosing tenosynovitis) are recommended to require surgical intervention. Otherwise, corticosteroid injection is recommended if splinting for 3 to 6 weeks fails [104]. Studies have shown that TF of the nodular type, in which a palpable nodule is clinically apparent on physical examination, responds better to local corticosteroid injection than if the TF is of a more diffuse type (Fig. 6) [96]. After a single injection of corticosteroids, most cases of TF resolve, and 97% of TF has been shown to resolve after two injections [105]. Efficacy of injection may be linked to duration of symptoms with higher success rates in patients who report symptoms for less than 4 months [106]. Advocates of non-operative treatment of TF cite fewer complications, lack of required immobilization and dressing changes, decreased cost of injection, and no loss time from work as benefits of injection over surgical treatment [96].

In the 1950s, Lapidus [103] reported surgical transection of the A1 pulley as the treatment of choice for stenosing tenosynovitis. This open operative procedure, although successful, is not without complications, including infection, digital nerve injury, incomplete release of the A1 pulley, transection of the A2 pulley, scar tenderness, stiffness, and weakness [96,107,108]. Later researchers recommend percutaneous release of the A1 pulley because of its simplicity, ability to be performed as an office procedure, and relative lack of complications [107–110]. Some controversy exists regarding efficacy of percutaneous release

Table 3
Six stages of digital stenosing tenosynovitis

Stage	Finger movements
1	Normal
2	Uneven
3	Triggering, clicking, catching
4	Locking of finger in flexion or extension unlocked by active finger movement
5	Locking of finger in flexion or extension unlocked by passive finger movement
6	Locked finger in flexion or extension

Each stage may be painless or painful.

From Patel MR, Bassini L. Trigger fingers and thumb: when to splint, inject or operate. J Hand Surg [Am] 1992;17A:110; ©1992, with permission from the American Society for Surgery of the Hand.

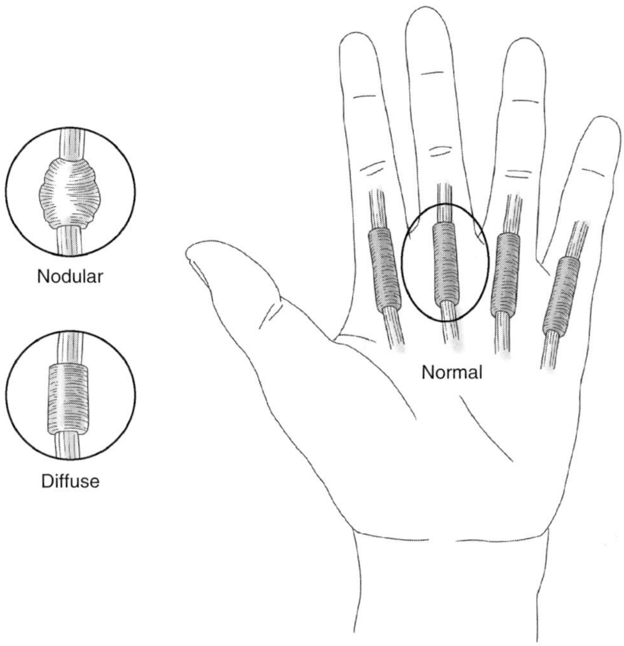

Fig. 6. Two types of TF: nodular and diffuse. (*From* Freiberg A, Mulholland RS, Levine R. Nonoperative treatment of trigger fingers and thumbs. J Hand Surg [Am] 1989;19A:555; © 1989, with permission from the American Society for Surgery of the Hand.)

for treatment of trigger thumb [110]. Wilhelmi and colleagues [111] recently identified surface landmarks that prevent neurovascular injury to the thumb and fifth digits, which makes percutaneous release a viable option. Patients with longstanding TF and persistent fixed flexion deformity have been shown to benefit from resection of the ulnar slip of the flexor digitorum superficialis tendon in the ulnar superficialis slip resection technique [112].

Summary

Tendinopathy in the upper extremity continues to be a source of morbidity and disability in the working population despite a benign clinical course. Many of these cases are preventable, and effective management requires identifying and managing risk factors at the workplace. Risk factors include high force, repetition, and awkward positions. Causation has not been established firmly. An understanding of the pertinent anatomy and pathophysiology should help clinicians in the management of these conditions. Tension overload and shear stress are the two mechanisms most likely responsible for most upper extremity tendinopathies. Clinical presentation includes localized pain and tenderness.

Swelling, crepitus, and triggering may be present depending on the location and severity of the condition. Most treatment options have yet to undergo evaluation for efficacy in well-designed clinical trials, yet there is a generally favorable response to nonoperative or conservative management. Cases resistant to conservative treatment may require surgical intervention.

References

[1] Gordon L. Hand and wrist disorders. In: Herrington TN, Morse LH, editors. Occupational injuries: evaluation, management, and prevention. St. Louis: Mosby; 1995. p. 103–24.

[2] Puddu G, Ippolito E, Postacchini F. A classification of Achilles tendon disease. Am J Sports Med 1976;4(4):145–50.

[3] Khan KM, Cook JL, Bonar F, et al. Histopathology of common tendinopathies: update and implications for clinical management. Sports Med 1999;27(6):393–408.

[4] Maffulli N, Wong J, Almekinders LC. Types and epidemiology of tendinopathy. Clin Sports Med 2003;22(4):675–92.

[5] Bureau of Labor Statistics. Statistics. 2003.

[6] Bystrom S, Hall C, Welander T, et al. Clinical disorders and pressure-pain threshold of the forearm and hand among automobile assembly line workers. J Hand Surg [Br] 1995;20:782–90.

[7] Battevi N, Menoni O, Vimercati C. The occurrence of musculoskeletal alterations in worker populations not exposed to repetitive tasks of the upper limbs. Ergonomics 1998;41(9):1340–6.

[8] Tanaka S, Petersen M, Cameron L. Prevalence and risk factors of tendinitis and related disorders of the distal upper extremity among US workers: comparison to carpal tunnel syndrome. Am J Ind Med 2001;39(3):328–35.

[9] Vender MU, Kasdan ML, Trupps KL. Upper extremity disorders: a literature review to determine work relatedness. J Hand Surg [Am] 1995;20:534–41.

[10] Armstrong TJ, Fine LJ, Goldstein SA, et al. Ergonomics considerations in hand and wrist tendinitis. J Hand Surg [Am] 1987;12(5 Pt 2):830–7.

[11] McCormack Jr RR, Inman RD, Wells A, et al. Prevalence of tendinitis and related disorders of the upper extremity in a manufacturing workforce. J Rheumatol 1990;17(7):958–64.

[12] Kurppa K, Viikari-Juntura E, Kuosma E, et al. Incidence of tenosynovitis or peritendinitis and epicondylitis in a meat-processing factory. Scand J Work Environ Health 1991;17(1):32–7.

[13] Roto P, Kivi P. Prevalence of epicondylitis and tenosynovitis among meatcutters. Scand J Work Environ Health 1984;10(3):203–5.

[14] Kivi P. Rheumatic disorders of the upper limbs associated with repetitive occupational tasks in Finland in 1975–1979. Scand J Rheumatol 1984;13(2):101–7.

[15] Ohlsson K, Attewell RG, Palsson B, et al. Repetitive industrial work and neck and upper limb disorders in females. Am J Ind Med 1995;27(5):731–47.

[16] Latko WA, Armstrong TJ, Franzblau A, et al. Cross-sectional study of the relationship between repetitive work and the prevalence of upper limb musculoskeletal disorders. Am J Ind Med 1999;36(2):248–59.

[17] Luopajarvi T, Kuorinka I, Virolainen M, et al. Prevalence of tenosynovitis and other injuries of the upper extremities in repetitive work. Scand J Work Environ Health 1979;5(Suppl 3): 48–55.

[18] Hakkanen M, Viikari-Juntura E, Martikainen R. Incidence of musculoskeletal disorders among newly employed manufacturing workers. Scand J Work Environ Health 2001;27(6): 381–7.

[19] Moore JS, Garg A. Upper extremity disorders in a pork processing plant: relationships between job risk factors and morbidity. Am Ind Hyg Assoc J 1994;55(8):703–15.

[20] Pedersen LK, Jensen LK. [Relationship between occupation and elbow pain, epicondylitis]. Ugeskr Laeger 1999;161(34):4751–5 [in Danish.].

[21] Piligian G, Herbert R, Hearns M, et al. Evaluation and management of chronic work-related musculoskeletal disorders of the distal upper extremity. Am J Ind Med 2000;37(1):75–93.
[22] Leclerc A, Landre MF, Chastang JF, et al, Study Group on Repetitive Work. Upper-limb disorders in repetitive work. Scand J Work Environ Health 2001;27(4):268–78.
[23] Tanaka S, Petersen M, Cameron L. Prevalence and risk factors of tendonitis and related disorders of the distal upper extremity among US workers: comparison to carpal tunnel syndrome. Am J Ind Med 2001;39(3):328–35.
[24] Fine LJ, Silverstein BA. Work-related disorders of the neck and upper extremity. In: Rom WN, editor. Environmental and occupational medicine. 3rd edition. Philadelphia: Lippincott-Raven; 1998. p. 959–69.
[25] Bongers PM, de Winter CR, Kompier MA, et al. Psychosocial factors at work and musculoskeletal disease. Scand J Work Environ Health 1993;19:297–312.
[26] Werner RA, Franzblau A, Gell N, et al. A longitudinal study of industrial and clerical workers: predictors of upper extremity tendonitis. J Occup Rehabil 2005;15(1):37–46.
[27] Derebery VJ. Etiologies and prevalence of occupational upper extremity injuries. In: Kasdean ML, editor. Occupational hand and upper extremity injuries and diseases. 2nd edition. Philadelphia: Hanley and Belfus; 1998. p. 49–58.
[28] Malmivaara A, Viikari-Juntura E, Huuskonen M, et al. Rheumatoid factor and HLA antigens in wrist tenosynovitis and humeral epicondylitis. Scand J Rheumatol 1995;24(3):154–6.
[29] Kay NR. Litigants' epicondylitis. J Hand Surg [Br] 2003;28(5):460–4.
[30] Glass LS, editor. Elbow complaints. In: Occupational medicine practice guidelines. 2nd edition. Beverly Farms (MA): OEM Press; 2004. p. 227–50.
[31] Bisset L, Paungmali A, Vicenzino B, et al. A systematic review and meta-analysis of clinical trials on physical interventions for lateral epicondylalgia. Br J Sports Med 2005;39:411–22.
[32] Runge F. Zur genese und behandlung des schreibekramfes. Borl Klin Wochanschr 1873;10: 245–8.
[33] Canale ST, editor. Shoulder and elbow injuries. In: Campbell's operative orthopedics. 10th edition. St. Louis: Mosby; 2003. p. 2361–6.
[34] Nirschl RP, Pettrone FA. Tennis elbow: the surgical treatment of lateral epicondylitis. J Bone Joint Surg Am 1979;61(6A):832–9.
[35] Nirschl RP, Ashman ES. Elbow tendinopathy: tennis elbow. Clin Sports Med 2003;22(4): 813–36.
[36] Potter HG, Hannafin JA, Morwessel RM, et al. Lateral epicondylitis: correlation of MR imaging, surgical, and histopathologic findings. Radiology 1995;196:43–6.
[37] Rempel DM, Harrison RJ, Barnhart S. Work-related cumulative trauma disorders of the upper extremity. JAMA 1992;267(6):838–42.
[38] Bennett JB. Lateral and medial epicondylitis. Hand Clin 1994;10(1):157–63.
[39] Korthals-de Bos IB, Smidt N, van Tulder MW, et al. Cost effectiveness of interventions for lateral epicondylitis: results from a randomised controlled trial in primary care. Pharmacoeconomics 2004;22(3):185–95.
[40] Allander E. Prevalence, incidence, and remission rates of some common rheumatic diseases or syndromes. Scand J Rheumatol 1974;3(3):145–53.
[41] Gabel GT. Acute and chronic tendinopathies at the elbow. Curr Opin Rheumatol 1999;11(2): 138–43.
[42] Hagberg M, Silverstein B, Wells R, et al. Evidence of the association between work and selected tendon disorders: shoulder tendinitis, epicondylitis, de Quervain's tendinitis, Dupuytren's contracture, Achilles tendinitis. In: Kuorinka I, Forcier L, editors. Work related musculoskeletal disorders (WMSDs): a reference book for prevention. New York: Taylor & Francis; 1995. p. 24–58.
[43] Bernard B, editor. Musculoskeletal disorders and workplace factors: a critical review of epidemiologic evidence for work-related musculoskeletal disorders of the neck, upper extremity and low back. Cincinnati (OH): National Institute for Occupational Health and Safety, US Department of Health and Human Services; 1997.

[44] Silverstein B, Viikari-Juntura E, Kalat J. Use of a prevention index to identify industries at high risk for work-related musculoskeletal disorders of the neck, back, and upper extremity in Washington State, 1990–1998. Am J Ind Med 2002;41(3):149–69.
[45] Haahr JP, Andersen JH. Prognostic factors in lateral epicondylitis: a randomized trial with one-year follow-up in 266 new cases treated with minimal occupational intervention or the usual approach in general practice. Rheumatology (Oxford) 2003;42(10):1216–25.
[46] Binder AI, Hazleman BL. Lateral humeral epicondylitis: a study of natural history and the effect of conservative therapy. Br J Rheumatol 1983;22(2):73–6.
[47] Khan KM, Cook JL, Kannus P, et al. Time to abandon the "tendinitis" myth. BMJ 2002; 324(7338):626–7.
[48] Jensen B, Bliddal H, Danneskiold-Samsoe B. [Comparison of two different treatments of lateral humeral epicondylitis: "tennis elbow." A randomized controlled trial]. Ugeskr Laeger 2001;163(10):1427–31 [in Danis].
[49] Van De Streek MD, Van Der Schans CP, De Greef MH, et al. The effect of a forearm/hand splint compared with an elbow band as a treatment for lateral epicondylitis. Prosthet Orthot Int 2004;28(2):183–9.
[50] Derebery J, Novotny J, Giang G, et al. The effects of splinting on outcomes for epicondylitis. Arch Phys Med Rehabil 2005;86:1081–8.
[51] Newcomer KL, Laskowski ER, Idank DM, et al. Corticosteroid injection in early treatment of lateral epicondylitis. Clin J Sport Med 2001;11(4):214–22.
[52] Brosseau L, Casimiro L, Milne S, et al. Deep transverse friction massage for treating tendinitis. Cochrane Database Syst Rev 2002;4:CD003528.
[53] Assendelft WJ, Hay EM, Adshead R, et al. Corticosteroid injections for lateral epicondylitis: a systematic overview. Br J Gen Pract 1996;46(405):209–16.
[54] Verhaar JA. Tennis elbow: anatomical, epidemiological and therapeutic aspects. Int Orthop 1994;18(5):263–7.
[55] Smidt N, van der Windt DA, Assendelft WJ, et al. Corticosteroid injections, physiotherapy, or a wait-and-see policy for lateral epicondylitis: a randomised controlled trial. Lancet 2002; 359(9307):657–62.
[56] Smith AG, Kosygan K, Williams H, et al. Common extensor tendon rupture following corticosteroid injection for lateral tendinosis of the elbow. Br J Sports Med 1999;33(6):423–4 [discussion: 424–5].
[57] Boisaubert B, Brousse C, Zaoui A, et al. Nonsurgical treatment of tennis elbow. Ann Readapt Med Phys 2004;47(6):346–55.
[58] Chung B, Wiley JP. Effectiveness of extracorporeal shock wave therapy in the treatment of previously untreated lateral epicondylitis: a randomized controlled trial. Am J Sports Med 2004;32(7):1660–7.
[59] Bennett JB. Lateral and medial epicondylitis. Hand Clin 1994;10(1):157–63.
[60] Ollivierre CO, Nirschl RP, Pettrone FA. Resection and repair for medial tennis elbow: a prospective analysis. Am J Sports Med 1995;23(2):214–21.
[61] Pienimaki TT, Siira PT, Vanharanta H. Chronic medial and lateral epicondylitis: a comparison of pain, disability, and function. Arch Phys Med Rehabil 2002;83(3):317–21.
[62] Ciccotti MC, Schwartz MA, Ciccotti MG. Diagnosis and treatment of medial epicondylitis of the elbow. Clin Sports Med 2004;23(4):693–705.
[63] Nicholas JA, Hershman EB, Posner MA. In: Nicholas JA, Herschmann EB, editors. The upper extremity in sports medicine. 2nd edition. St. Louis: Mosby; 1995. p. 317–9.
[64] Descatha A, Leclerc A, Chastang JF, et al, The Study Group on Repetitive Work. Medial epicondylitis in occupational settings: prevalence, incidence and associated risk factors. J Occup Environ Med 2003;45(9):993–1001.
[65] Stahl S, Kaufman T. The efficacy of an injection of steroids for medial epicondylitis: a prospective study of sixty elbows. J Bone Joint Surg Am 1997;79(11):1648–52.
[66] De Quervain F. Uber eine form von chronischer tendovaginitis. Korrespondenz-Blatt fur Schweiz Aertze 1895;25:389–94.

[67] Moore JS. De Quervain's tenosynovitis: stenosing tenosynovitis of the first dorsal compartment. J Occup Environ Med 1997;39(10):990–1002.
[68] Kay NR. De Quervain's disease: changing pathology or changing perception? J Hand Surg [Br] 2000;25(1):65–9.
[69] Clarke MT, Lyall HA, Grant JW, et al. The histopathology of de Quervain's disease. J Hand Surg [Br] 1998;23(6):732–4.
[70] Finklestein H. Stenosing tendovaginitis at the radial styloid process. J Bone Joint Surg Am 1930;12:509–40.
[71] Canale ST. Carpal tunnel, ulnar tunnel and stenosing tenosynovitis. In: Campbell's operative orthopedics. 10th edition. St. Louis (MO): Mosby; 2003. p. 3773–4.
[72] Faithfull DK, Lamb DW. De Quervain's disease: a clinical review. Hand 1971;3(1):23–30.
[73] Turek S, Weinstein S, Buckwalter J. Turek's orthopedics: principles and their application. 5th edition. Philadelphia: Lippincott; 1994.
[74] Putz-Anderson V. Cumulative trauma disorders: a manual for musculoskeletal diseases of the upper limbs. National Institute for Occupational Safety and Health; 1988.
[75] Mani L, Gerr F. Work-related upper extremity musculoskeletal disorders. Prim Care 2000; 27(4):845–64.
[76] Greene WB, editor. Essentials of musculoskeletal care. 2nd edition. Rosemont (IL): American Academy of Orthopedic Surgeons; 2001. p. 232–4.
[77] Weiss AP, Akelman E, Tabatabai M. Treatment of de Quervain's disease. J Hand Surg [Am] 1994;19(4):595–8.
[78] Michlovitz S, Hun L, Erasala GN, et al. Continuous low-level heat wrap therapy is effective for treating wrist pain. Arch Phys Med Rehabil 2004;85(9):1409–16.
[79] Anderson BC, Manthey R, Brouns MC. Treatment of de Quervain's tenosynovitis with corticosteroids: a prospective study of the response to local injection. Arthritis Rheum 1991; 34(7):793–8.
[80] Harvey FJ, Harvey PM, Horsley MW. De Quervain's disease: surgical or nonsurgical treatment. J Hand Surg [Am] 1990;15(1):83–7.
[81] Richie III CA, Briner Jr WW. Corticosteroid injection for treatment of de Quervain's tenosynovitis: a pooled quantitative literature evaluation. J Am Board Fam Pract 2003;16(2):102–6.
[82] Zarin M, Ahmad I. Surgical treatment of de Quervain's disease. J Coll Physicians Surg Pak 2003;13(3):157–8.
[83] Hanlon DP, Luellen JR. Intersection syndrome: a case report and review of the literature. J Emerg Med 1999;17(6):969–71.
[84] Pantukosit S, Petchkrua W, Stiens SA. Intersection syndrome in Buriram Hospital: a 4-yr prospective study. Am J Phys Med Rehabil 2001;80(9):656–61.
[85] Grundberg AB, Reagan DS. Pathologic anatomy of the forearm: intersection syndrome. J Hand Surg [Am] 1985;10(2):299–302.
[86] Parmelee-Peters K, Eathorne SW. The wrist: common injuries and management. Prim Care 2005;32(1):35–70.
[87] Bishop AT, Gabel MD, Carmichael SW. Flexor carpi radialis tendonitis. I. Operative anatomy. J Bone Joint Surg Am 1994;76A(7):1009–14.
[88] Bishop AT, Gabel MD, Carmichael SW. Flexor carpi radialis tendonitis. II. Results of operative treatment. J Bone Joint Surg Am 1994;76A(7):1015–8.
[89] Cannon NM, editor. Diagnosis and treatment manual for physicians and therapists upper extremity rehabilitation. 4th edition. Hand Rehabilitation Center of Indiana; 2001. p. 221.
[90] Budoff JE, Kraushaar BS, Ayala G. Flexor carpi ulnaris tendinopathy. J Hand Surg [Am] 2005;30A:125–9.
[91] Rettig AC. Wrist and hand overuse syndromes. Clin Sports Med 2001;20(3):591–611.
[92] Allan CH. Flexor tendons: anatomy and surgical approaches. Hand Clin 2005;21:151–7.
[93] Notta A. Recherches sur une affection particuliere des gaines tendincuscs de la main, characterisee par le development d'une nodosite sur le trajet des tendons fleschisseurs des doigts et par l'empechement de leurs mouvements. Arch Gen Med 1850;24:142–61.

[94] Nelaton A, Depres A, Jamain A. Tumeurs des doigts. Elements de Pathologic Chirurgicale 1859;5:953–6.
[95] Murphy D, Failla JM, Koniuch MP. Steroid versus placebo injection for trigger finger. J Hand Surg [Am] 1995;20A:628–31.
[96] Freiberg A, Mulholland RS, Levine R. Nonoperative treatment of trigger fingers and thumbs. J Hand Surg [Am] 1989;19A:553–8.
[97] Moore SJ. Flexor tendon entrapment of the digits (trigger finger and trigger thumb). J Occup Environ Med 2000;42(5):526–45.
[98] Johnson TR, Anderson W, Gorsuch WL, et al. Trigger finger. In: Greene WB, editor. Essentials of musculoskeletal care. 2nd edition. Rosemont (IL): American Academy of Orthopedic Surgeons; 2001. p. 249–51.
[99] Anderson BC. Trigger finger. In: Office orthopedics for primary care: diagnosis and treatment. 2nd edition. Philadelphia: WB Saunders; 1999. p. 86–8.
[100] Gottlieb NL. Digital flexor tenosynovitis: diagnosis and clinical significance. J Rheumatol 1991;18:954–5.
[101] Sperling WP. Snapping finger: roentgen treatment and experimental production. Acta Radiol 1951;37:74–80.
[102] Gorsche R, Wiley JP, Renger R, et al. Prevalence and incidence of stenosing flexor tenosynovitis (trigger finger) in a meat-packing plant. J Occup Environ Med 1998;40(6):556–60.
[103] Lapidus PW. Stenosing tenovaginitis. Surg Clin North Am 1953;33:1317–47.
[104] Patel MR, Bassini L. Trigger fingers and thumb: when to splint, inject or operate. J Hand Surg [Am] 1992;17A:110–3.
[105] Marks MR, Gunther SF. Efficacy of cortisone injection in treatment of trigger finger. J Hand Surg [Am] 1989;14:722–7.
[106] Rhoades CE, Gelberman RH, Manjarris JF. Stenosing tenosynovitis of the fingers and thumb: results of a prospective trial of steroid injection and splinting. Clin Orthop Relat Res 1984;190: 236–8.
[107] Bain GI, Turnbull J, Roth JH, et al. Percutaneous A1 pulley release: a cadaveric study. J Hand Surg [Am] 1995;20A:781–4.
[108] Pope DF, Wolfe SW. Safety and efficacy of percutaneous trigger finger release. J Hand Surg [Am] 1995;20A:280–3.
[109] Tanaka J, Muraji M, Negoro H, et al. Subcutaneous release of trigger thumb and fingers in 210 fingers. J Hand Surg [Am] 1990;15A:463–5.
[110] Dunn MJ, Pess GM. Percutaneous trigger finger release: a comparison of a new push knife and a 19-gauge needle in a cadaveric model. J Hand Surg [Am] 1999;24A:860–5.
[111] Wilhelmi BJ, Mowlawi A, Neumeister MW, et al. Safe treatment of trigger finger with longitudinal and transverse landmarks: an anatomic study of the border finger for percutaneous release. J Plast Reconstr Surg 2003;112:993–9.
[112] LeViet I, Tsionos M, Boulouednine M, et al. Trigger finger treatment by ulnar superficialis slip resection (USSR). J Hand Surg [Am] 2004;29A:368–73.

ELSEVIER
SAUNDERS

Clin Occup Environ Med
5 (2) 323–331

CLINICS IN
OCCUPATIONAL AND
ENVIRONMENTAL
MEDICINE

Ligament Injuries of the Hand and Wrist

Bruce F. Hermann, MD

Department of Surgery, University of Louisville, 605 Wallace Avenue, Louisville, KY 40207, USA

Ligament injuries of the hand

The design and function of the human hand allow for amazing feats of manual dexterity for daily activities and occupational tasks. Hand injuries that may involve damage to the ligamentous attachments of the carpometacarpal (CMC), metacarpophalangeal (MP), and interphalangeal joints require prompt evaluation and treatment, because these patients often can have function restored if the injury is diagnosed and treated promptly and correctly.

Normal structural anatomy

The five metacarpal bones are miniature long bones that extend from the wrist at the CMC joint to the fingers at the MP joint. The metacarpals and phalanges are properly numbered starting on the radial border, or they can be named as thumb, index, middle, ring, and little. The ligamentous attachments of the CMC joint include interosseous, dorsal and palmar components, which offer strong stability with limited mobility. The fingers have a proximal interphalangeal joint and a distal interphalangeal joint, whereas the thumb has only a single interphalangeal joint.

Types of injuries

The type of injury and comorbidities dictate the severity of the injury and the probable outcome of hand function. Twisting and longitudinal force injuries frequently involve ligamentous injury, which can vary from simple sprains to complex fracture dislocations. Injuries to the ligamentous structures of the hand,

E-mail address: tamias2@yahoo.com

1526-0046/06/$ – see front matter
doi:10.1016/j.coem.2005.12.001

although never life threatening by themselves, can have disabling complications, such as deformity, loss of range of motion, chronic pain limiting mobility and function, and permanent joint instability.

Evaluation

With each hand injury, a complete evaluation should be completed to assess the structural function of the hand. Initial assessment should start with the history of the injury. Information about the specific task being performed at time of injury and any prior injuries or limitations of hand function are all details that should be included in the history. The potential normal function of the hand, including passive and active range of motion, usually can be evaluated by assessing the noninjured hand. When evaluating the upper extremity, it is important to assess for pain, point tenderness, deformity, erythema, swelling, and range of motion.

Diagnostic medical imaging plays a large role in the evaluation of hand injuries and diseases. In addition to standard radiographs of the hand, specialized plain radiograph views, CT, MRI, and three-phase bone scans can provide additional information. CT scans give excellent three-dimensional images of the hand, which allow for diagnosis of subtle fractures and dislocations where standard radiographs could be insufficient. MRI scans provide good three-dimensional images but also provide more detail of possible soft tissue injuries.

Carpometacarpal joints of the fingers

Anatomy and function

The metacarpal bones of the fingers (ie, index, middle, ring, and little) form a plane synovial joint with the distal row of carpal bones, and they share a common joint cavity with the intercarpal joints. The interlocking skeletal configuration combines with the soft tissue support of the ligamentous attachments to ensure stability while allowing little mobility.

The CMC joints can be subdivided into radial and ulnar subsets based on their anatomy and function. The radial (ie, index and middle finger) CMC joints are exceptionally stable because of the interdigitating articulations of the skeletal joint and the thickness of the ligamentous attachments. Although somewhat stable, the ulnar (ie, ring and little) CMC joints are more mobile by comparison, which makes them somewhat more susceptible to injury [1].

Evaluation and treatment

Injuries to the CMC joints occur most frequently to the thumb and little finger. Patients frequently have pain and point tenderness at the joint accompanied by swelling, which is most often seen on the dorsum of the hand. If the joint is dislocated, physical examination may reveal loss of the outline of the metacarpal head.

After the physical examination, plain radiograph films should be taken. Assessment of the CMC joint can be difficult with plain radiographs because fracture lines are often subtle and superimposition of the noninjured metacarpal bones makes visualization even more challenging. Radiographs for assessment of the CMC joint should include nonstandard views, such as oblique angles, forearm in 30° pronation, Brewerton views (ie, tangential radiographs used to detect occult fractures), or even CT scans if previous plain films are indeterminate [2].

Once the diagnosis of dislocation with or without fracture to the CMC joint is made, focus should be turned to proper treatment. Initial therapy includes elevation to reduce swelling and analgesia for comfort. Definitive treatment involves reduction of the dislocation. If acute injuries are treated promptly, treatment can be accomplished via closed reduction plaster immobilization, closed reduction with percutaneous K-wires, or open reduction and internal fixation depending on severity [3]. Consultation with a hand surgeon is recommended.

Carpometacarpal joint of the thumb

Anatomy and function

The metacarpal of the thumb articulates with the trapezium, which is composed of two perpendicular reciprocally interlocking saddles. Mostly because of the design of the volar ligament, the CMC joint of the thumb allows not only for flexion and extension but also for more precise functions, such as pinch and opposition.

Evaluation and treatment

Injuries to the CMC joint of the thumb occur when there is significant axial loading to the partially flexed thumb metacarpal. Although isolated injury to the ligaments with simple dislocation is possible, injuries sustained are most often fracture dislocation injuries [4]. Bennett's fracture dislocation is the most common type of injury seen, and these injuries involve intra-articular fracture of the base of the metacarpal bone with the fragment still attached to the volar ligament. Symptoms include severe pain at the base of the thumb, significant tenderness to palpation, and swelling. Appropriate radiographs should include posteroanterior, lateral, and oblique films, and pronation of the hand and wrist can aid in visualizing the CMC joint.

Treatment of thumb CMC injuries centers on reduction of the dislocation and internal stabilization. Improper reduction of this injury results in chronic pain and loss of motion of the joint. Because this joint allows for much of the thumb's functional ability, prompt and proper evaluation and treatment are a necessity.

Metacarpophalangeal joints of the fingers

Anatomy and function

The metacarpals of the fingers adjoin to the proximal phalanges of the fingers in a condyloid-type (ball and socket) joint, which allows not only flexion and extension but also up to 30° of lateral motion while the joint is in extension. The ligamentous attachments of these joints include the volar plate, a specialized thickening of the joint capsule, and the radial and ulnar collateral ligaments, which each have an accessory ligament to add to their strength.

Evaluation and treatment

The MP joint is resistant to ligamentous injury. All of the MP joints are most stable while in flexion; most injuries to this joint system are seen with hyperextension injuries.

Isolated hyperextension injuries to the ligaments without dislocation do occur. Patients present with pain, ecchymosis, and swelling of the affected joint; physical examination reveals tenderness at the MP joint, and there may be some instability of joint depending on the severity of the injury. Radiographs usually are normal; Brewerton views should be obtained to rule out small bone fragments [5]. Isolated hyperextension injuries usually can be treated initially with a splint with subsequent referral to a hand specialist.

Dislocation injuries of the MP joint are seen most frequently in the index finger, followed by the little finger. The dislocations are almost always dorsal and are a result of rupture of the volar plate. These injuries can be divided into two types: simple and complex. Simple MP dislocations involve a partial or complete tear of the volar plate from its proximal insertion on the metacarpal. Complex MP dislocations result when the disrupted volar plate is interposed into the MP joint space. Patients who have MP dislocations present with pain, ecchymosis, and swelling of the joint, and complex dislocations often result in a palpable, prominent metacarpal head in the palm.

Radiographs demonstrate obvious dislocations in the lateral view and posteroanterior views. Simple dislocations normally can be reduced by closed methods with subsequent buddy taping or splinting. Postreduction films always should be obtained. Complex dislocations almost always require open operative repair [6].

Collateral ligament injuries to the MP joint are classified as first-degree sprains with minimal ligament injury and tenderness without laxity, second-degree sprains with partial ligament tear and tenderness with some laxity, or third-degree sprains with complete ligament rupture, swelling, severe pain, and gross instability of the joint with ulnar deviation. Treatment for less severe injuries includes immobilization followed by therapy, whereas more severe injuries usually necessitate operative intervention.

Metacarpophalangeal joint of the thumb

Anatomy and function

Although the ligamentous structure of the MP joint of the thumb is significantly stronger than finger MP joints, the thumb's vulnerable position makes it account for five times the injuries of all other MP joints combined [7]. Because the common hand functions of pinch and grasp rely on a stable thumb MP joint, injuries to this area should be evaluated promptly and treated to prevent chronic loss of function.

Evaluation and treatment

Injuries to the thumb can include partial or complete tears of the volar plate or radial or ulnar collateral ligament systems. The examination should include gentle palpation of the thumb along with the standard radiographs to rule out fracture, and the noninjured thumb should be assessed to evaluate a patient's normal range of motion, because the MP joint of the thumb carries the most variability of any joint [3]. The injured joint should be assessed, and gentle stress testing in flexion and extension give insight into the stability of the collateral ligament structures [8].

Injuries to the volar plate of the thumb MP joint are caused by hyperextension forces. For simple sprains without dislocations, immobilization for 3 to 4 weeks is usually sufficient for treatment. Simple dorsal dislocations normally can be treated with closed reduction followed by immobilization. Similar to finger complex dorsal dislocations, closed reduction is rarely successful, and operative intervention is usually required.

The ulnar collateral ligament is frequently injured via forced abduction of the MP joint. This injury is known as skier's thumb or gamekeeper's thumb, and it is a frequently misdiagnosed injury [9]. Examination reveals pain, tenderness, and occasionally ecchymosis over the ulnar aspect of the joint. Radiographs should be obtain to rule out fracture, and stress testing should be performed to access the laxity of the joint. Complete rupture of the ligament results in obvious laxity during stress testing, and operative intervention is necessary. Partial ruptures of the ligament with concomitant fracture likewise should be repaired operatively if postreduction films demonstrate separation of the fragments. For incomplete ligament rupture without fracture, proper immobilization is adequate treatment [10].

Radial collateral ligament injuries are significantly less common. Similar to other ligament injuries, pain, swelling, tenderness, ecchymosis, and joint laxity can be found. After normal radiographs rule out fracture, stress testing should be performed. Partial disruptions can be treated with immobilization, whereas complete disruptions should be addressed by operative intervention and repair.

Interphalangeal injuries

Anatomy and function

The proximal interphalangeal and distal interphalangeal joints of the fingers and the interphalangeal joint of the thumb are hinge-type joints that are strong. The ligaments form a three-sided box around the joints, comprised of a thick volar plate and laterally positioned collateral ligaments. This design allows the joint up to 100° of flexion and some hyperextension.

Evaluation and treatment

The proximal interphalangeal joint is recognized as the most commonly dislocated joint of the hand. Proximal interphalangeal and distal interphalangeal injuries can range from a "jammed" finger or thumb to complex fracture dislocations, but most injuries result in partial ligament injuries, which cause pain and swelling while retaining joint stability. The joint is most frequently injured secondary to forced hyperextension with axial loading.

When proximal interphalangeal and distal interphalangeal injuries are suspected, a thorough history of the injury should be obtained. Anteroposterior, oblique, and lateral radiographs of the injured digits should be taken to evaluate for fracture or dislocation. The clinical examination should include gentle palpation of the affected digit and evaluation of passive and active range of motion. The contralateral hand and digits can be evaluated for comparison.

After the history and physical examination and radiographs are complete, the clinician should be able to determine the extent of the injury: minor ligament injury without instability, moderate ligament injury with some laxity of the joint, or severe injury with joint dislocation with or without fracture. Nondislocated sprains with or without some aspect of joint instability are fairly minor injuries and can be treated with immobilization for 2 to 4 weeks followed by return of active motion to prevent stiffness and contracture. Dorsal dislocations without fracture are treated with closed reduction (postreduction radiographs should be obtained).

Unstable dorsal fracture dislocations are severe injuries, because long-term sequelae are frequently encountered even with proper treatment. Closed reduction can be successful, but prompt referral to a hand specialist is recommended.

Ligament injuries of the wrist

Injuries to the wrist are fairly common and are frequently encountered after a fall on an outstretched hand. The anatomy, function, and possible injuries of the wrist could fill volumes of text. This section seeks to cover the basics of wrist anatomy and function and discuss common injuries and how to diagnose and treat them properly.

Basic wrist anatomy and function

The foundation of the wrist joint system is the skeletal bones that form the link between the forearm and the hand. The distal radius and ulna make up the most proximal border of the wrist, and they join with the proximal row of carpal bones, which consists of (from radial to ulnar side) the scaphoid, lunate, triquetrum, and pisiform, although the pisiform bone is best described as a sesamoid bone that acts as a lever arm for the flexor carpi ulnaris tendon [11]. The proximal carpals join to the distal row of carpal bones, which consist of (from radial to ulnar side) the trapezium, trapezoid, capitate, and hamate bones. The distal row of carpals adjoins tightly to the proximal bases of the five metacarpal bones through strong ligamentous attachments.

The centrally located lunate bone acts as a separate intercalated segment. The lunate acts as an anchor between the scaphoid and triquetrum bones, which have significant movement with wrist flexion and extension. The stability of the proximal carpals relies heavily on the scapholunate and triquetrolunate ligaments, which makes the lunate an excellent indicator of carpal stability.

Carpal instability

Carpal instability can be defined as a carpal injury that involves fracture or ligament damage that disturbs the normal balance of carpal anatomy and function. Carpal instabilities can be given a measure of severity by determining if they are either dynamic, in which the malalignment is only detected when the wrist is loaded or moving, or static, in which the abnormality is detectable when the wrist is at rest [12].

When the lunate or proximal carpals angulate into flexion, the instability is called volar intercalated segment instability; when they angulate into extension, the instability is known as dorsal intercalated segment instability [13]. These terms do not give a specific diagnosis for the injury; they merely give a description of the carpal system's reaction to the injury received.

Evaluation of the injured wrist

Any evaluation of a wrist injury should start with a thorough history, because the mechanism of injury can give insight into which ligaments may be injured. Most injuries to the wrist are received after a fall on an outstretched hand, and differentiating point of impact with careful history taking and examination can suggest possibly injured structures. Thenar eminence impact suggests scaphoid and supporting ligament injuries, whereas hypothenar eminence impact suggests triquetrum, pisiform, and supporting ligament injuries [14]. Conversely, a fall sustained on a palmar flexed wrist is more likely to injure the dorsal radioulnar ligaments [15]. The history also should include specific questioning about symptoms such as popping, clicking, clunking, or onset of pain with wrist movement, which can be indicators of carpal instability. Evaluation of the noninjured wrist gives a comparison of wrist function. Neurovascular evaluation should not be forgotten, because fractures and dislocations can compromise these structures.

Palpation of the wrist for areas of maximal tenderness should be performed in a systematic and methodical manner. One suggestion for systematic palpation of the wrist involves dividing the wrist into five zones: radial dorsal, central dorsal, ulnar dorsal, radial volar, and ulnar volar [16]. Using this systematic approach, the major landmarks of the wrist can be evaluated thoroughly. The radial dorsal region includes the anatomic snuff box, in which the scaphoid can be palpated. Just distal to this point, the scaphotrapezial joint and trapezium can be assessed, and distal to this location the CMC joint can be evaluated. The major landmarks in the central dorsal region include the scapholunate joint (just ulnar to the scaphoid) and adjoining lunate bone, which can be palpated most easily with the wrist in flexion. Significant tenderness at this location or widening of the joint space can be an indication of scapholunate ligament injury. The capitate bone is located distally to the lunate. The ulnar dorsal region contains the ulnar snuff box, in which palpation of the triquetrum and pisotriquetral joint can be performed; tenderness in this region may indicate triquetrum or triangular fibrocartilage injury, or most significantly, midcarpal instability.

Significant information can be obtained from the radial volar zone by performing the scaphoid shift test [17]. This test is considered positive when a painful snap is elicited while applying pressure to the volar aspect of the scaphoid while moving the wrist from ulnar to radial deviation, which suggests a scapholunate ligament injury. The trapezium also can be palpated in this zone distal to the scaphoid. The ulnar volar zone contains several structures that should be evaluated, such as the pisiform, which is found at the base of the hypothenar eminence, and the hook of the hamate.

After the history and physical examination are complete, the clinician should have enough information to decide whether a significant carpal injury or carpal instability may exist. Using this information can direct which radiographic studies could confirm the diagnosis. Plain radiographic films should include anteroposterior, lateral, oblique, and ulnar anteroposterior views. These films are obtained with the elbow at 90° and the forearm in midpronation and supination. If a static carpal instability is present, the resting radiographs show loss of normal alignment of the carpal bones [18]. When the initial films are normal and there is a suspicion of carpal instability, dynamic radiographs or cineradiography can confirm the diagnosis. Other radiographic studies that have been shown to be useful in diagnosing subtle or dynamic instability injuries include three-phase bone scans, arthrograms, CT, and MRI scans [19].

Treatment of common specific wrist ligament injuries

Scapholunate injuries

Scapholunate instability is the most common type of carpal instability encountered [20]. It involves injury to the scapholunate ligaments and, if the injury is static, the palmar radiocarpal ligaments. Adequate treatment of simple acute dynamic scapholunate ligament injuries usually can be accomplished with cast immobilization for 6 to 8 weeks [21], although recent studies have shown excellent results treating these injuries using operative radioscaphoid capsulodesis [22].

For acute static or dynamic scapholunate instability, treatment focuses on reduction of the injury, which requires referral to a specialist. When any of the internal wrist injuries are suspected, it is good judgment to refer to a hand or orthopedic surgeon.

Summary

Ligament injuries to the hand and wrist are common occupational injuries. These injuries can be diagnosed using thorough history and physical examination skills in conjunction with diagnostic imaging. Prompt diagnosis and treatment of these injuries are crucial, because many of the injuries will heal with minimal decrease in function if they are treated early without allowing them to become chronic. When these injuries are discovered late, not only does treatment become more difficult but also traumatic arthritis frequently develops.

References

[1] Greene TL, Strickland JW. Carpometacarpal dislocations (excluding the thumb). In: Strickland JW, Steichen JB, editors. Difficult problems of the hand. St Louis (MO): CV Mosby; 1982. p. 189–95.
[2] Gurland M, et al. Carpometacarpal joint injuries of the fingers. Hand Clin 1992;8:733.
[3] Green DP. Green's operative hand surgery. 5th edition. Philadelphia: Elsevier; 2005.
[4] Chen VT. Dislocation of the carpometacarpal joint of the thumb. J Hand Surg Br 1987; 12:246.
[5] Wilson RL, et al. Complications following small joint injuries. Hand Clin 1986;2:329.
[6] Barry K, et al. Complex dislocation of the metacarpophalangeal joint of the index finger, a comparison of surgical approaches. J Hand Surg Br 1988;13(4):466–8.
[7] The hand. In: Rosen, Barkin, editors. Emergency medicine: concepts and clinical practice. 4th edition. St. Louis (MO): Mosby; 1998. p. 625–68.
[8] Palmer AK, et al. Assessing ulnar instability of the metacarpophalangeal joint of the thumb. J Hand Surg 1978;3:542–6.
[9] Musharafieh R, et al. Ulnar collateral ligament rupture of the first metacarpophalangeal joint: a frequently missed injury in the emergency department. J Emerg Med 1997;15(2):193–6.
[10] Heyman P, et al. Injuries to the ulnar collateral ligament of the thumb metacarpophalangeal joint. J Am Acad Orthop Surg 1997;5(4):224–9.
[11] Laude M, et al. Valeur fonctionelle du pisiforme dans les mecanismes de preehension. Bull Acad Natl Med 1981;165:479–83.
[12] Amadio PC. Carpal kinematics and instability: a clinical and anatomic primer. Clin Anat 1991; 4:1–12.
[13] Linscheid RL, et al. Traumatic instability of the wrist: diagnosis, classification, and pathomechanics. J Bone Joint Surg Am 1972;54:1612–32.
[14] Ritchie JV. Emergency department evaluation and treatment of wrist injuries. Emerg Med Clin North Am 1999;17:823.
[15] Beckenbaugh RD, et al. Accurate evaluation and management of the painful wrist following an injury: an approach to carpal instability. Orthop Clin North Am 1984;15:289–306.
[16] Honing EW. Wrist injuries. Part 1: Pinpointing pathology in a complex joint. Phys Sportsmed 1998;26(9).
[17] Watson HK, et al. Examination of the scaphoid. J Hand Surg 1988;13(5):657–60.
[18] Taleisnik J. Current concepts review: carpal instability. J Bone Joint Surg Am 1988;70:1252–68.
[19] Kuschner SH, Lane CS. Evaluation of the painful wrist. Am J Orthop 1997;26(2):95–102.
[20] Bozentka DJ. Scapholunate instability. Univ Penn Ortho J 1999;12:27–32.
[21] Palmer AK, et al. Management of the post-traumatic instability of the wrist secondary to ligament rupture. J Hand Surg 1978;3:507–32.
[22] Wintman BI, et al. Dynamic scapholunate instability: results of operative treatment with dorsal capsulodesis. J Hand Surg 1995;20(6):971–9.

ELSEVIER
SAUNDERS

Clin Occup Environ Med
5 (2) 333–352

CLINICS IN
OCCUPATIONAL AND
ENVIRONMENTAL
MEDICINE

Compression Neuropathies of the Upper Extremity

Hal M. Corwin, MD

Division of Physical Medicine and Rehabilitation, University of Louisville Health Sciences Center, 3900 Kresge Way, Suite 56, Louisville, KY 40207, USA

Patients who have upper extremity compression neuropathy may seek medical attention because of pain, weakness, numbness, tingling, fatigue, dysautonomia, or loss of coordination. The diagnosis of a compression neuropathy must be based on objective findings, including neurologic deficits such as weakness, atrophy, or reflex asymmetry and abnormal electrodiagnostic studies.

The standard for evaluation of any neurologic complaint is a complete neurologic examination. Neurologic injuries manifest as loss of function (exemplified by the claw hand deformity of peripheral neuropathy), release phenomena (eg, spasticity and hyperreflexia), neuronal excitation (including seizures and movement disorders), and the compensatory mechanism of partial assumption of function [1]. Positional and postural paresthesias and pain are not objective indicators of a disease process. Electrodiagnostic tests support the diagnosis of compression neuropathy but cannot replace the neurologic examination. Misdiagnosis stems from inaccurate observation, insufficient examination, or false conclusions concerning the results of the neurologic or electrodiagnostic examinations. The most frequent error is incomplete examination. Neurologic examination techniques are discussed elsewhere [2,3].

Compressive neuropathy

Compression neuropathy refers to nerve damage from applied pressure of any source. The diagnosis of compression mononeuropathy implies a neurologic deficit in the distribution of a single nerve. The term "entrapment" implies a

E-mail address: halcorwin@pol.net

1526-0046/06/$ – see front matter
doi:10.1016/j.coem.2006.01.002 ***occmed.theclinics.com***

mononeuropathy caused by pressure exerted by an anatomic or pathologic structure. All entrapment neuropathies are compression neuropathies, but not all compression neuropathies are caused by entrapment. A nerve may be compressed because of abnormal enlargement. A nerve of normal dimensions may be compressed from a narrowed space, however. The site of compression may be a static or dynamic structure, such as the pronator teres muscle [4]. Compression neuropathy may develop acutely, as with tourniquet paralysis, or chronically. Entrapment neuropathies are all chronic conditions. In the absence of trauma, the relation of the disorder to work or other activity must be supported by the medical literature.

Minimal nerve compression causes a familiar falling asleep sensation because nerve ischemia results in an acute physiologic block of nerve conduction. The symptoms are transient and reversible. Most of the clinical symptoms of entrapment are caused by direct effects of pressure on the myelin sheath or axon, however. Saltatory conduction is facilitated by myelin. Ionic current flows inward at the node of Ranvier, which is activated by action current. If the myelin is disrupted, the action current dissipates to adjacent tissue spaces, which prolongs the internodal conduction time and slows the conduction velocity. Severe demyelination causes failure of nerve conduction, which is observed as conduction block during nerve conduction studies (NCS). Remyelination after purely demyelinating processes occurs over several weeks and is usually completed within 12 weeks. The new internodes are abnormally short and conduct slower than normal.

Wallerian degeneration of the distal nerve segment occurs after axonal injury. The axons may conduct normally for 5 days after axonal disruption. The axon recovers by a process of sprouting from the intact peripheral axons and formation of a growth cone from the injured axon stump. Axons that do not reach their target tissue successfully may form a traumatic neuroma or may show clinical signs of aberrant reinnervation [5].

Electrodiagnosis: nerve conduction studies and needle examination

Electrodiagnostic studies play a crucial role in the diagnosis of compression neuropathies by expanding the neurologic examination into an electrophysiologic evaluation. The pairing of NCS and the needle examination of the muscles is termed electromyography (EMG). These studies serve to evaluate the peripheral nervous system, including the motor unit: anterior horn cell, axon, neuromuscular junction, and muscle fibers (Fig. 1). The electromyographer uses extensive knowledge of neurophysiology and neuroanatomy to assemble the EMG study that is suitable for the situation. The EMG report, which includes an impression, constitutes the practice of electrodiagnostic medicine and may assist in the diagnosis of disorders of the nerve roots, brachial or lumbar plexus, sensory, motor or autonomic nerves, neuromuscular junction, or muscle.

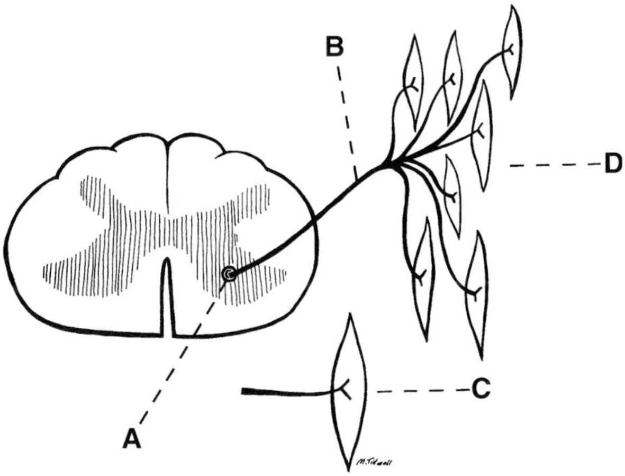

Fig. 1. The motor unit. (*A*) Anterior horn cell. (*B*) Axon. (*C*) Neuromuscular junction. (*D*) Muscle fiber. (*From* Corwin HM. Neurologic evaluation of the upper extremity. In: Kasdan ML, editor. Occupational hand and upper extremity injuries and diseases. 2nd edition. Philadelphia: Hanley & Belfus; 1998. p. 296; with permission.)

A physician trained in electrodiagnostic medicine should perform the needle examination. The physician should have special training in the diagnosis of neurologic and neuromuscular diseases as part of a residency or fellowship program. Because the test is designed around a patient's history and examination, there is no standard test but rather an extensive array of studies that may be chosen for any particular situation. Nonphysicians may assist in data collection but do not have the necessary background to make a diagnosis [6].

The American Association of Neuromuscular and Electrodiagnostic Medicine develops practice parameters and position statements concerning the practice of electrodiagnostic medicine. The practice parameters are based on literature review and clinical experience and outline the process of diagnosing some of the disorders discussed in this article.

Misdiagnosis of compression neuropathy caused by electrodiagnostic errors

Errors in electrodiagnosis are common [7]. Nerve conduction velocities are calculated using a simple formula (Fig. 2). If the length of the nerve segment under consideration is measured improperly, the nerve velocity may be calculated incorrectly, which implies a diagnosis of nerve compression. Limb temperature affects nerve conduction. Cool extremities should be warmed before testing to avoid factitious results. Distal latencies may increase, nerve conduction velocities slow, and nerve amplitudes increase because of cooling (Fig. 3). False slowing of nerve conduction velocities of 1.5 to 2 m/sec/1°C caused by low limb tem-

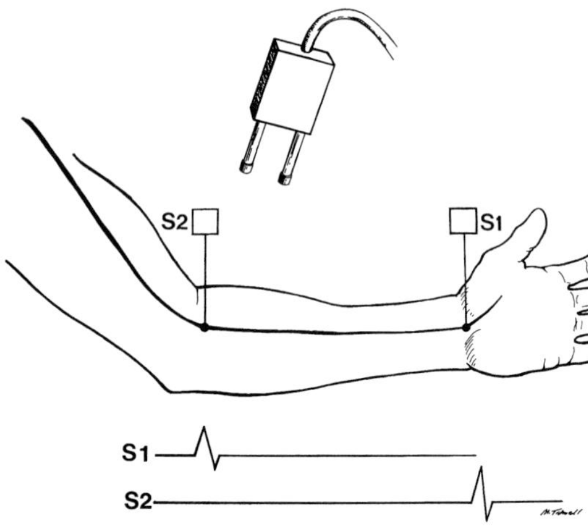

Fig. 2. Calculating nerve conduction velocity. S1, distal latency (msec); S2, proximal latency (msec); D, distance between S1 and S2 stimulation sites (cm); NCV (meters/sec), (S2-S1/D). (*From* Corwin HM. Neurologic evaluation of the upper extremity. In: Kasdan ML, editor. Occupational hand and upper extremity injuries and diseases. 2nd edition. Philadelphia: Hanley & Belfus; 1998. p. 295; with permission.)

perature may lead to an incorrect diagnosis of entrapment neuropathy. Unnecessary splinting, steroid injections, or surgery may be ordered as a consequence of testing errors. Cold temperatures may enhance transmission at the neuromuscular junction, the structure affected in myasthenia gravis and Lambert-Eaton myasthenic syndrome [8].

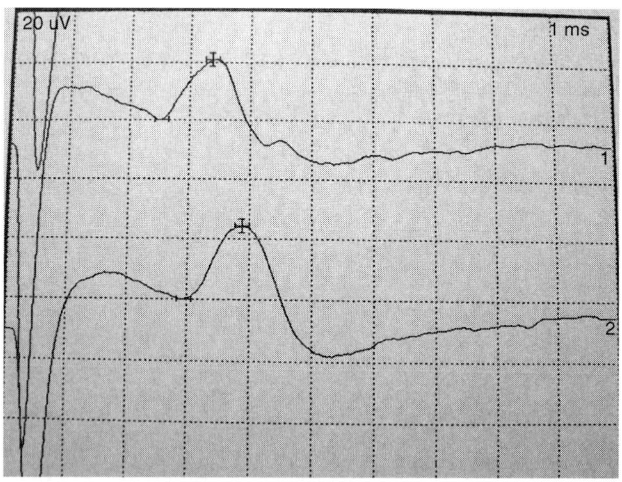

Fig. 3. The effects of cooling on nerve conduction. Trace 1, median distal sensory latency is 3.4 msec; hand temperature of 33°C. Trace 2 (same patient), median distal sensory latency is 3.9 msec; hand temperature of 29°C. (Normal median distal sensory latency value is <3.6 msec at distance of 14 cm, at hand temperature of 32°C or higher.)

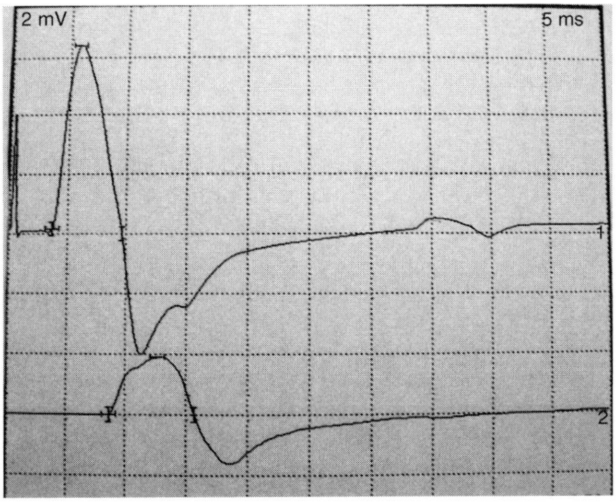

Fig. 4. Conduction block. Trace 1, ulnar motor nerve stimulated at the wrist. Amplitude of CMAP is 6.3 mV. Trace 2 (same patient), ulnar nerve stimulated at the elbow. Amplitude of CMAP is 1.9 mV. There is an amplitude drop >50%. CMAP, compound muscle action potential.

NCS reports that do not include the amplitudes of the sensory nerve action potential and compound muscle action potential are erroneous. Axonal degeneration may be caused by nerve transection or axonopathy. Both types of disorders may reduce nerve amplitude without nerve slowing. The diagnosis of these and other disorders depends on proper amplitude measurement [9]. Chronic nerve compression may injure the myelin at specific nerve segments. This segmental demyelination may cause conduction block with or without slowing of the velocity. Conduction block is diagnosed by comparing amplitude values after stimulating proximal and distal to the site of compression and is missed if amplitudes are not measured (Fig. 4). Submaximal nerve stimulation during the testing process may falsely imply the presence of conduction block and nerve compression [9]. Submaximal stimulation yields unreliable nerve amplitude and latency values.

The diagnosis of compression mononeuropathy includes the exclusion of alternate diagnoses of polyneuropathy and plexopathy. To prevent these diagnostic errors, all abnormal nerve conduction test results are compared with the same nerve in the opposite limb and to another nerve in the affected limb [10–12].

Thoracic outlet syndrome

The term thoracic outlet syndrome (TOS) was introduced in 1956 by Peet and colleagues [13] in an attempt to group conditions in which nerves or vessels or both are compressed in the root of the neck or in the axilla. It is currently known that this expression links four medical conditions that differ in fundamental ways: the structure compromised, the clinical presentation, the path to correct diagnosis, and the proper treatment.

Muscle wasting caused by a cervical rib (neurogenic thoracic outlet syndrome) (cervical rib and band syndrome)

The first report of brachial plexopathy caused by a cervical rib was by Thomas and Cushing in 1903 [14]. The genesis of all neurogenic thoracic outlet compressive disorders is the cervical rib or a deformed first rib at the base of the scalene triangle. The subclavian artery and the brachial plexus pass through the scalene triangle, which is bounded by scalenus anterior, scalenus medius, and the first rib. A cervical rib, if present, is at the base of the triangle. The cervical rib may be a fully formed rib or the enlarged transverse process of C7.

Muscle wasting caused by a cervical rib has an incidence of slightly more than 1 per million. The disorder usually presents in young and middle-aged women who may have bilateral cervical ribs. The larger rib is often on the asymptomatic side. A ligamentous band stretches between the cervical rib and the first thoracic rib (Fig. 5). The C8 and T1 anterior primary rami pass over this radiotranslucent band and join to form the lower trunk of the brachial plexus. These fibers—T1 more so than C8—are vulnerable to entrapment from the fibrous band, which causes the cervical band and rib syndrome. The signs and symptoms of this disorder include intermittent aching of the medial forearm, forearm wasting, weakness of intrinsic hand muscles, atrophy of the lateral thenar muscles, and variable sensory loss in the T1 dermatome.

The absence of some clinical signs is important in differentiating this disorder from carpal tunnel syndrome (CTS), ulnar neuropathy, and vascular disorders of

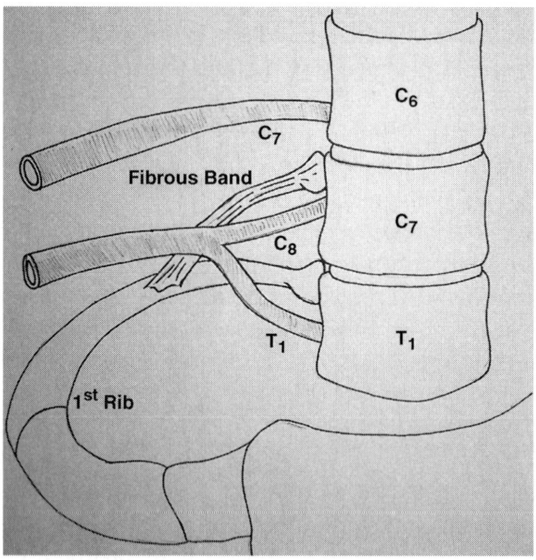

Fig. 5. Neurogenic TOS. Drawing shows a small cervical rib and the fibrous band that arises from the tip of the cervical rib to attach to the first rib. The lower trunk (C8 and T1) of the brachial plexus is angulated over the band.

the thoracic outlet. Nocturnal exacerbations are infrequent, as are complaints of numbness and tingling. Discoloration of the hand is not present. Deep tendon reflexes are normal. Sensory loss does not divide the ring finger. Positional tests for bruits are not helpful in making the diagnosis.

Cervical band and rib syndrome behaves as a severe, chronic lower trunk brachial plexopathy. The diagnosis is suspected clinically and confirmed with electrodiagnostic studies. The median motor, ulnar sensory, and medial antebrachial cutaneous sensory nerve amplitudes are reduced. Chronic denervation is found during the needle examination of muscles receiving C8 and T1 motor fibers. A sharp fibrous band that extends from the tip of the C7 transverse process or cervical rib to the first rib is discovered at surgery. Successful surgery alleviates arm pain, but atrophy, wasting, and weakness are little changed because of the chronicity of the condition [15–19].

Subclavian artery compression with a fixed lesion

Cervical ribs causing upper extremity ischemia were first described in 1818. The bony anomaly compresses the subclavian artery and causes poststenotic dilatation with thrombus formation. Patients present with ischemic pallor of the hand and exercise-induced pain with coolness in the arm or a diminution of the radial pulse. Distal embolization to the digits may occur with Raynaud's phenomenon, subungual hemorrhages, and ulceration of the fingertips. Arteriography or magnetic resonance angiography is diagnostic and surgical treatment is definitive [16].

Subclavian and axillary venous thrombosis

Effort thrombosis (Paget-von Schroetter disorder)

Spontaneous thrombosis of the subclavian and axillary veins occurs more often in young persons and frequently follows vigorous arm use. Presenting symptoms are abrupt onset of cyanosis, swelling, ache, and exercise-induced fatigue. Dilated collateral veins are evident on the upper chest and shoulders. There is no root, trunk, or nerve compression; neither is a bony anomaly present. Thrombosis may be iatrogenic or caused by vascular compression at the thoracic outlet, hypercoagulable states, or luminal webs. The diagnosis is made by venography. Treatment depends on the cause. Complications may include residual extremity edema, pain, and pulmonary embolism [16].

Pain plus sensory symptoms without a fixed lesion

Disputed thoracic outlet syndrome

Patients who have disputed TOS do not have cervical ribs, muscle wasting, or other neurologic deficits. The symptoms are protean and range from arm pain and dysesthesia to shoulder dysfunction, headaches, and chest pain. Neurologic complaints often do not follow known neuroanatomic patterns. The physical examination demonstrates only soft nonquantifiable findings, such as tenderness and collapsible weakness [17–19].

Mild positional paresthesias caused by physiologic compression of the lower trunk of the brachial plexus during sleep or with occupational hyperabduction of the arm are not harbingers of a disease process and should not be construed as the intermittent positional effects of fibrous bands in the scalene triangle. Various provocative tests, such as the Adson maneuver, the costoclavicular maneuver, the hyperabduction maneuver, and the Roos test, must be interpreted with caution because they are often positive with pulse reduction or even pulse obliteration in normal asymptomatic individuals. These positional tests have never received universal acceptance [16,20,21].

Routine electrodiagnostic studies are normal in disputed TOS but are useful in eliminating a diagnosis of true nerve compression neuropathy. Somatosensory evoked potentials are of limited value in the evaluation of muscle wasting caused by a cervical rib and of no established value in the diagnosis of disputed TOS [22].

Patients who have disputed TOS should be evaluated thoroughly for psychogenic, vascular, muscular, and other pathologic conditions. Neurogenic or vascular forms of TOS may be ruled out with the proper tests. Identifying the presence or absence of litigation is critical. Pain may be caused by muscle imbalance in the neck, shoulders, and upper back. Physiatrists can design a program to improve posture, including strengthening of the elevators of the shoulder or various conservative treatments modalities. The psychological component of pain and associated behavioral responses needs consideration in some cases [23].

Median neuropathies

In the forearm the median nerve passes beneath the lacertus fibrosus, the aponeurotic band of the biceps. The nerve enters the pronator teres, where numerous fibrous bands may exist in the vicinity of the two heads of the muscle (Fig. 6). The anterior interosseous nerve has its origin from the median nerve at this location. Leaving the pronator teres, the median nerve passes below the proximal edge of the flexor digitorum sublimes. At the wrist the median nerve crosses into the palm through the carpal tunnel. The roof of this canal is the transverse carpal ligament, and a concave arch of carpal bones constitutes the floor.

Pronator syndrome

Pronator syndrome is caused by entrapment of the median nerve between the humeral and ulnar heads of pronator teres because of hypertrophy, trauma, fibrous bands, or anomalous structures. Symptoms include pain in the proximal forearm during pronation or other forearm exercise and paresthesias in the median distribution of the hand. Tinel's sign and tenderness at the site of entrapment

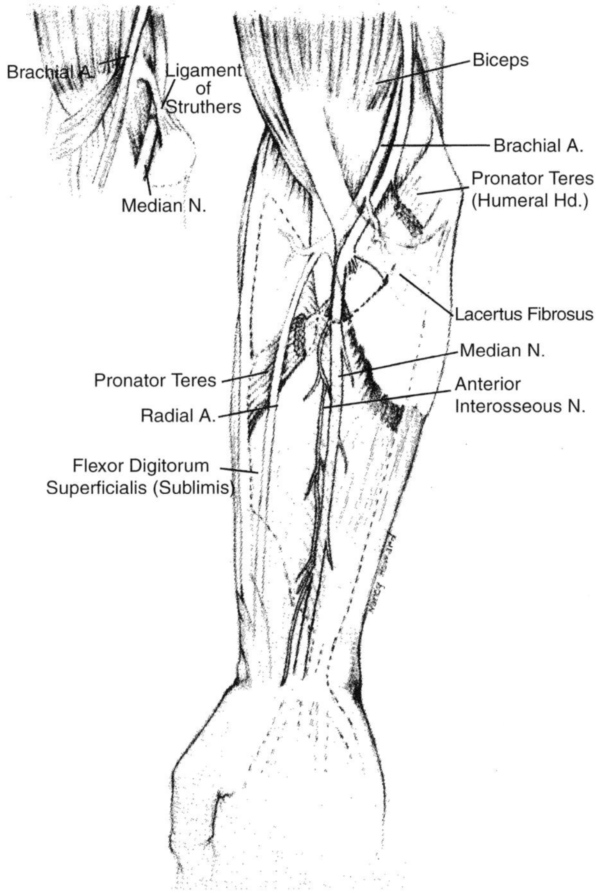

Fig. 6. Anatomy of the median nerve in the proximal forearm with detail of the anterior interosseous nerve. (*From* Mosely LH, Kalafut RM, Levinson PD, et al. Cumulative trauma disorders and compression neuropathies of the upper extremities. In: Kasdan ML, editor. Occupational hand and upper extremity injuries and diseases. Philadelphia: Hanley & Belfus; 1991. p. 373; with permission.)

are subjective findings in some patients. Similar complaints may occur with nerve compression beneath the lacertus fibrosus or as the nerve passes beneath the proximal edge of flexor digitorum sublimes (Fig. 6).

Objective findings include weakness of flexor pollicis longus and the lateral thenar muscles with demonstrable atrophy in chronic cases. The presence of a sensory deficit in the proximal palm in the territory of the palmar cutaneous branch, the absence of nocturnal exacerbation, and lack of improvement with wrist splinting differentiate pronator syndrome from CTS.

Electrodiagnostic studies of severe cases of pronator syndrome with axon loss of the median nerve may localize the site of compression to the forearm. The needle examination of chronic median nerve compression with axon loss reveals denervation in median-innervated muscles of the forearm and hand. If the entrapment is less severe, the needle examination is normal and NCS demonstrate partial or complete conduction block caused by demyelination. EMG also rules out CTS and other forms of neuropathy.

Pronator syndrome is rare and overdiagnosis is common. Most patients who complain of forearm pain and tingling in the arm or hand do not have nerve entrapment in the proximal forearm. Conservative treatment measures for pronator syndrome include restricting specific upper extremity activities, medications, injections, and splinting. Decompression of the median nerve is considered when there are objective findings, including wasting and definitive electrodiagnostic tests [24–29].

Anterior interosseous nerve entrapment

Anterior interosseous nerve entrapment at the level of the pronator teres or flexor digitorum sublimis from fibrous bands, anomalies, or trauma also causes proximal forearm pain that increases with exercise (Fig. 6). Anterior interosseous nerve syndrome causes weakness of thumb and index flexion at the distal interphalangeal joints demonstrated by an abnormal pinch. Weakness of wrist pronation also may be present. There is no sensory loss in the hand or weakness of the lateral thenar muscles, which differentiates this disorder from pronator syndrome and CTS. Routine NCS are normal. Median conduction to pronator quadratus may be delayed. Needle examination reveals denervation in the flexor pollicis longus, pronator quadratus, and flexor digitorum profundus I and II with sparing of the thenar muscles [30].

Anterior interosseous nerve entrapment may occur spontaneously. Brachial plexopathy that affects the medial cord may masquerade as anterior interosseous syndrome with similar electrodiagnostic findings. Surgical exploration is required if rest, immobilization, and other conservative measures do not improve motor function [24].

Carpal tunnel syndrome

CTS is the most common entrapment neuropathy in the upper extremity. It is a symptom complex caused by compression of the median nerve in the carpal tunnel with pain and burning or tingling paresthesias in the fingers and hand, sometimes extending to the elbow [2]. Any process that compromises the size of the carpal canal predisposes an individual to CTS (Fig. 7). Systemic disorders that predispose an individual to develop CTS include hypothyroidism, pregnancy, diabetes mellitus, amyloid disease, systemic lupus erythematosus, hyperthyroidism, Lyme disease, and multiple myeloma [31]. Acute CTS may follow wrist trauma.

Patients who have CTS complain of intermittent tingling in the hand in the distribution of the median nerve but with sparing of the palm (Fig. 7). The symptoms are usually worse at night or during gripping activities and are relieved by shaking the hand vigorously. These intermittent, reversible symptoms are

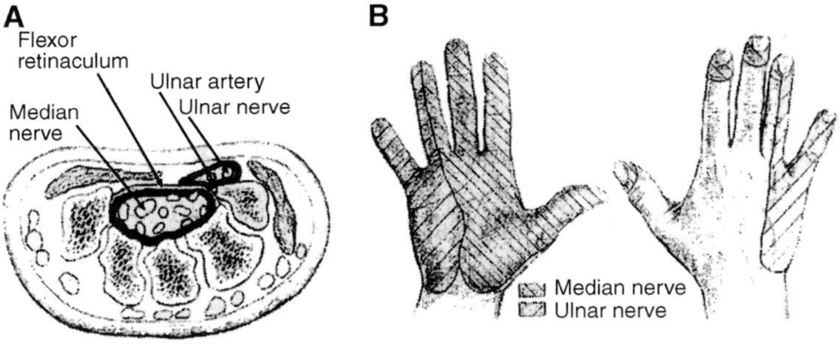

Fig. 7. (*A*) Wrist anatomy shows the median nerve through the carpal tunnel in close proximity to Guyon's canal, where the ulnar nerve passes. (*B*) Median and ulnar nerve sensory distribution. (*From* West SG, editor. Rheumatology secrets. Philadelphia: Hanley & Belfus; 1997; with permission.)

caused by hypovascularity of the median nerve. There may be sensory loss in the distal median territory, sparing the palm. As the neuropathy progresses, the sensory symptoms become more prolonged and pain accompanies the tingling. The pain may radiate to the forearm, elbow, or shoulder. Some patients may describe vasospastic symptoms. Loss of grip strength or dexterity may occur at any stage of the illness but more often as the process worsens. Atrophy of the lateral thenar muscles occurs in the later stages and is caused by physical compression of the median nerve with axonal degeneration [24]. Tinel's sign and Phalen's test are too insensitive to serve as reliable diagnostic maneuvers.

The differential diagnosis of CTS is broad. Numbness and tingling in the hand may be described in peripheral neuropathy, cervical radiculopathy, poliomyelitis, amyotrophic lateral sclerosis, and central nervous system disorders, including infections, trauma, seizures, tumors, vascular disorders, and psychiatric illness. Raynaud's syndrome, angina pectoris, arthritis, tenosynovitis, and other musculoskeletal conditions may mimic CTS. Atrophy of the lateral thenar muscles is not unique to CTS and may be seen with proximal median neuropathy, brachial plexus disorders, cervical radiculopathy, multifocal motor neuropathy, and syringomyelia [32].

Electrodiagnostic studies are the mainstay in the diagnosis of CTS. EMG may verify the diagnosis in atypical cases, establish a baseline for comparison to future examinations, guide decision making concerning surgical treatment, and detect underlying peripheral neuropathy or other disorders that mimic CTS [3].

A literature-based practice parameter concerning the electrodiagnosis of CTS has been approved by the American Academy of Neurology and endorsed by the American Academy of Physical Medicine and Rehabilitation [33]. The practice standard for testing workers with suspected CTS is a median sensory NCS across the wrist at a distance of 13 to 14 cm with comparison of abnormal findings to one other adjacent sensory in the symptomatic limb (Fig. 8). Median motor NCS and needle EMG are also reviewed in this parameter. The EMG should be fashioned to rule out other common disorders, including cervical radiculopathy and peripheral neuropathy.

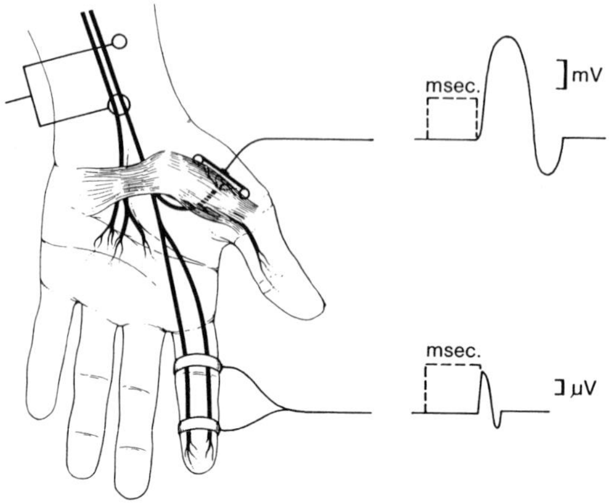

Fig. 8. Ring electrodes around the index finger record the sensory response, and surface electrodes over the abductor pollicis brevis record the motor response after electrical stimulation of the median nerve at the wrist. (*From* Chaplin E, Kasdan M, Corwin H. Occupational neurology and the hand: differential diagnosis. Hand Clinics 1986;2(3):515; with permission.)

Conservative treatment measures include splinting and oral or injected steroids. Activity modifications may reduce symptoms, but epidemiologic studies have not isolated the contribution (if any) of wrist position, repetition, or force from intrinsic risk factors, including use of hormonal medications, smoking, obesity, and sedentary lifestyle [34]. Open carpal tunnel surgical release is preferable to endoscopic surgery to decrease the risk of complications and incomplete release [24].

Ulnar neuropathies

There are multiple potential areas of ulnar nerve entrapment or injury (Fig. 9). The ulnar nerve passes between the medial border of the triceps and the intermuscular septum (arcade of Struthers) and may be compressed by the edge of the septum. The nerve passes posterior to the medial epicondyle and lies in the condylar groove, where it is palpable on clinical examination (Fig. 10). If the groove is shallow or the medial epicondyle is small, the ulnar nerve may sublux during elbow flexion. When the nerve is translocated from the groove it is more vulnerable to trauma. Passing between the medial epicondyle and the olecranon the ulnar nerve enters the forearm between the heads of the flexor carpi ulnaris, which it innervates. The deep fascia forms a fibrous arcade that serves as the roof of a structure termed the cubital tunnel, which is another potential site of entrapment [35,36]. The ulnar nerve also innervates the medial head of flexor digitorum profundus in the proximal forearm. The dorsal ulnar cutaneous sensory nerve arises from the ulnar trunk 5 to 6 cm proximal to the wrist and transmits sensation from the dorsoradial hand.

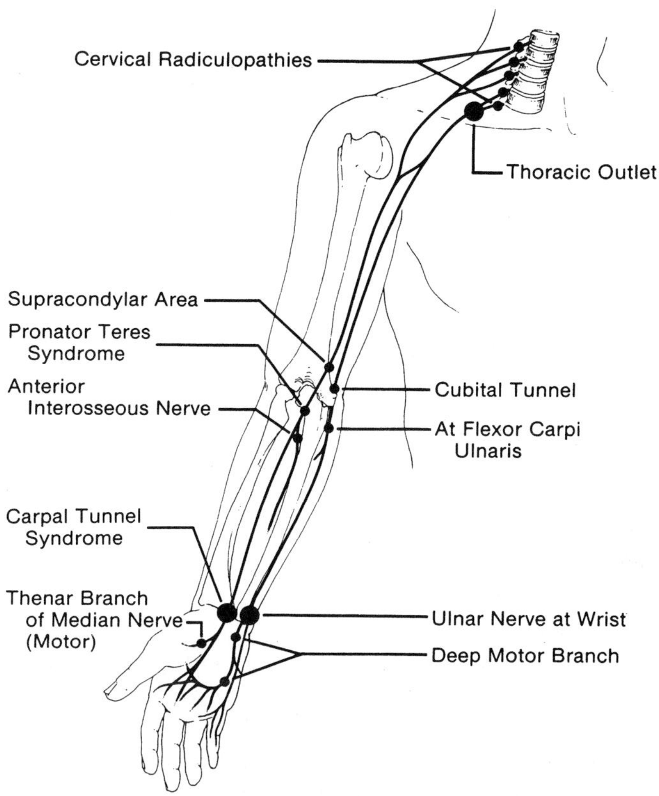

Fig. 9. Common areas of median and ulnar nerve compression in the upper arm, elbow, forearm, wrist, and hand. (*From* Chaplin E, Kasdan M, Corwin H. Occupational neurology and the hand: differential diagnosis. Hand Clinics 1986;2(3):517; with permission.)

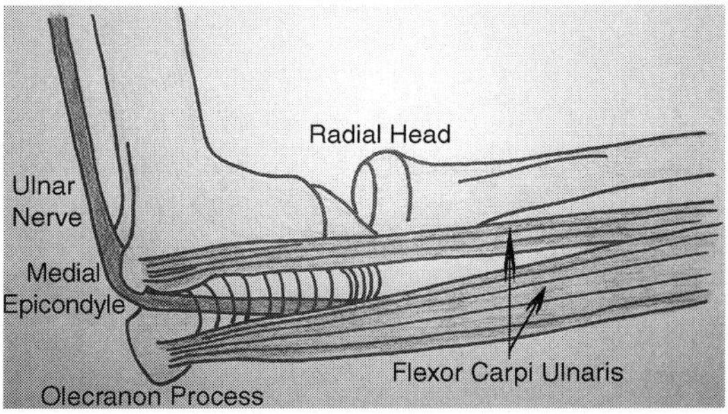

Fig. 10. Detail of the ulnar nerve at elbow.

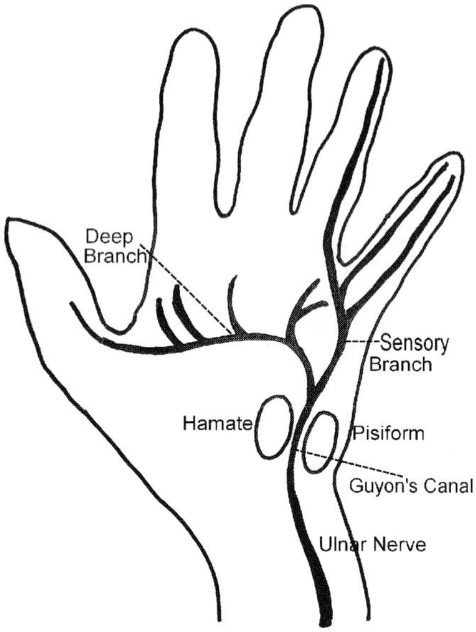

Fig. 11. Detail of the ulnar nerve at wrist.

In the palm, the ulnar nerve enters Guyon's canal (the ulnar tunnel) between the pisiform and the hook of the hamate (Fig. 11). Within Guyon's canal the superficial sensory branch innervates palmaris brevis and supplies sensation to the fifth digit and the medial half of the fourth digit. The deep motor branch supplies the hypothenar muscles before exiting the ulnar tunnel to innervate the interossei, ulnar lumbricals, adductor pollicis, and deep head of flexor pollicis brevis (Fig. 11).

Ulnar neuropathy at the elbow

Ulnar neuropathy at the elbow (UNE), the second most common upper extremity mononeuropathy, is a group of conditions. The mechanics of nerve injury likely include external compression, traction, or entrapment at the arcade of Struthers, condylar groove, or flexor carpi ulnaris. Space-occupying lesions, elbow deformity, arthritis, and peripheral neuropathy may predispose to UNE. Cubital tunnel syndrome is UNE distal to the condylar groove where the nerve enters flexor carpi ulnaris and is probably the most frequent of these conditions.

Individuals who have UNE commonly complain of tingling of the ring and fifth fingers because of ulnar nerve ischemia. In mild cases the clinical findings are restricted to hypesthesia or sensory loss over the fifth and medial half of the ring fingers, ulnar palm, and dorsum of the hand. Forearm dysesthesias, elbow aching, pain at the cubital tunnel, or reduced grip strength may be described. The ulnar nerve may be palpably thickened at the condylar groove and sublux with elbow flexion. A positive elbow flexion test or a painful Tinel's sign at the elbow is too insensitive to serve as a reliable diagnostic maneuver and must be supported by electrodiagnostic studies. Reduced grip associated with atrophy of the interosseous or hypothenar muscles is the most common motor sign. Less often there is weakness of flexion of the distal interphalangeal joints of the ring and fifth fingers and wrist flexion. Wartenburg's sign, decreased adduction of the small finger caused by weakness of the third palmar interosseous, may indicate the presence of ulnar neuropathy. Denervation of the first dorsal interosseous and adductor pollicis muscles because of ulnar neuropathy causes weakness when grasping paper between the thumb and radial index finger. A patient may compensate for this deficit by using the flexor pollicis longus to preserve pinch strength (Froment's sign) [37].

The differential diagnosis of UNE includes cervical radiculopathy, neurogenic TOS, Pancoast tumor and other brachial plexus disorders, ulnar tunnel syndrome, amyotrophic lateral sclerosis, multifocal motor neuropathy, and peripheral neuropathy. Some central nervous system and musculoskeletal disorders (see the discussion on CTS) also may mimic the symptoms of UNE.

Electrodiagnostic testing remains the gold standard for the diagnosis of UNE. The interpretation of the tests for ulnar neuropathy is complex, with frequent errors of omission. The goal of the electromyographer is to localize anatomically the area of nerve compression and grade the severity of the process. A literature-based practice parameter concerning the electrodiagnosis of UNE has been approved by the American Academy of Neurology and endorsed by the American Academy of Physical Medicine and Rehabilitation. The NCS are performed with the elbow at moderate flexion using a 10-cm across-elbow distance. Slowing of ulnar conduction velocity of less than 50 m/s should be combined with other abnormalities to strengthen the diagnosis of UNE. The needle examination must include ulnar-innervated muscles and other muscles to exclude a diagnosis of brachial plexopathy or radiculopathy [38]. Abnormal NCS of the dorsal ulnar cutaneous branch suggest that the lesion is proximal to the wrist.

Treatment of mild symptoms of UNE is conservative and may include activity modification and splinting. Surgery is indicated in cases of a space-occupying lesion or progressive cases that fail conservative management. Ulnar nerve decompression may be accomplished with various nerve transposition procedures, medial epicondylectomy, and microneural dissection [35].

Ulnar tunnel syndrome

Ulnar tunnel syndrome is compression of the ulnar nerve at the wrist and may involve sensory or motor fibers or both. Shea and McClain [39] classified the ulnar tunnel syndrome into a pure motor, a pure sensory, or combined motor and sensory neuropathy. The clinical presentation of the three types of ulnar tunnel syndrome varies depending on the location of the lesion. Clinical findings that differentiate ulnar tunnel syndrome from UNE include normal sensation on the dorsum of the hand and normal strength of flexor carpi ulnaris and flexor digitorum profundus. Ulnar compression at the wrist from ganglion cysts and other space-occupying lesions, occupational injuries, trauma, bicycling, and congenital anomalies has been described. Modification of hand use with avoidance of pressure on the wrist or splinting is tried in cases in which no surgical lesion is found [39,40].

Radial neuropathy

Radial nerve compression is less common than median or ulnar nerve compression. The main trunk of the radial nerve courses between the lateral and medial heads of the triceps then lies along the spiral groove of the humerus (Fig. 12). The spiral groove is a potential site of radial nerve injury. The nerve runs anterior to the lateral epicondyle before supplying brachioradialis and extensor carpi radialis longus. The main trunk then divides into a superficial sensory and terminal deep motor branch. The superficial sensory branch descends the radial aspect of the forearm and supplies the dorsal radial aspect of the hand. The terminal motor branch, the posterior interosseous nerve, passes through the supinator and enters the extensor compartment where it supplies supinator, adductor pollicis longus, and all of the extensors of the forearm. The fibrous edge of the supinator, the arcade of Frohse, is a potential site of entrapment of the posterior interosseous nerve.

Posterior interosseous syndrome

Posterior interosseous syndrome is a mononeuropathy of the posterior interosseous nerve usually at the arcade of Frohse from trauma, inflammation, or space-occupying lesions. Tenderness over the lateral aspect of the elbow may be present but is not the most prominent symptom. Patients complain of gradual

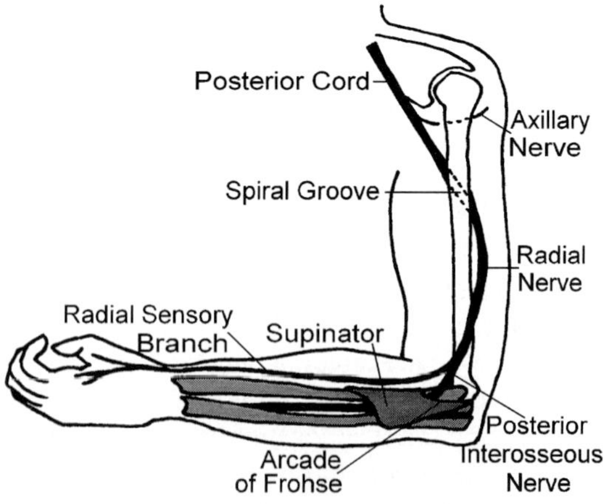

Fig. 12. Detail of the radial nerve and the arcade of Frohse.

or sudden onset of wrist and finger weakness. Examination reveals partial weakness or paralysis of wrist and finger extensors. Supinator and extensor carpi radialis longus function are normal, and the wrist may be radially deviated. There is no sensory loss. EMG differentiates posterior interosseous nerve compression from extensor tendon rupture with denervation in radial innervated muscles distal to the lesion and slowing of conduction across the supinator. Surgery is indicated if there is progression of motor loss or lack of response to activity modification and splinting [24,41].

Localized tenderness at the region of common extensor tendon insertions at the humeral lateral epicondyle has been termed "tennis elbow." The pain is aggravated by certain forearm movements but is not associated with weakness and typically responds to conservative management. Resistant cases that respond to surgery have been termed radial tunnel syndrome with compression of the posterior interosseous nerve at the level of extensor carpi radial brevis and supinator from fibrous bands, recurrent vessels, or thickening of the fascia. Despite surgical observations, no clinical or electrodiagnostic evidence indicates that radial tunnel syndrome is a motor entrapment neuropathy [41,42].

Wartenberg's syndrome

Wartenberg's syndrome is entrapment of the radial sensory nerve between the tendons of extensor carpi radialis longus and brachioradialis in the distal forearm. Various causes have been described, including trauma, fascial bands and space-occupying lesions, tight jewelry, and handcuffs. Forearm pain and numbness in the radial sensory territory sometimes provoked by ulnar deviation of the hand or percussion of the nerve at the level of entrapment are noted. Immobilization and removing tightly fitting wristbands are preferred to surgery [43].

Unusual disorders that mimic upper extremity nerve compression

Multifocal motor neuropathy with conduction block

Multifocal motor neuropathy with conduction block, reported initially in 1988, is an idiopathic purely motor multineuropathy that consists of progressive weakness of the upper extremities, usually asymmetric, without sensory loss. The disorder frequently masquerades as entrapment neuropathy. More than 80% of patients present with weakness of forearm and hand muscles, and more than 50% note fasciculations and muscle cramps with mild atrophy. The disease may be marked by slow or stepwise progression and may be differentiated from amyotrophic lateral sclerosis by the absence of typical upper motor neuron signs, including extensor plantar response, spasticity, and hyperreflexia. Multifocal motor neuropathy with conduction block has mimicked CTS, anterior interosseous nerve, and radial nerve compression [44–46].

Electrodiagnostic criteria for multifocal motor neuropathy with conduction block have been outlined [47]. The key feature is partial conduction block of motor nerves. Motor NCS usually show other features of demyelination, whereas sensory NCS are normal. Needle examination reveals reduced recruitment in weak muscles that are otherwise normal in appearance. Sparing of the paraspinous muscles differentiates the disorder from cervical radiculopathy. The most important laboratory finding is an increased level of serum IgM antibodies to GM1 ganglioside found in approximately half of the patients. These antibodies are not specific for this disorder. Creatine kinase is normal or minimally elevated. Nerve biopsy of sensory nerves is not useful. MRI of the brachial plexus may show abnormal findings [48]. Most patients respond to treatment with intravenous infusion of immunoglobulin but fail to improve or worsen with steroids [44].

Inclusion body myositis

Inclusion body myositis is an inflammatory myopathy with onset after age 50. Slowly progressive, asymmetric distal weakness of wrist and finger extensors may masquerade as radial nerve compression or clenched fist syndrome. MRI has demonstrated patchy involvement of forearm muscles [49]. Quadriceps muscle and ankle dorsiflexor weakness are also common. Creatine kinase may be normal or elevated. Motor and sensory NCS are normal, but the needle examination of involved muscles reveals a myopathic pattern. Muscle biopsy is diagnostic of inclusion body myositis [50].

Summary

Nerve compression and entrapment syndromes of the upper extremity occur at predictable locations. Diagnostic errors are often caused by limited neurologic examinations, overreliance on nonobjective data, and errors on EMG testing. Familiarity with the neuroanatomy and physiology of nerve compression enables the physician to formulate the correct diagnosis. The treatment of compression neuropathy varies with causation or the response to conservative management.

References

[1] DeJong RN. The neurologic examination. In: Magee KR, editor. The neurologic examination. 4th edition. Hagerstown (MD): Harper & Row; 1979. p. 3–6.

[2] Corwin HM. Neurologic evaluation of the upper extremity. In: Kasdan ML, editor. Occupational hand and upper extremity injuries and diseases. 2nd edition. Philadelphia: Hanley & Belfus; 1998. p. 287–302.

[3] Wilbourn A. Electrodiagnosis with entrapment neuropathies. In: American Association of Electrodiagnostic Medicine. 1992 Plenary session I: entrapment neuropathies. Rochester (NY): Custom Printing; 1992. p. 23–37.

[4] Lundborg G, Dahlin LB. The pathophysiology of nerve compression. Hand Clin 1992;8(2):215–27.
[5] Campbell W. Focal neuropathies. In: Mitchell CW, editor. Essentials of electrodiagnostic medicine. Baltimore: Williams & Wilkins; 1999. p. 255–78.
[6] American Association of Neuromuscular and Electrodiagnostic Medicine. Who is qualified to practice electrodiagnostic medicine? Position statement. Rochester (MN): American Association of Neuromuscular and Electrodiagnostic Medicine; 1999.
[7] Corwin H, Kasdan M. Electrodiagnostic reports of median neuropathy at the wrist. J Hand Surg [Am] 1998;23A:55–7.
[8] Rutkove S. AAEM minimonograph #14. The effects of temperature in neuromuscular electrophysiology. Muscle Nerve 2001;24:867–82.
[9] Albers JW. The influence of electrodiagnosis on the evaluation and management of peripheral neuropathy. In: American Association of Electrodiagnostic Medicine. 1997 AAEM Course B: Using electrodiagnosis in clinical decision making. Rochester (NY): Johnson Printing Company; 1997. p. 25–35.
[10] Brumback RA, Bobele GB, Rayan GM. Electrodiagnosis of compressive nerve lesions. Hand Clin 1992;8(2):241–54.
[11] Griffin JW, Hsieh ST, McArthur JC, et al. Laboratory testing in peripheral nerve disease. Neurol Clin 1996;14(1):119–33.
[12] Swenson MR, Vilasana DR. Neurologic evaluation of the upper extremity. In: Kasdan ML, editor. Occupational hand and upper extremity injuries and diseases. Philadelphia: Hanley & Belfus; 1991. p. 115–30.
[13] Peet RM, Henrickson JD, Anderson TP, et al. Thoracic outlet syndrome: evaluation of a therapeutic exercise program. Staff Meet Mayo Clin 1956;31:281–7.
[14] Thomas HM, Cushing HG. Exhibition of two cases of radicular paralysis of the brachial plexus: one from the pressure of a cervical rib with operation, the other of uncertain origin. Johns Hopkins Hosp Bull 1903;14:315.
[15] Levin K, Wilbourn A, Maggiano H. Cervical rib and median sternotomy-related brachial plexopathies. Neurology 1998;50:1407–13.
[16] Cuetter A, Bartoszek D. The thoracic outlet syndrome: controversies, overdiagnosis, overtreatment, and recommendations for management. Muscle Nerve 1989;12:410–9.
[17] Wilbourn AJ. Disease of the peripheral nervous system. In: Dyck P, Thomas DK, Lambert EH, et al, editors. Peripheral neuropathy. 3rd edition. Philadelphia: WB Saunders; 1993. p. 936–40.
[18] Gilliatt RW. Thoracic outlet syndromes. In: Dyck P, Thomas DK, Lambert EH, et al, editors. Peripheral neuropathy. 2nd edition. Philadelphia: WB Saunders; 1984. p. 1409–19.
[19] Wilbourn AJ, Porter JM. Thoracic outlet syndrome. Spine: State of the Art Reviews 1988;2: 597–626.
[20] Poole G, Thomas K. Thoracic outlet syndrome reconsidered. Am Surg 1996;62:287–91.
[21] Rayan G, Jensen C. Thoracic outlet syndrome: provocative examination maneuvers in a typical population. J Shoulder Elbow Surg 1995;4:113–7.
[22] Aminoff M, Eisen A. AAEM minimonograph #19: somatosensory evoked potentials. Muscle Nerve 1998;21:277–90.
[23] Mosley LH, Kalafut RM, Levinson PD, et al. Cumulative trauma disorders and compression neuropathies of the upper extremities. In: Kasdan ML, editor. Occupational hand and upper extremity injuries and diseases. Philadelphia: Hanley & Belfus; 1991. p. 353–402.
[24] Vendor MI, Ruder JR, Pomerance J, et al. Upper extremity compressive neuropathies. In: Kasdan ML, editor. Occupational hand and upper extremity injuries and diseases. 2nd edition. Philadelphia: Hanley & Belfus; 1998. p. 83–96.
[25] Wilbourn AJ. The pronator syndrome. In: American Association of Electrodiagnostic Medicine. 1991 AAEM Course D: Focal peripheral neuropathies: selected topics. Rochester (NY): Johnson Printing Company; 1991. p. 29–32.
[26] Johnson R, Spinner M, Shrewsbury M. Median nerve entrapment in the proximal forearm. J Hand Surg [Am] 1979;4A:48–51.
[27] Jones N, Ming N. Persistent median artery as a cause of pronator syndrome. J Hand Surg [Am] 1988;13A:728–32.

[28] Morris H, Peters B. Pronator syndrome: clinical and electrophysical features in seven cases. J Neurol Neurosurg Psychiatry 1976;36:461–4.
[29] Seyffarth H. Primary myoses in the m. pronator teres as cause of lesion of the n. medianus (the pronator syndrome). Acta Psychiatr Neurol Scand 1951;74(Suppl):251–4.
[30] Nakano K, Lundergan C, Okihiro M. Anterior interosseous nerve syndromes: diagnostic methods and alternative treatments. Arch Neurol 1977;34:477–80.
[31] Kimura J. Mononeuropathies and entrapment syndromes. In: Electrodiagnosis in diseases of nerve and muscle: principles and practice. 2nd edition. Philadelphia: FA Davis; 1989. p. 495–516.
[32] Corwin HM. Neurologic evaluation of cumulative trauma disorders. In: Asfour SS, editor. Trends in ergonomics/human factors IV. Amstersdam: Elsevier Science; 1987. p. 1005–11.
[33] Jablecki C, Andary M, Floeter M, et al. Practice parameter: electrodiagnostic studies in carpal tunnel syndrome. Neurology 1998;88:1447–51.
[34] Szabo RM. Occupational carpal tunnel syndrome. In: Kasdan ML, editor. Occupational hand and upper extremity injuries and diseases. 2nd edition. Philadelphia: Hanley & Belfus; 1998. p. 113–27.
[35] Rayan G. Proximal ulnar nerve compression. Hand Clin 1992;8(2):325–35.
[36] Feindel W, Stratford J. The role of the cubital tunnel in tardy ulnar palsy. Can J Surg 1958;1: 287–300.
[37] Chung KC. Tendon transfers. In: Jebson PJL, Kasdan ML, editors. Hand secrets: questions you will be asked on rounds, in the clinic, on oral exams. Philadelphia: Hanley & Belfus; 1998. p. 227–8.
[38] American Association of Electrodiagnostic Medicine, American Academy of Neurology, and American Academy of Physical Medicine and Rehabilitation. Practice parameter: electrodiagnostic studies in ulnar neuropathy at the elbow. Neurology 1999;52:688–90.
[39] Shea J, McClain E. Ulnar nerve compression syndromes at and below the wrist. J Bone Joint Surg Am 1969;51A:1095–103.
[40] Moneim M. Ulnar nerve compression at the wrist: ulnar tunnel syndrome. Hand Clin 1992; 8(2):337–44.
[41] Markiewitz A, Merryman J. Radial nerve compression in the upper extremity. J Am Soc Surg Hand 2005;5(2):87–99.
[42] Elleler MG. Resistant tennis elbow: a posterior interosseous entrapment neuropathy? In: American Association of Electrodiagnostic Medicine. 1991 AAEM Course D: Focal peripheral neuropathies: selected topics. Rochester (NY): Johnson Printing Company; 1991. p. 33–6.
[43] Gabriel TM. Compression neuropathies of the upper extremity. In: Jebson PJL, Kasdan ML, editors. Hand secrets: questions you will be asked on rounds, in the clinic, on oral exams. 2nd edition. Philadelphia: Hanley & Belfus; 2002. p. 239.
[44] Nobile-Orasia E, Cappellari A, Priori A. Multifocal motor neuropathy: current concepts and controversies. Muscle Nerve 2005;31:663–80.
[45] Seror P, Leger J, Maisonobe T. Anterior interosseous nerve and multifocal motor neuropathy. Muscle Nerve 2002;26:841–4.
[46] Beydoun S. Multifocal motor neuropathy with conduction block misdiagnosed as multiple entrapment neuropathies. Muscle Nerve 1998;21:813–5.
[47] Olney R, Lewis R, Putnam T, et al. Consensus criteria for the diagnosis of multifocal motor neuropathy. Muscle Nerve 2003;27:117–21.
[48] Es H, Van den Berg L, Franssen H, et al. Magnetic resonance imaging of the brachial plexus in patients with multifocal motor neuropathy. Neurology 1997;48:1218–24.
[49] Takamure M, Murata K, Kaiwahara M, et al. Finger flexor weakness in inclusion body myositis. Neurology 2005;64(2):389.
[50] Amato A, Gronseth G, Jackson C, et al. Inclusion body myositis: clinical and pathological boundaries. Ann Neurol 1996;40(4):581–6.

ELSEVIER
SAUNDERS

Clin Occup Environ Med
5 (2) 353–367

CLINICS IN
OCCUPATIONAL AND
ENVIRONMENTAL
MEDICINE

Work-Related Carpal Tunnel Syndrome: The Facts and the Myths

Jane Derebery, MD, FACOEM

Concentra Health Services, 10200 Broadway Boulevard, Suite 201, San Antonio, TX 78217, USA

Carl Zenz's 1988 second edition of "Occupational Medicine: Principles and Practical Applications" contains only two citations on carpal tunnel syndrome in the index and includes only one brief paragraph on the subject in the entire volume [1]. By contrast, the 1994 third edition (the latest) of Zenz's text cites carpal tunnel syndrome 20 times in the index and covers the subject in depth [2].

In Austin, Texas, a neurologist currently advertises the opening of a carpal tunnel clinic, and in Houston, a hand surgeon has spent approximately $200,000 annually to place a monthly ad in Southwest airline's magazine to entice patients who have carpal tunnel syndrome to his clinic for surgical treatment. A subject that was deemed barely worth mentioning in the occupational medicine textbooks of the 1980s has become big business.

Carpal tunnel syndrome currently accounts for more lost time than any other work-related malady. According to the US Bureau of Labor Statistics, since 1994, the median lost days average for carpal tunnel syndrome was the highest of all claims. For example, in 2000, the carpal tunnel syndrome median average was 27 days off, compared with 20 days for a fracture and 18 days for an amputation [3]. Although it still accounts for a relatively small percentage of occupationally related claims filed, carpal tunnel syndrome has gained substantial media attention and accounts for substantial disability. What has happened in the interim since the 1980s—when carpal tunnel syndrome was barely more than mentioned in occupational medicine textbooks—that has brought about the idea that a chief cause of carpal tunnel syndrome is repetitive workplace activities?

E-mail address: Jane.derebery@concentra.com

doi:10.1016/j.coem.2005.11.014 ***occmed.theclinics.com***

A review of the literature regarding the potential for work activities to cause carpal tunnel syndrome reveals wide variation in opinion on the matter, ranging from "almost never" to up to 90% of cases being caused by workplace activities [4–7]. The wide variation in opinions on the matter suggests multifactorial causation and the fact that there is much variability in criteria used to determine work relatedness. Little consistent scientific evidence supports the idea that routine physical activities of the modern American workforce are a major cause of carpal tunnel syndrome. Most studies find no consistent relationship between carpal tunnel syndrome and workplace activities, and studies that do find relationships have been criticized for having serious methodologic flaws [5,8–11]. In most states, however, carpal tunnel syndrome is still commonly attributed to repetitive work activities from a legal standpoint.

All cultures develop myths that reflect deeply entrenched beliefs and ideas, and the culture of the medical profession is no exception. Established medical myths can be difficult to discredit, even sound scientific evidence refutes them. The workers' compensation system in particular has promulgated numerous myths and societal expectations regarding causation and management of injuries perceived to be caused by workplace exposures and activities. The common aches and pains of everyday living that would be accepted as a normal condition of aging or lack of conditioning often are attributed to the work environment.

Patients, doctors, insurance carriers, employers, and the legal system have some vested or self-serving interest in supporting given cultural beliefs and expectations regarding illness and management, and these strongly held beliefs and expectations greatly influence the medical management and outcome of a given case. A Medline search on carpal tunnel syndrome–related medical articles published between 1997 and 2005 is revealing regarding where the areas of interest regarding carpal tunnel syndrome lie for the medical profession. There were 531 citations, with the highest number (177) focusing on surgical aspects of treatment. Eighty-seven citations addressed electrodiagnostic testing and imaging, 57 focused on issues of diagnosis, 50 focused on nonsurgical treatments, 30 discussed causation determination, 22 involved workers' compensation issues, 4 focused on psychosocial aspects, and two articles addressing the issue of return to work.

The lack of focus on subject areas that provide little financial incentive to physicians, such as areas that deal with psychosocial issues or return-to-work issues, is compelling. According to US Bureau of Labor Statistics data, not only has the median lost days average been highest for carpal tunnel syndrome than all other claims but also it has been increasing. In 2000, the average time off for carpal tunnel syndrome was 27 days; in 2003 it was 32 [3].

The current controversy regarding carpal tunnel syndrome work causation may embroil treating physicians in conflict regarding work relatedness, treatment, and the need for work restrictions and disability in a venue in which medically it is arguable at best that the job is causative but in which the legal and social constructs deem it work related. This article discusses those controversies and suggests ways of managing carpal tunnel syndrome cases.

Causation

The status of being designated work related is in itself a risk for disability [12]; logically, a primary means of minimizing the risk of disability from carpal tunnel syndrome is to avoid classifying a case as work related when no good evidence supports it as being caused by the job. When the causation of a given disorder is misdirected, then too might be the direction and content of care and the outcome of the case. For instance, a clerical worker who has carpal tunnel syndrome is restricted from the job because of an erroneous assumption that the condition was work related, when in actuality a 25-pound weight gain and hormonal problems are the cause. Not only does the patient suffer financially and emotionally from loss of work but also treatment is not likely to address the true causes. The patient is at risk of gaining even more weight when off work, which further contributes to the problem.

SYSTEMIC	ANATOMIC	ERGONOMIC
Flexor tendinitis	Osteoarthritis	Awkward posture
Rheumatoid diseases	Anomalous muscles	+
Diabetes	Small wrist dimension	High repetition
Collagen-vascular &	Neoplasms	+
Thyroid disease	Tubercular granuloma	High force
Gout	Radial head fracture	+
Renal disease	Hematoma	Vibration
Long term Dialysis	Volkman's ischemia	
Gynecological disorders	Carpal bone fracture with dislocation	
Amyloidosis		
Pregnancy	High pressure injection injury	
Obesity	Burn injuries	
Alcoholism		High force
Dupuytren's disease		+
Hereditary Neuropathy with liability to pressure palsies		High repetition
		+
Genetic (trisomy of chromosome 8)		Cold work environment
Endocrinopathies		
Use of certain medications		
Cigarette smoking		
High caffeine consumption		
Aerobic deconditioning		
Congestive heart failure		
Infection (33 agents		
Nutritional deficiency		
Vitamin toxicity		
Exposure to Neurotoxins		
Ingestion of rapeseed oil		
Multiple myeloma		
Raynauds syndrome		

Fig. 1. Causation of carpal tunnel syndrome is difficult to determine, and work relatedness is controversial. Causation is believed to be multifactorial in many cases and often may be idiopathic, with no apparent associated risk factors.

Carpal tunnel syndrome is an illness, not an injury, and health factors such as obesity, smoking, heavy alcohol consumption, diabetes, and thyroid disease are much more likely to contribute substantially to the onset of carpal tunnel syndrome than workplace activities. Carpal tunnel syndrome can be caused or associated with many systemic diseases and conditions, and it also occurs in patients with no identifiable risk factors. Tendonitis, pregnancy, and hormonal disorders are just a few more of the medical conditions that have been associated with carpal tunnel syndrome. The tendency to develop carpal tunnel syndrome has even been found to be genetic [4,6,8,11,13]. Numerous associated conditions must be considered in the assessment of patients who have carpal tunnel syndrome (Fig. 1).

Although there is a prevailing cultural perception that carpal tunnel syndrome is often caused by physical activities, the combination of a sedentary lifestyle and being overweight has been identified as one of the most significant risk factors [14]. Association with carpal tunnel syndrome has been found most consistently found with obesity, advanced age, small wrist dimensions, and lack of exercise [8,14]. Long-term periodic follow-up of patients who have prolonged median nerve latency at the wrist has indicated that latency and nerve pathology tend to remain and increase with aging. Symptoms tend to fluctuate through the years, however, but in most cases do improve. Most workers with median nerve latency who initially are asymptomatic do not develop clinical carpal tunnel syndrome [8].

Work-related carpal tunnel syndrome

Although there are numerous associations with other medical conditions, many—if not most—cases of carpal tunnel syndrome occur with no clear-cut cause or association in presumably perfectly healthy individuals, and establishing causation is often not possible. Patients without clear medical associations are more likely to be presumed to have work-related carpal tunnel syndrome by misinformed administrators, employers, and physicians, even when no identifiable activity at work would be expected to promote symptoms. Generally, in the workers' compensation arena the decision of work relatedness may be more of a legal one than a medical one. In most cases it is an administrative decision made by an insurance company using input from a patient, the employer, and the treating physician.

National Institute of Occupational Safety and Health (NIOSH) reviewed the literature on causation, and the analysis suggested that for work activity to be considered significantly causative, high repetition, high force, awkward posture, and vibration exposure all must be present [15]. An analysis conducted by New Zealand researchers suggested that a combination of performing highly repetitive and forceful arm activity while in a cold environment seems to be the most significant work risk. In fact, the only two occupations that seem to have a higher risk ratio for developing carpal tunnel syndrome are boners who work in a cold (refrigerated) environment and frozen food workers who perform highly repetitive, forceful work [16].

Routine occupational activities sometimes may unmask rather than actually cause carpal tunnel syndrome. If a data entry worker's job requires prolonged sedentary work and the workload is excessive because of layoffs, the worker may be more bothered by intermittent numbness and tingling from carpal tunnel syndrome while performing that task than he or she would be by comparison if performing the varied tasks of a warehouse worker. Consequently, the data entry worker might be more likely to seek treatment and believe that the work caused the problem than would the warehouse worker.

Because the symptoms and signs associated with carpal tunnel syndrome are nonspecific and occur in unaffected persons on a frequent and regular basis, the disorder is commonly overdiagnosed, particularly in the workers' compensation arena [4,14]. One study found that only 17% of patients who were diagnosed with work-related carpal tunnel syndrome actually had symptoms and objective evidence [17]. Consequently, it is possible that most patients who present to an occupational medicine clinic with classic symptoms of carpal tunnel syndrome do not actually have carpal tunnel syndrome, because the symptoms occur commonly and transiently in people who, if tested, have normal nerve conduction studies [4,18]. Typical symptoms may be brought on by muscle tension caused by work in static postures, fatigue, stress, or poor conditioning [6,8]. Although from a medical causation standpoint there is good reason to argue that carpal tunnel syndrome is rarely substantially caused by the workplace, many cases still are being designated as work related because the job duties, although not causative, are believed to exacerbate the symptoms of the disease.

Carpal tunnel syndrome and trauma at work

Uncommonly, carpal tunnel syndrome can develop from trauma at work. Carpal tunnel syndrome can occur as sequelae from a radial fracture, traumatic tenosynovitis, carpal bone fracture with dislocation, Volkman's ischemic contracture, traumatic ganglion, or a carpal tunnel hematoma [19]. Symptoms may occur acutely or may be delayed.

Carpal tunnel syndrome and keyboarding

A 2004 NIOSH report of job activities associated with carpal tunnel syndrome listed computer use as the primary cause and indicated that it accounted for one half of all cases [20]. To quote Brandt Steele, a renowned psychiatrist, "statistics are like bikinis—what they reveal is quite interesting, but what is concealed is vital." Although it may be true that computer workers file claims for carpal tunnel syndrome, it is also true that the three most common occupations listed by people with carpal tunnel syndrome consistently have been homemaker, unemployed, and retired [20–22]. The NIOSH report could lead one to assume erroneously by association that computer work was causative. According to the NIOSH report, the other most commonly associated activities noted were reaching and twisting, followed by lifting and loading. To a much lesser degree the report related customer service, handwriting, and cashier work to carpal tunnel syndrome. The implication of the NIOSH report is that these job tasks largely caused the carpal tunnel syndrome cases.

The NIOSH report does not reflect the considerable controversy regarding work causation and carpal tunnel syndrome within the medical and scientific community, nor does it reflect that sound studies do not support a causal relationship between carpal tunnel syndrome and repetitive physical activity. All of these activities, including keyboard activities, are common, routine activities of daily living, regardless of job duties, performed by a large segment of the population at work and away from work, and although a person who has carpal tunnel syndrome may become more aware of symptoms during certain activities (including sleeping), that does not mean that the activity was causative.

No scientific evidence supports the fact that carpal tunnel syndrome can be caused or aggravated by prolonged keyboard use, yet it has been reported regularly as fact in such widely read periodicals as *TIME*, *Newsweek*, and the *New York Times*, and consequently the predominant public perception is that keyboarding is causative. Major manufacturers of computers commonly include a safety manual with each new computer that warns that prolonged use of a computer keyboard may cause serious injury, despite the lack of scientific evidence substantiating this commonly held belief. Currently a preponderance of evidence indicates that carpal tunnel syndrome is not caused by keyboarding and no sound scientific supports that finding [23–33].

Although keyboarding does not cause carpal tunnel syndrome, it is still not uncommon for an occupational medicine practitioner to be asked to assess and treat patients who have carpal tunnel syndrome presumed to be caused by keyboarding. Because work causation is a legal determination in most states despite a medical opinion to the contrary, carpal tunnel syndrome that develops in a computer worker may be deemed work related. For instance, an insurance company may have incorrectly accepted culpability initially and may be required to continue coverage. Some companies may request that all carpal tunnel syndrome cases of their computer workers be treated as work related by the company physician to ensure that appropriate care is delivered by a knowledgeable physician. Occasionally, because of individual circumstances, a physician may feel that work-related keyboarding substantially exacerbates a carpal tunnel syndrome condition and should be treated as work related.

Most patients with the diagnosis of carpal tunnel syndrome are able to work at a keyboard for prolonged periods without experiencing significant problems. Staying physically fit, using proper body mechanics and frequent brief postural breaks, and having a well-situated workstation increase the likelihood that a patient who has carpal tunnel syndrome can perform job tasks, such as keyboarding, without particular discomfort. The focus of management of workers who have carpal tunnel syndrome and use a keyboard extensively should be educating patients about the disorder, allaying any fears and misapprehensions about keyboarding and carpal tunnel syndrome, and promoting improved fitness to improve work tolerance.

Carpal tunnel syndrome and neurotoxin exposures

A Medline search failed to identify any articles that confirmed neurotoxin exposure as a work-related cause of carpal tunnel syndrome. The National Institutes of Health website on toxicologic hazards of the workplace listed 557 references to carpal tunnel syndrome and toxins [34]. Almost none of these articles referred to chemical neurotoxin exposures but instead focused on the physical and ergonomic aspects of the workplace relative to carpal tunnel syndrome. There were individual references to possible increased associations of carpal tunnel syndrome and exposures to mercury, radiofrequency electromagnetic fields, and chlorpyrifos, although the supporting evidence was isolated and limited [35–37]. There were also two case reports regarding patients who developed carpal tunnel syndrome within a few weeks of receiving a vaccination (one rubella and the other influenza) [38,39]. The associations seemed limited.

Diagnosis

The diagnosis of carpal tunnel syndrome can be made in patients who have symptoms and signs typical of median nerve entrapment or ischemia that is confirmed by electrodiagnostic testing that demonstrates median nerve latency at the wrist [6,31]. In cases that involve symptoms without electrodiagnostic abnormalities or electrodiagnostic latency without symptoms, neither situation confirms carpal tunnel syndrome; both must be present. A careful history and examination should indicate cases in which patients need further medical evaluation to exclude an associated medical condition.

Typical symptoms may include intermittent numbness and tingling of the hand and the thumb, index, and middle finger (or some combination of those three and occasionally the ring finger), which generally cause nocturnal awakening. Symptoms may be brought on by routine activities of daily living and often manifest with static postures, such as when driving or reading the newspaper. Patients may experience paresthesias or pain proximally in the forearm, sometimes even extending to the shoulder and neck areas.

The history should assess for symptoms that suggest any of the large number of medical conditions known to be associated with carpal tunnel syndrome, including diabetes, hypothyroidism, hormonal conditions, and obesity [32,33]. Cigarette smoking, ingestion of caffeine, and excessive alcohol consumption are also associated risks [40]. Recent weight gain, dry skin, constipation, and fatigue can suggest hypothyroidism. Cyclical fluid retention and weight gain in middle-aged women can suggest perimenopause. Use of certain medications (such as nonsteroidal anti-inflammatory drugs) can cause fluid retention and exacerbate symptoms. Certain antibiotics, such as cipro derivatives, can cause tendonitis, which in turn can cause carpal tunnel syndrome. Carpal tunnel syndrome may result from a recent wrist or carpal bone fracture [32]. One also should ask about pain, numbness, and tingling of the lower extremities to exclude peripheral neuritis. Peripheral neuritis generally involves the feet before the hands, and patients who present with hand symptoms may not mention lower extremity symptoms unless asked. Patients also should be asked about the presence of neck or shoulder symptoms.

It is important to document patients' exercise status, because carpal tunnel syndrome is more common in individuals with a sedentary lifestyle [41]. Carpal tunnel syndrome can present after recent weight gain. Patients should be asked about problems with sleeping, which can indicate depression and hormonal deficiency and can be a cause of increased muscle tension that contributes to symptoms. Patients also should be asked about other symptoms of anxiety, depression, and increased recent stress, because they can contribute to increased musculoskeletal symptoms and may impede recovery [6,42].

Job history is important to assess job requirements and a patient's perception of it. Just as pain is more accurately described as a perceptual phenomenon rather than a purely sensory one, a patient's perception of how dangerous or noxious a job is can have significant impact on how he or she perceives any physical symptoms. What is a patient's understanding of what is causing the problem? What activities of daily living cause symptoms? Specifically, one should ask about job title, length of time on the job, and relation of physical symptoms to work activity. Do they only occur at work or at home? Do they occur on off days or at night? Can the patient specify what aspect of the job is associated with onset of symptoms? Have any family members had carpal tunnel syndrome? The tendency to develop carpal tunnel syndrome can be inherited, including such diagnoses as Dupuytren's contracture, hereditary neuropathy with liability to pressure palsies, and even a genetic defect (eg, trisomy of chromosome eight) [13,43].

Physical examination should include height and weight. A thorough neck and bilateral upper extremity examination should be performed. Axial compression of the neck should be done to assess for cervical root compression. Research has estimated that 92% of all carpal tunnel syndromes may involve a double crush syndrome in the median nerve distribution [44]. The Spurling test is also helpful. The neck and trapezius areas should be palpated for spasm (which can contribute to paresthesias and pain symptoms in the arms and hands), and the thyroid should be examined for enlargement or nodularity. Shoulder retraction can help identify contributing muscle spasm in the shoulders and upper back. Shoulder retraction is performed by having a patient lift both arms to shoulder height with both elbows flexed to 90° and the wrists in a neutral position. Passive retraction of the shoulders posteriorly that causes paresthesias in the hand within 10 to 20 seconds suggests that muscle spasm/tension is contributing to hand symptoms.

The skin around the elbow should be felt to identify dryness from hypothyroidism. In patients who present with any symptoms in the lower extremity (eg, paresthesias, edema), the lower extremity should be inspected for edema and tested for sharp dull sensation on the feet. Reflexes of the upper and lower extremity also should be tested. Physical examination may reveal a decrease in two-point discrimination ($>$10 mm) in the thumb, index, and possibly the middle finger. Only rarely does motor involvement occur, in which case there may be thenar atrophy and weakness to testing of thumb opposition. The Phalen and Tinel tests are generally performed to provoke symptoms, although neither test has high reliability [45,46].

The flexor fingers should be assessed for evidence of Dupuytren's disease or flexor tendonitis, both of which can bring about symptoms of carpal tunnel syndrome [13]. The finger joints should be palpated for tenderness and observed for swelling and arthritis. Grip strength should be assessed by a dynomometer, and wrist strength should be tested for. Grip strength should not be affected by carpal tunnel syndrome, although discomfort caused by carpal tunnel syndrome may prevent good effort and can give a good indication of a patient's fitness level.

Diagnostic tests

Because there is no valid clinical test to confirm the diagnosis of carpal tunnel syndrome, electrodiagnostic studies are needed to confirm the diagnosis. If a patient's symptoms improve substantially with conservative treatment and do not impair function, electrodiagnostic testing is not necessary. If there is conservative treatment failure, motor weakness, or uncertainty about the diagnosis or if surgery is being considered, however, electrodiagnostic testing is recommended. Ideally, bilateral nerve conduction velocity should be obtained, even when symptoms are unilateral, and it is recommended that the ulnar and radial nerves be included to rule out a polyneuropathy [11].

A substantial number of people over age 40 (reported by some researchers as up to 40%) may have median nerve slowing but be entirely asymptomatic [8]. Most patients who have median nerve latency who are asymptomatic do not develop symptoms of carpal tunnel syndrome according to studies of long-term follow-up [8,47]. Conversely, less than 50% of women younger than 40 years who had been given the diagnosis of carpal tunnel syndrome actually had median nerve latency [18].

Identify underlying contributing health conditions

Treatment focus should be on identifying any underlying health condition that may contribute to symptoms. When historical or physical evidence suggests that patients need a further medical evaluation to exclude systemic disease, patients should be advised of that and told to follow-up with a personal physician.

In some instances the workers' compensation insurance company may approve a limited systemic evaluation to clarify the issue of work causation.

Management

Although a case may be designated as work related by a given legal or administrative action, in many cases it is unlikely that the workplace activities contribute substantially to causation. Such knowledge enables a physician to avoid unnecessary disability during treatment, because in almost all cases—even when some aspects of work tend to bring about symptoms—patients may remain at work, generally at full duty, during conservative care. If substantial exacerbation of symptoms occurred with overtime work, then patients should be advised not to work overtime until symptoms abate. Although the condition is not work related, patients should be given advice on how to minimize symptoms at work and should be encouraged to promote blood supply to the upper extremity by strengthening, stretching, reducing muscle tension, and improving aerobic fitness.

Provide a conceptual model in the explanation of causation

A key aspect of management often involves explaining to patients' satisfaction that in all likelihood the symptoms of carpal tunnel syndrome that they experience are not caused by the workplace activities. Giving patients a conceptual model may help them to understand the condition and its relationship to activity. For example, the association between data entry, reaching, twisting, loading, lifting, and handwriting and carpal tunnel syndrome is analogous to a comparison that an increased number of poisonous snake bites has been associated with an increased consumption of ice cream in a population. One should not assume that the association means that snakes are more likely to bite people who eat ice cream but rather that snakebites occur primarily in the summer months, which is the peak time of ice cream consumption. A high percentage of workers perform keyboard tasks or data entry as routine parts of their jobs, and a worker who has carpal tunnel syndrome might experience some symptoms while performing routine tasks of all kinds. Workers also read the newspaper, use a steering wheel, and perform housekeeping tasks, but that does not mean that any of these tasks caused carpal tunnel syndrome. Even while sleeping, patients may experience symptoms of carpal tunnel syndrome.

In cases in which it seems that certain job activities substantially exacerbate carpal tunnel syndrome, physicians should explain to patients that although the job did not cause the condition, it seems to exacerbate the condition; consequently, short-term treatment to improve job tolerance is indicated. If patients should decide to have surgery at a later date, however, that generally would not be considered work related. The decision regarding whether an exacerbation of carpal tunnel syndrome is covered by workers' compensation generally is made by the insurance company but may vary in different states.

Surgery

For true carpal tunnel syndrome that persists after conservative care, surgery is generally successful. Patients who have work-related carpal tunnel syndrome claims may not fare as well, however [36]. During the Australian repetitive strain injury epidemic of the 1970s and 1980s, surgery rarely benefited workers diagnosed with carpal tunnel syndrome [47]. A 1999 review of the literature on surgical outcomes found that one third of patients continued to experience pain and functional loss after surgery, and work-related cases were much more likely to have poor outcomes. In a 3-year follow-up, 41% had complete relief of symptoms, 45% had moderate relief, and 14% had no improvement [48].

These findings can be compared with patients who receive no treatment for carpal tunnel syndrome. An Italian study followed 196 untreated patients who had carpal tunnel syndrome and abnormal median nerve conduction velocities. After 10 to 15 months with no treatment, 27% of the subjects had improved, 57% remained the same, and 16% experienced worsening of their condition [49]. When a patient who has carpal tunnel syndrome does not respond well to surgical treatment, it may indicate that the patient did not actually have the diagnosis, because many of the mildly positive nerve conduction cases involve false-positive results.

Patients older than age 50 who experience constant paresthesias and have an accompanying stenosynovitis are most likely to benefit from surgery. Rarely, carpal tunnel syndrome occurs acutely because of a rapid, sustained rise in carpal tunnel pressure that occurs over a period of hours. Unremitting and severe symptoms occur, and in such cases, emergent surgery should be performed within 40 hours of the onset to avoid poor clinical outcome caused by intraneural scarring. Acute carpal tunnel syndrome reportedly has occurred after trauma to the wrist, infections, rheumatologic diseases, hemmorhage, vascular disorders, burns, and high-pressure injection injuries [23,50].

Conservative treatment

Limited data are available on conservative treatment success, and long-term data are lacking on most treatments. A systematic review of nonsurgical treatment of carpal tunnel syndrome indicated that 50% of patients who had carpal tunnel syndrome improved with placebo [51]. A 2005 Cochrane Database concluded that oral steroids gave short-term benefit only and the use of splints (at night) was equivocal, as was ultrasound. One trial that comparing yoga to splinting found that yoga was better than splinting. Another trial suggested that carpal bone mobilization could be effective. No good evidence supports exercise, magnets, lasers, or medication use. The conclusion of the review was that more studies are needed and that the effectiveness and duration of benefit from nonsurgical treatment for carpal tunnel syndrome remain unknown. [52].

Patients who have carpal tunnel syndrome symptoms should be educated regarding weight reduction or at least control, aerobic fitness, and smoking cessation. Perimenopausal women who are retaining fluids may be helped by salt restriction and an aerobic exercise program [53]. Key to management is educating patients regarding the natural course of the disease and allaying fears and reassuring patients that the condition will not become disabling.

Work status

Temporary restrictions from performing highly repetitive and forceful hand work in a cold environment may be indicated because of subjective intolerance by the worker, as would be jobs in which there is substantial vibration exposure to the arm. Using the arm while held in an awkward posture, performing highly repetitive and forceful work, and avoiding compressive forces on the volar wrist should be restricted initially until the symptoms are treated successfully [15,54,55]. Persons with more severe carpal tunnel syndrome may require work limitations because of loss of hand dexterity, as measured with the Perdue Peg Board Test. Grip strength is generally not affected, although discomfort may decrease gripping tolerance early in treatment [15,23].

Expected duration of disability days for conservative treatment of persons who work sedentary and light jobs ranges from 0 to 7 days, whereas persons who perform heavy work have expected disability days of 0 to a maximum of 28 days. Patients who undergo surgical treatment who work at light office jobs are expected to miss 0 to 7 days of work, and persons who work heavy jobs miss from 21 to 61 days, according to Hand Center data [56]. Despite the recommended best practices, the US Bureau of Labor Statistics reported in 2003 that the average median of lost days for carpal tunnel syndrome was 32 days, which indicates that there is much room for improvement regarding disability for carpal tunnel syndrome [3].

Summary

The concept of work-related carpal tunnel syndrome has grown to such proportions as to be problematic for society, having spawned health care industries to support a cultural concept and a largely mythical medical paradigm. This in turn provides an economic benefit to health care providers and hospitals and may provide a simplistic, albeit unhealthy, solution for patients in the midst of difficult life situations. Because of these social and economic reinforcements, cultural perceptions and expectations have adjusted to this flawed medical model.

Carpal tunnel syndrome is a medical disease, not an injury, although symptoms may occur in association with certain physical activities of the upper extremity. Success in improving patient management and making the best use of sound medical evidence depends on the concurrent use of educational strategies that address social influences and attitudinal changes of practicing physicians, patients, and third-party administrators. To change culture requires changing the public perception and, no doubt, legislation. Key is the promotion of evidence-based medicine. Such a change for the better in what is a flawed medical paradigm is a tall order. Economic necessity, along with increased concern about health and the health care industry, may be sufficient to foster such change.

References

[1] Zenz C, editor. Occupational medicine. 2nd edition. Chicago (IL): Year Book Medical Publishers; 1988.
[2] Zenz C, editor. Occupational medicine. 3rd edition. St. Louis (MO): Mosby Year Book; 1994.
[3] US Bureau of Labor Statistics. Survey of occupational injuries and illnesses: nonfatal (OSHA recordable) injuries and illnesses. Case and demographic characteristics. Available at www.bls.gov/iif/oshcdnew.htm. Accessed July 12, 2005.
[4] Hadler N. Is carpal tunnel syndrome a consequence of the physical demands of work tasks? OEM Report 2003;17(8):53–7.
[5] Hapberg M, Morgenstern H, Kelsh M. Impact of occupations and job tasks on the prevalence of carpal tunnel syndrome. Scand J Work Environ Health 1992;18:337–45.
[6] Nathan P, Keniston R. Carpal tunnel syndrome: personal risk profile and role of intrinsic and behavioral factors. In: Kasdan M, editor. Occupational hand and upper extremity injuries and diseases. 2nd edition. Philadelphia: Hanley & Belfus; 1998. p. 129–39.
[7] Silverstein M, Silverstein B, Franklin G. Evidence for work-related musculoskeletal disorders: a scientific counterargument. J Occup Environ Med 1996;38:477–84.
[8] Nathan P, Meadows K, Istvan J. Predictors of carpal tunnel syndrome: an 11 year study of industrial workers. J Hand Surg [Am] 2002;27A:644–51.
[9] Nilsson T, Hapberg M, Berstrom L, et al. A five-year follow-up of nerve conduction over the carpal tunnel: Stockholm workshop 1994. Arbete Och Halsa Vetenskaplig Skriftserie 1995; 5:117–20.
[10] Kasdan M, Lewis K. Management of carpal tunnel syndrome in the working population. Hand Clin 2002;18(2):325–30.
[11] Szabo R. Occupational carpal tunnel syndrome. In: Kasdan M, editor. Occupational hand and upper extremity injuries and disease. 2nd editor. Philadelphia: Hanley & Belfus; 1998. p. 113–27.
[12] Katz J, Amick B, Keller R, et al. Determinants of work absence following surgery for carpal tunnel syndrome. Am J Ind Med 2005;47(2):120–30.
[13] Bonnici A, Birjandi J, Spencer J, et al. Chromosomal abnormalities in Dupuytren's contracture and carpal tunnel syndrome. J Hand Surg [Br] 1992;17B:349–55.
[14] Nathan P, Keniston R, Meadows K, et al. Longitudinal study of median nerve sensory conduction in industry: relationship to age, gender, hand dominance, occupational hand use, and clinical diagnosis. J Hand Surg [Am] 1992;17A:850–7.
[15] US Department of Health and Human Services. Publication No. 2004–146. Available at: www.cdc.gov/niosh. Accessed July 12, 2005.
[16] Falkiner S, Myers S. When exactly can carpal tunnel syndrome be considered work-related? Aust N Z J Surg 2002;72:204–9.
[17] Kirschberg G, Fillingim R, Davis V, et al. Carpal tunnel syndrome: clinical symptoms and electrodiagnostic studies in poultry workers with hand, wrist, and forearm pain. South Med J 1994;87:328–31.

[18] Nathan P, Keniston R, Meadows K, et al. Predictive values of nerve conduction measurements at the carpal tunnel. Muscle Nerve 1993;16:1377–82.
[19] Shuman S, Osterman L, Bora F. Compression neuropathies. Semin Neurol 1987;7:76–87.
[20] Stevens J, Sun S, Beard C, et al. Carpal tunnel syndrome in Rochester, Minnesota, 1961–1980. Neurology 1988;38:134–8.
[21] Miller R, Iverson D, Fried R, et al. Carpal tunnel syndrome in primary care: a report from ASPN. J Fam Pract 1994;38:337–44.
[22] Atroshi I, Gummersson C, Johnson R, et al. Prevalence of carpal tunnel syndrome in a general population. JAMA 1999;282:153–9.
[23] Michelson H, Posner M. Medical history of carpal tunnel syndrome. Hand Clin 2002;18:257–68.
[24] Andersen J, Thomsen J, Overgaard E, et al. Computer use and carpal tunnel syndrome: a 1-year follow up study. JAMA 2003;289(22):2963–70.
[25] Clarke Stevens J, Witt J, Smith B, et al. The frequency of carpal tunnel syndrome in computer users at a medical facility. Neurology 2001;56:1568–70.
[26] Nordstrom D, Vierkant R, DeStefano F, et al. Risk factors for carpal tunnel syndrome in a general population. Occup Environ Med 1997;54:734–40.
[27] Hadler NM. A keyboard for "Daubert." J Occup Environ Med 1996;38:469–76.
[28] Lo SL, Raskin K, Lester H, et al. Carpal tunnel syndrome: a historical perspective. Hand Clin 2002;18:211–7.
[29] Kryger A, Andersen J, Lassen C, et al. Does computer use pose an occupational hazard for forearm pain; from the NUDATA study. Occup Environ Med 2003;60:14–7.
[30] Rempel D, Tittiranonda P, Burastero S, et al. Effect of keyboard keyswitch design on hand pain. J Occup Environ Med 1999;41:111–9.
[31] Vender M, Kasdan M, Truppa K. Upper extremity disorders: a literature review to determine work-relatedness. J Hand Surg [Am] 1995;20A:534–41.
[32] Derebery J. Determination of causation. In: Derebery J, Kasdan M, editors. Occupational upper extremity and hand disorders. State of the art review: occupational medicine. Philadelphia: Hanley & Belfus; 1997. p. 569–82.
[33] Stevens J, Witt J, Smith B, et al. The frequency of carpal tunnel syndrome in computer users at a medical facility. Neurology 2001;56:1568–70.
[34] US National Library of Medicine. Available at: tox.net.nlm.nih.gov. Accessed July 5, 2005.
[35] Shapiro I, Ship I. Preventing mercury poisoning in dental practice. J Mass Dent Soc 1980;33(2): 72–4.
[36] Burns C, Cartmill J, Powers B, et al. Update of the morbidity experience of employees potentially exposed to chlorpyrifos. Occup Environ Med 1998;55(1):65–70.
[37] Kolmodin-Hedman B, Hansson M, Hagberg M, et al. Health problems among operators of plastic welding machines: exposure to radiofrequency electromagnetic fields. Int Arch Occup Environ Health 1988;60(4):243–7.
[38] Ray P, Black S, Shinefield H, et al. Risk of chronic arthropathy among women after rubella vaccination. JAMA 1997;278:551–6.
[39] Hasselbacher P. Neuropathy after influenza vaccination. Lancet 1977;1:551–2.
[40] Nathan P, Keniston R, Meadows K, et al. Tobacco, caffeine, alcohol, and carpal tunnel syndrome in American Industry. J Occup Environ Med 1996;38:290–8.
[41] Nathan PA, Keniston R. Carpal tunnel syndrome and its relation to general physical condition. Hand Clin 1993;9:253–61.
[42] Amick B, Habeck R, Ossmann J, et al. Predictors of successful work role functioning after carpal tunnel release surgery. J Occup Environ Med 2004;46(5):490–500.
[43] Shuman S, Osterman L, Bora F. Compression neuropathies. Semin Neurol 1987;7:76–87.
[44] Pope D, Croft P, Pritchard C, et al. Occupational factors related to shoulder pain and disability. Occup Environ Med 1997;54:316–21.
[45] Marx R, Hudak P, Bombardier C, et al. The reliability of physical examination for carpal tunnel syndrome. J Hand Surg [Br] 1998;23B:499–502.
[46] Katz J, Larson M, Sabra A, et al. The carpal tunnel syndrome: diagnostic utility of the history and physical exam findings. Ann Intern Med 1990;112:321–7.

[47] Lucire Y. Constructing RSI: belief and desire. Sydney (Australia): UNSW Press; 2003.
[48] Feuerstein M, Burrell L, Miller V, et al. Clinical management of carpal tunnel syndrome: a 12-year review of outcomes. Am J Ind Med 1999;35:232–45.
[49] Padua L, Padua R, Aprile I, et al. Multiperspective follow-up of untreated carpal tunnel syndrome. Neurology 2001;56:1459–66.
[50] Szabo R, Madison M. Carpal tunnel syndrome. Orthop Clin North Am 1992;23:103–9.
[51] Goodyear-Smith F, Arroll B. What can family physicians offer patients with carpal tunnel syndrome other than surgery? A systematic review of nonsurgical management. Ann Fam Med 2004;2:267–73.
[52] O'Connor D, Marshall S, Massy-Westropp N. Non-surgical treatment (other than steroid injection) for carpal tunnel syndrome. Cochrane Database Syst Rev 2005;1:1–5.
[53] Nathan P, Wilcox A, Emerick P, et al. Effects of an aerobic exercise program on median nerve conduction and symptoms associated with carpal tunnel syndrome. J Occup Environ Med 2001; 43(10):840–3.
[54] US Department of Health and Human Services. Musculoskeletal disorders and workplace factors: a critical review of epidemiologicial evidence for work-related musculoskeletal disorders of the neck, upper extremity, and low back. Cincinnati (OH): NIOSH; 1997.
[55] Talmage J, Melhorn J. Carpal tunnel syndrome. In: A physician's guide to return to work. Washington, DC: AMA Press; 2005. p. 197–202.
[56] Melhorn J. Work guides, functional capacity, work restrictions used by the hand center. Wichita (KS): Hand Center; 2003.

ELSEVIER
SAUNDERS

Clin Occup Environ Med
5 (2) 369–380

CLINICS IN
OCCUPATIONAL AND
ENVIRONMENTAL
MEDICINE

Occupational Hand Infections

Earl Gaar, MD, FACS*

Department of Surgery, University of Louisville School of Medicine, 529 South Jackson Street, Louisville, KY 40202, USA

Types of hand infections

Paronychia

Paronychia is one of the most common infections encountered in the hand and comprises some 30% of all septic lesions of the hand. The thumb and the index finger are the digits mostly commonly involved. It has been associated with nail biting and overzealous manipulation during manicure. It is often a tender superficial infection that consists of a small abscess in the epidermis about the base of the nail fold. Any disruption of the seal between the proximal nail fold and the nail plate can cause acute infections of the eponychial space by providing a portal of entry for bacteria. Haircutters and meat handlers are prone to getting punctures between the nail plate and the eponychium. Acute paronychia may develop over a few hours. The nail fold becomes red, swollen, and tender, or chronic paronychia may develop in a more insidious fashion. Yellow pus may appear under the cuticle. Fever and ipsilateral lymphadenopathy may be present in particularly virulent cases. Acute cases are generally the result of staphylococcus, whereas chronic paronychia may involve gram-negative bacilli and yeast. Definitive treatment of acute paronychia is drainage via lifting of the nail fold or removal of the nail, which can act as a foreign body. With chronic paronychia, contact avoidance of the offending irritant in combination with an antifungal agent or steroid cream may suffice [1]. Patients with chronic paronychias that are unresponsive to therapy should be checked for unusual causes. Chemotherapeutic agents may induce a wide variety of adverse mucocutaneous effects, including

* Louisville Veterans Administration Medical Center (112), 800 Zorn Avenue, Louisville, KY 40206.

E-mail address: earl.gaar@med.va.gov

1526-0046/06/$ – see front matter
doi:10.1016/j.coem.2005.11.004

nail changes [2]. Rarely, papillary adenocarcinoma or squamous cell carcinoma of the digit may present as paronychia [3,4].

Paronychia has been associated with rare early manifestations of pemphigus vulgaris [5] and protein contact dermatitis associated with latex [6]. There are reports of association with sculptured nails, especially if concomitant diabetes is present [7]. For severe infections, an antistaphylococcal penicillin or a first-generation cephalosporin should be given. Clindamycin or amoxicillin-clavulanate potassium may be considered if anaerobes and *Escherichia coli* are suspected organisms. A tetanus booster should be administered when appropriate (this holds true for all infections).

Felon

Fingertip pulp is divided into some 15 to 20 small compartments by vertical septa that stabilize the pad. Infection that occurs within these compartments can lead to abscess formation, edema, and rapid development of increased pressure in a closed space. This increased pressure may compromise blood flow and lead to skin necrosis, septic arthritis, or osteomyelitis of the phalanx [8,9]. Common predisposing causes include splinters, bits of glass, abrasions, and minor puncture wounds, although in more than half of cases, no predisposing event can be identified. Infection also may spread from paronychia. Patients present with rapid onset of severe throbbing pain with associated redness and swelling of the fingertip. The pain caused by a felon is usually more intense than that caused by paronychia.

An early felon (cellulitis) may be amenable to elevation, oral antibiotics, and warm water or saline soaks. A true felon requires incision and drainage. Drainage is best accomplished via longitudinal incision over the area that is pointing. Care should be taken to look for a foreign body, invaginated skin, and the neurovascular bundles. An index of suspicion always should be kept in mind for the occult presentation of malignant disease [10]. *Staphylococcus aureus* is the most common cause. Gram-negative organisms have been reported with immunosuppressed patients. Trauma from diabetic glucose finger checks also has been implicated. *Eikenella corrodens* has been reported in persons with diabetes who bite their fingernails. Antimicrobial treatment usually consists of a first-generation cephalosporin or antistaphylococcal penicillin.

Cellulitis

Cellulitis of the hand may be a consequence of a closed space infection or may be a serious condition. The word cellulitis literally means inflammation of the cells. It generally indicates an acute spreading infection of the dermis and subcutaneous tissues that results in pain, erythema, edema, and warmth. Associated lymphadenopathy and ascending lymphangitis are indicators of serious advanced infection. In the absence of fluctuance or abscess, treatment consists of elevation, heat, and appropriate antibiotic therapy directed at *S aureus* and Group A streptococcus, usually achieved with a first-generation cephalosporin. A small fusiform biopsy may be valuable in identifying the offending organism. Sweet's syndrome, originally described as an acute febrile neutrophilic dermatosis, belongs to a class of skin lesions that histologically have intense epidermal or dermal inflammatory infiltrate of neutrophils without evidence of infection or vasculitis. Skin lesions of Sweet's syndrome most commonly present on the face, trunk, upper extremities, and hands. The presenting lesions are often confused with infections because of their clinical appearance. As physicians responsible for the treatment of hand lesions, it is important to consider the diagnosis of Sweet's syndrome because these wounds are unresponsive to antibiotics, do not benefit from débridement, and require treatment with steroids [11].

High-pressure injection injuries

In 1937, Rees described a series of patients who had been injured by the fuel injection system of diesel engines [2]. It was not until the 1960s, however, when the world was more highly industrialized, that high-pressure injection injuries were more frequently encountered. Although innocuous at initial presentation, these injuries have the potential for considerable morbidity, especially when underappreciated by the uninformed. A high-pressure injection injury always should be considered a potential surgical emergency. Significant delay in diagnosis and treatment may result in severe tissue necrosis and limb gangrene. The incidence of ultimate amputation approaches 50% [12]. Ultimate recovery depends directly on the length of time from injury to definitive treatment. Immediate decompression and thorough cleansing and débridement of the offending material from the tissue are required to preserve optimal function. Acute injury is caused by introduction of a foreign material under high pressure between 2000 and 10,000 psi into the poorly distensible digital or palmar tissues. The pathophysiology involves acute and chronic inflammation and foreign body granuloma formation. Damage results from the impact; ischemia is caused by vascular compression, chemical inflammation, and secondary infection. Highly viscous substances (eg, grease) require higher injection pressures than paint or solvents. Fuel and paint injections lead to the most severe inflammatory response with a high incidence of subsequent amputation. Grease- and oil-based compounds may lead to oleogranulomas with chronic fistula formation, scarring, and eventual loss of digit function. Expression of the wound can yield foreign material, and radiographs may reveal the presence of gas in the flexor tendon sheaths and soft tissues.

Gudair ovine paratuberculosis vaccine can cause prolonged granulomatous inflammation if inadvertently injected into human tissue and as been reported in the farm industry [13]. Similar reports of injection of fish vaccines have been reported in the fish industry. After self-inoculation, early surgical débridement of the damaged tissue and drainage to remove the vaccine material is advised to avoid progression to extensive necrosis. Air and clear water injections may be treated in a modified manner with elevation, splinting, and the administration of broad-spectrum antibiotics, provided that clear air or water was definitely the injected substance.

The most common injection site is the tip of the nondominant index finger proximal to the terminal crease. Other common injection sites are the long finger, thumb, and palm. Delay in treatment likely compromises the outcome; in some cases steroids may be effective in reducing eventual impairment. Early recognition of the gravity of these wounds is of the utmost importance, and early decompression, tetanus prophylaxis, antibiotics, and judicious steroid use are advocated [14]. The extent of injury cannot be determined simply by examining the wound in the office or the emergency department. Even if the digit survives the injury, ultimate result may be that of a stiff, painful, atrophic digit, which may result in the digit being more of a hindrance than having functional importance.

Collar button infection

Collar button infections are multilayered and communicating abscesses that involve plantar and dorsal sides, and they usually involve a web space. This infection frequently evolves from a distal plantar callus but spreads to the dorsal side. The spread of infection is usually limited in the palmar region by the adherence of the palmar skin to the underlying fascia. Palmar abscesses begin as intense throbbing pain with swelling and severe tenderness to touch. The infection proceeds dorsally just distally to the bifurcation of the common digital vessels and proceeds to involve the dorsal subcutaneous tissues. On examination, the fingers may lie in an abducted position. Upon exploration, care should be taken to protect the digital vessels and nerves. *Mycobacterium marinum* infections of unusual aggressiveness have been described [15]. *S aureus* and *Streptococcus* species are often the offending organisms. Cultures should be obtained at the time of drainage. As with any hand infection, the abscess cavity should be explored thoroughly to find a sinus tract that extends to another abscess. Dorsal and palmar incisions may be required for adequate wide drainage.

Herpetic whitlow

Herpetic whitlow is an infection of the fingertip. As opposed to the bacterial origin of most infections seen in the hand, herpetic whitlow is the result of herpes simplex virus type I or II. Infections by either type I or II are clinically indistinguishable. The fingertip is painful and swollen but is not as firm as in a felon. The appearance of tiny fluid-filled blebs (vesicles) on the fingers is diagnostic. Although health care workers are at high risk, herpetic whitlow is most commonly reported in children who have coexistent herpetic gingivostomatitis and in adult women who have genital herpes [16]. The index finger and thumb are most often involved. Professionals at particular risk include dentists, hygienists, physicians, nurses, and other persons who may have contact with saliva or body fluids that contain the virus. People who have oral or genital herpes also may infect their own fingers [17]. Prevention is best ensured by using universal precautions with examination.

The diagnosis is usually apparent on physical examination. Herpetic whitlow may present with a prodrome of tingling, itching, and burning before vesicle formation in 24 hours. Typically the area of infection and sensory nerve distribution is painful out of proportion to the clinical findings. Multinucleate giant cells may be seen on a Tzanck smear prepared from the base or margins of the vesicles. The vesicles are highly infective. Alternatively, the definitive test is viral culture, although the time required for culture results in most laboratories is 5 to 7 days. Acute and convalescent serum antibody titers also can be used for diagnosis. As with other manifestations of herpes, it is believed that the virus may remain dormant in the ganglia, which results in recurrent manifestations. Surgical treatment is not indicated, and as with other herpes attacks, the process is self-limited. These lesions should not be confused with a bacterial felon.

Treatment of herpetic whitlow includes symptomatic relief with oral analgesics and cool compresses. Acyclovir, an antiviral medication active against herpes, decreases viral excretion, new lesion formation, and promotes rapid healing, although unfortunately it is not curative. It is beneficial if started in the prodromal phase or within 2 days of vesicle formation. Unfortunately, it has not been proven to influence the recurrence rate. Herpetic whitlow can last anywhere from 2 to 6 weeks. Consideration should be given as to whether herpetic whitlow may be an initial manifestation of HIV infection [17,18].

Suppurative tenosynovitis

Kanaval's four cardinal signs are diagnostic hallmarks of pus in the tendon sheath: (1) Pain along the course of the involved flexor tendons with passive extension. In the case of local furuncle, the finger can be extended passively without significant pain. (2) Flexed position that is held for comfort. (3) Uniform edema that involves the entire digit. (4) Tenderness along the course of the involved tendon sheath. All four signs may not be immediately apparent early in the course of the infection. Associated lymphangitis and lymphadenopathy may be present. These cases should be referred promptly to a hand surgeon if optimal outcome is to be expected. This is not a condition to be attended to solely in the industrial clinic. One should be alert to the fact that a midpalmar space abscess may elicit pain with passive motion of the ring and long fingers. Patients who are taking the anticoagulant warfarin may present with localized bleeding within the tendon sheath, which gives the exact appearance of tenosynovitis on clinical examination. Infection within a tendon sheath, as in other infections of the hand, usually is the result of direct inoculation of bacteria from penetrating trauma.

A common cause is the result of one person striking another person in the mouth, which results in a human bite. "Fish tank finger" may be the result of *M marinum* infection [19]. *S aureus* and streptococcus are the usual isolates, although *Neisseria gonorrhoeae* should be considered a potential pathogen until excluded by culture. Infection with *E corrodens* may be seen after human bites. *Pasteurella multocida* and capnocytophaga infections caused by cat and dog bites can progress rapidly to septic shock and death.

Infection typically follows the course of the tendon sheath, which results in the spread of infection into the radial or ulnar bursae, depending on the primary tendon sheath involved. The tenosynovial coverings of the second, third, and fourth digits do not communicate with either the radial or ulnar bursae in most individuals. Elevated pressure within the tendon sheath caused by infection may impair nutrient flow to the tendon. Tendon necrosis or impaired function is a disastrous sequela of untreated elevated tendon sheath pressure. Suspicion of the clinical diagnosis may be substantiated with ultrasonography. Definitive treatment is accomplished via incision and drainage in the operating room by an experienced hand surgeon. Radiographs are important adjuncts to rule out the presence of a retained foreign body. Intraoperative culture and sensitivity are a must to direct appropriate antibiotic therapy.

Long-term sequelae may include tendon destruction with resultant functional disability, sepsis/septic shock, skin loss, osteomyelitis, loss of the extremity, and death. Ultimate prognosis is fair, depending on the extent of tissue destruction, bony involvement, pre-existing vascular insufficiency, and systemic complications (eg, bacteremia, sepsis).

Septic arthritis

Acute septic arthritis should be viewed as a drainable abscess [20]. Staphylococcus and streptococcus remain the most common involved pathogens. *N gonorrhoeae* is seen in young, sexually active individuals with no history of previous joint pathology. Gram-negative bacilli may be seen in immunocompromised individuals, persons who have diabetes, intravenous drug users, and patients with pre-existing arthritis. Lesser common organisms, including *Haemophilus influenzae*, *Pseudomonas aeruginosa*, *Serratia* species, *N gonorrhoeae*, *P multocida*, *E corrodens*, and *M marinum*, also may occur in specific clinical settings [21]. Particular care should be taken with older workers who present with a laceration over the dorsum of the distal interphalangeal joint. Mucoceles are ganglion cysts that arise from degenerative arthritis in that joint. Even a small puncture wound can result in severe joint infection. In general, patients present with pain and limited motion of the involved joint. The joints of the hand are involved with traumatic and bite wounds. Although low grade, fever is present in 60% to 80% of cases. Definite diagnosis is usually based on Gram stain and culture of the synovial fluid.

The goals of treatment are twofold: removal of the infectious process and restoration of function. The best clinical results occur after an accurate diagnosis, prompt surgical drainage, and débridement in concert with appropriate antibiotics and early postoperative range of motion. A delay in diagnosis or treatment is associated with an unsatisfactory outcome [22].

Animal bites

Animal bites may be associated with significant morbidity if not tended to appropriately. Of all bite injuries seen in emergency departments, dog bites account for approximately 60% to 90% of cases and cat bites account for 15% of cases [23]. A dog bite can generate pressure up to 200 psi, although their teeth in general are not sharp and they produce more of a crush injury; cat bites produce more of a puncture wound. More than 100 different organisms have been cultured from dog bites, including streptococci, staphylococci, *Capnocytophaga canimorsus*, *Klebsiella*, *Bacillis subtilis*, *Pseudomonas*, and *Enterobacteriaceae*. Some organisms, such as *P multocida*, are slightly infectious; others, such as *C canimorsus*, may cause serious complications, including hypotension with septic shock with multiorgan system failure and disseminated intravascular coagulation. With cat bites, *P multocida* and staphylococal and streptococcal infections are common.

On presentation, these wounds should be elevated. A thorough history and physical examination are in order, including status of prior tetanus immunizations. Radiographs should be obtained as indicated. Open wounds should be irrigated copiously with normal saline. Exploration and débridement are indicated depending on the extent and severity of the wound. Prophylactic antibiotic treatment is considered by many as controversial, with most studies showing no benefit, although certainly it is indicated for severe injuries [24]. Antibiotic prophylaxis for human bites has been shown to be efficacious. Most physicians recommend a first-generation cephalosporin or amoxicillin-clavulante [25].

Human bites

A fight bite is a clenched fist injury in which a tooth penetrates the metacarpal phalangeal joint. These injuries are notorious for being the worst human bites. Appropriate treatment is imperative because these injuries may have long-term medical and legal ramifications. Although at initial presentation the small puncture wound may appear unremarkable, the penetration often injures the soft tissues and extensor tendon and may disrupt the metacarpal phalangeal joint itself. It is often important to examine the wound in the position in which the injury occurred to appreciate the full extent of injury (eg, fully flexed or extended). Prophylactic high-dose antibiotic therapy is indicated with all human bites. This is also true with injuries from toothpicks, which should be considered and treated as a human bite [26]. Radiographs are indicated to rule out foreign bodies, identify soft tissue injury, and identify fractures. Staphylococcus and streptococcus are often offending organisms [27,28].

Principles of antibiotic use in hand infections

S aureus is still the most common organism involved with infections of the hand. Certainly this fact suggests inoculation of skin flora at the time of injury.

Other organisms include beta-streptococcus and various gram-negative organisms (*E coli*, *Klebsiella*, *Enterobacter*). Anaerobes are common in instances of intravenous drug abuse, in patients who have diabetes, and in bite wounds. *E corrodens,* an anaerobic gram-negative rod, is part of the normal human oral flora and is recovered in many human bite wounds in the hand. *P multocida,* a facultative gram-negative anaerobe, is recovered from many cat and dog bites.

Mycobacterium tuberculosis is responsible for a small percentage of acute and chronic hand infections. *M marinum* is found in warm water environments and is responsible for some infections in people who come in contact with marine life, boating equipment, piers, fish tanks, and swimming pools. Other bacteria that have been cultured from hand wounds include enterococci, *N gonorrhoeae*, *E coli*, *P aeruginosa*, and *Proteus mirabilis.* Gram-negative organisms frequently are cultured in patients who have diabetes and persons who abuse intravenous drugs. Puncture wounds from the environment in general tend to be gram negative. Cultures from hand infections often show multiple organisms or mixed bag infections, which may be particularly true in persons who have diabetes and small vessel disease or immunocompromised persons. Injuries sustained during the handling of seafood may develop atypical mycobacterial infection.

Early tissue culture and sensitivity are vital for the successful management of these infections that may have started as seemingly trivial wounds and may have been neglected. Empiric antibiotics may be started based on the likelihood of one organism or another in conjunction with Gram stain, if possible. Adjustments can be made once the results of the culture and sensitivity are known. The statement that "the surgeon is in his finest hour when draining laudable pus" still holds true despite the explosion in the number and types of new antibiotics on the market. Antibiotics, although often an important adjunct, are never a substitute for adequate drainage.

S aureus is responsible for 80% of hand infections. This normal resident of human skin flora historically was sensitive to penicillin. Through the years several resistant strains have emerged. Acceptable initial choices include a first- or second-generation cephalosporin or amoxicillin-clavulinic acid. Clindamycin is an acceptable alternative for penicillin-sensitive patients, with vanocmycin having emerged as a popular choice along with linezolid and daptomycin for methicillin-resistant strains. Tigecycline is a new semi-synthetic glycylcycline for the treatment of serious infections. Tigecycline has been designed to overcome many existing mechanisms of resistance among bacteria and confers broad antibiotic coverage against vancomycin-resistant enterococci, methicillin-resistant *S aureus*, and many species of multidrug-resistant gram-negative bacteria [29].

S pyogenes or group A beta-hemolytic streptococcus is responsible for the rapid and fulminating progress of streptococcal involved infections. Not uncommonly, patients are seen with an otherwise trivial wound with associated ascending lymphangitis accompanied by the systemic signs of chills, fever, and generalized malaise. This outcome is part the result of the bacterial production of hyaluronidase and streptokinase. Penicillin is still uniformly effective in treatment of group A streptococcal disease.

Pseudomonads are motile, gram-negative rods that use glucose oxidatively. Members of this genus are classified into five groups based on ribosomal RNA homology. These bacteria are clinically important because they are resistant to most antibiotics and are capable of surviving in conditions that few other organisms can tolerate. They also produce a slime layer that is resistant to phagocytosis. Pseudomonas is often encountered in hospital and clinical work because it is a major cause of hospital-acquired (nosocomal) infections. Gram-negative infections, such as those produced by *Pseudomonas* species, may be particularly difficult to manage. Pseudomonas in culture and in some wounds emits a sweet, grapelike odor [8]. Pseudomonas favors moist areas, such as sinks, toilets, pools, and hot tubs, and usually can withstand standard levels of pool chlorination. These bacteria have been known to live in antiseptic solutions. The basis of this organism's pathogenicity involves several toxins and chemicals that the bacterium secretes. The lipopolysaccharide layer helps the cell adhere to host tissues and prevents leukocytes from ingesting and lysing the organism. Lipases and exotoxins then proceed to destroy host cell tissue, which leads to the complications associated with infection.

Paronychia secondary to pseudomonas may result in a greenish discoloration of the nail secondary to pyocyanin pigmentation [30]. Healthy persons can develop a pseudomonas skin rash after exposure to the bacterium in contaminated hot tubs, water parks, whirlpools, or spas. This skin disorder is called pseudomonas or "hot tub" folliculitis and is often confused with chickenpox.

Because *Pseudomonas* is commonly resistant to antibiotics, severe infections are usually treated with two antibiotics at once. Pseudomonas infections may be treated with combinations of ceftazidime, ciprofloxacin, imipenem, gentamicin, tobramycin, ticarcillin-clavulanate, and piperacillin-tazobactam.

Aeromonas hydrophilia is a gram-negative organism that lives in water and soil. It is characterized by cellulitis, osteomyelitis, acute diarrhea, septicemia (ecthyma gangrenosum), and necrotizing myositis. The usual setting is a rapidly progressive cellulitis after a water-related injury. Leeches carry the *Aeromonas*, which has resulted in stoppage of the use of medical leeches because of the resultant surgical wound infections. Treatment of aeromonas infections involves use of sulfas, quinolones, aminoglycosides, and third-generation cephalosporins.

P multocida is a common organism found in the respiratory tracts of dogs and cats and is the most common organism that causes infections after animal bites. Two to 4.5 million animal bites occur each year in the United States; approximately 1% of these bites require hospitalization. Animal bites result in 334,000 emergency room visits per year, which represents approximately 1% of all emergency hospital visits, at an annual cost of approximately $100 million in health care expenses and lost income. *P multocida* is a common cause of infection after bites or scratches caused by dogs and (especially) cats. It is rarely reported, however, and apparently often overlooked as a pathogen. The typical clinical manifestation is a rapidly developing cellulitis at the site of injury. The infection is potentially dangerous and can lead to osteomyelitis and a chronic local infection of deep tissues [31]. Amoxicillin-clavulanate potassium and second-generation cephalosporins are recommended for prophylaxis and treatment of infection [32].

M marinum infections of the hand are seen in persons who handle fish, crabs, shrimp, and coral. Classic lesions develop after a 2- to 3-week incubation period. Clinical manifestations may vary, with the papulonodular form predominating (sometimes referred to as "swimming pool granuloma"), although the acquisition from a pool is rare because most pools are chlorinated. Infection may result in persistent ulceration, draining sinuses, and septic arthritis. Severe infection of the digit may result in severe osteomyelitis with ultimate amputation. Patients who have AIDS have been reported to have disseminated infection. In 25% to 50% of patients affected, the nodules proliferate along the path of lymphatic drainage in a sporotrichotic type of distribution. Patients also may present with an erythematous plaque on their hands. Ninety percent of all infections involve the upper extremities. Most patients have a tuberculosis test of less than 10 mm induration.

The laboratory must be informed of a physician's suspicions. The method of culturing for this organism requires a special media and temperature. Strains of *M marinum* are resistant to the antituberculosis medications isoniazid, streptomycin, and para-aminosalicylic acid. This organism is sensitive to rifampin, ethambutol, tetracyclines, trimethoprim-sulfamethoxazole, clarithromycin, and levofloxacin [33–35].

Clostridial myonecrosis is a true medical emergency with an associated high rate of morbidity and mortality. In addition to *Clostridium perfringens*, other organisms capable of producing a similar clinical scenario include *E coli*, *Klebsiella*, and *Pseudomonas*. The usual site for infection is a dirty wound that has been closed without adequate débridement. The toxins produced by these organisms destroy the cell wall and rapidly lead to tissue necrosis. Other *Clostridium* species can cause gas gangrene, including *Clostridium novyi* and *Clostridium septicum*.

Infection requires two conditions to coexist. First, organisms must be inoculated into the tissues. Second, oxygen tension must be low enough for the organisms to proliferate. These organisms are not strict anaerobes; 30% oxygen tension in the tissues allows for free growth of these bacteria, but 70% oxygen tension restricts their growth. Inoculation of organisms into low oxygen tension tissues is followed by an incubation period that usually ranges from 12 to 24 hours. This period can be as brief as 1 hour, however, or as long as several weeks. The organisms then multiply and produce exotoxins that result in myonecrosis. The process of myonecrosis can proceed at a pace of 2 cm/h.

Although not well understood, exotoxins seem to be tissue-destructive soluble antigens produced by clostridia. They include lecithinase, collagenase, hyaluronidase, fibrinolysin, hemagglutinin, and hemolysin toxins. *C perfringens* produces at least 17 identifiable exotoxins that are used for species typing (eg, type A, type B, type C).

Penicillin is the preferred drug for clostridial infections. Patients who are allergic to penicillin may be treated with clindamycin or chloramphenicol. Antibiotics are only adjunctive treatment after adequate surgical débridement of devitalized tissues. Tetanus immunization should be adequate. Mortality continues to be high in these cases.

References

[1] Tosti A, Piraccini BM, Ghetti E, et al. Topical steroids versus systemic antifungals in the treatment of chronic paronychia: an open, randomized double-blind and double dummy study. J Am Acad Dermatol 2002;47(1):73–6.

[2] Freiman A, Bouganim N, O'Brien EA. Case reports: mitozantrone-induced onycholysis associated with subungual abscesses, paronychia, and pyogenic granuloma. J Drugs Dermatol 2005;4(4):490–2.

[3] Gorva AD, Mohil R, Srinivasan MS. Aggressive digital papillary adenocarcinoma presenting as a paronychia of the finger. J Hand Surg Br 2005;30:534.

[4] High WA, Tyring SK, Taylor RS. Rapidly enlarging growth of the proximal nail fold. Dermatol Surg 2003;29(9):984–6.

[5] Engineer L, Norton LA, Ahmed AR. Nail involvement in pemphigus vulgaris. J Am Acad Dermatol 2000;43(3):529–35.

[6] Kanerva L. Occupational protein contact dermatitis and paronychia from natural rubber latex. J Eur Acad Dermatol Venereol 2000;14(6):504–6.

[7] Roberge RJ, Weinstein D, Thimons MM. Perionychial infections associated with sculptured nails. Am J Emerg Med 1999;17(6):581–2.

[8] Kasdan JL, Rogers JL. Hand infections seen in the industrial clinic. Occup Med 1989;4(3):463–71.

[9] Richard JC, Vilain R. Acute septic arthritis of the fingers: a clinical study of 87 cases. Ann Chir Main 1982;1(3):214–20.

[10] Rose BA, Wood FM. Metastatic bronchogenic carcinoma masquerading as a felon. J Hand Surg Am 1983;8(3):325–8.

[11] O'Halloran LE, Bennett LL, Grothaus PC, et al. Sweet's syndrome presenting as acute hand infection. Plast Reconstr Surg 2005;116(2):497–501.

[12] Luber KT, Rehm JP, Freeland AE. High-pressure injection injuries of the hand. Orthopedics 2005;28(2):129–32.

[13] Windsor PA, Bush R, Links I, et al. Injury caused by self-inoculation with a vaccine of a Freund's complete adjuvant nature (Gudair) used for control of ovine paratuberculosis. Aust Vet J 2005;83(4):216–20.

[14] Hayes CW, Pan HC. High-pressure injection injuries to the hand. South Med J 1982;75(12): 1491–8.

[15] Wendt JR, Lamm RC, Altman DI, et al. An unusually aggressive *Mycobacterium marinum* hand infection. J Hand Surg Am 1986;11(5):753–5.

[16] Gill MJ, Arlette J, Buchan K. Herpes simplex virus infection of the hand: a profile of 79 cases. Am J Med 1988;84:89–93.

[17] El Hachem M, Bernardi S, Giraldi L, et al. Herpetic whitlow as a harbinger of pediatric HIV-1 infection. Pediatr Dermatol 2005;22(2):119–21.

[18] Garcia-Plata MD, Moreno-Gimenez JC, Velez Garcia A, et al. Herpetic whitlow in an AIDS patient. J Eur Acad Dermatol Venereol 1999;12(3):241–2.

[19] Van Seymortier P, Verellen K, De Jonge I. *Mycobacterium marinum* causing tenosynovitis: fish tank finger. Acta Orthop Belg 2004;70(3):279–82.

[20] http://www.biomedcentral.com/content/pdf/cto-id3412.pdf. Accessed August, 2005.

[21] Murray PM. Septic arthritis of the hand and wrist. Hand Clin 1998;14(4):579–87.

[22] Boustred AM, Singer M, Hudson DA, et al. Septic arthritis of the metacarpophalangeal and interphalangeal joints of the hand. Ann Plast Surg 1999;42(6):623–8 [discussion 628–9].

[23] Daniels JM, Zook EG, Lynch JM. Hand and wrist injuries: Part II. Emergent evaluation. Am Fam Physician 2004;69(8):1941–8.

[24] Tuncali D, Bingul F, Terzioglu A, et al. Animal bites. Saudi Med J 2005;26(5):772–6.
[25] Maimaris C, Quinton DN. Dog-bite lacerations: a controlled trial of primary wound closure. Arch Emerg Med 1988;5(3):156–61.
[26] Chang MC, Huang YL, Liu Y, et al. Infectious complications associated with toothpick injuries of the hand. J Hand Surg Am 2003;28(2):327–31.
[27] Peeples E, Boswick Jr JA, Scott FA. Wounds of the hand contaminated by human or animal saliva. J Trauma 1980;20(5):383–9.
[28] Perron AD, Miller MD, Brady WJ. Orthopedic pitfalls in the ED: fight bite. Am J Emerg Med 2002;20(2):114–7.
[29] Noskin GA. Tigecycline: a new glycylcycline for treatment of serious infections. Clin Infect Dis 2005;41(Suppl 5):S303–14.
[30] Harter RT, Harter KC. High pressure injection injuries. Hand Clin 1986;2:547–52.
[31] Arons MS, Fernando L, Polayes IM. *Pasteurella multocida:* the major cause of hand infections following domestic animal bites. J Hand Surg Am 1982;7(1):47–52.
[32] Weber EJ, Callahan ML. Mammalian bites. In: Marx JA, Hockberger RS, Walls RM, et al, editors. Rosen's emergency medicine: concepts and clinical practice. 5th edition. St. Louis: Mosby; 2002. p. 774–80.
[33] Bhatty MA, Turner DP, Chamberlain ST. *Mycobacterium marinum* hand infection: case reports and review of literature. J Plast Surg 2000;53(2):161–5.
[34] Habif TP. Clinical dermatology. 2nd edition. St. Louis: CV Mosby; 1990. p. 213–99.
[35] Tsai MS, Liu JW, Chen WS, et al. Tuberculous wrist in the era of effective chemotherapy: an eleven-year experience. Int J Tuberc Lung Dis 2003;7(7):690–4.

ELSEVIER
SAUNDERS

Clin Occup Environ Med
5 (2) 381–396

CLINICS IN
OCCUPATIONAL AND
ENVIRONMENTAL
MEDICINE

Hand Dermatitis and Nail Disorders of the Workplace

Hari Dhir, MD, MPH, MBA[a,b,*]

[a]*University of Texas Health Center at Tyler, 11937 US Highway 271, Tyler, TX 75708-3154, USA*
[b]*Concentra Health Services, Ste. 601, 8868 Research Boulevard, Austin, TX 78758, USA*

Contact dermatitis of the hands is one of the commonest skin conditions caused or aggravated by the workplace. Approximately 90% to 95% of all skin diseases caused or aggravated by work are caused by contact dermatitis, which includes allergic and irritant types. Eighty percent of all work-related contact dermatitis is caused by irritants, and the remainder is caused by allergen contact [1]. An occupational medicine physician frequently is the only physician managing contact dermatitis, even in severe cases, because many dermatologists are unwilling to treat work-related disorders. Consequently, the occupational medicine physician must be well versed in management of this disorder. This article is restricted to a discussion of irritant and allergic dermatitis and nail and nail bed disorders that a physician may encounter in an occupational medicine practice.

Dermatitis can be caused by internal or exogenous factors. Atopic dermatitis and seborrheic dermatitis are examples of endogenous dermatitis and are caused by internal factors. Exogenous dermatitis is caused by contact with substances that are irritants or allergens, which are often found in the workplace. Irritants cause dermatitis by nonimmunologic reactions, whereas allergens cause dermatitis by delayed hypersensitivity immunologic reactions. It is difficult to differentiate irritant from allergic contact dermatitis clinically. Chemicals are the most important cause of occupational skin disease followed by mechanical, physical, and biologic agents. Individuals may develop contact dermatitis to most chemicals if they are exposed to a chemical in a sufficient strength for an adequate period of time. Chemicals cause approximately 53% of work-related dermatitis [2].

* 9917 Pumpkin Ridge Court, Austin, TX 78717.
E-mail address: hdhir@msn.com

1526-0046/06/$ – see front matter
doi:10.1016/j.coem.2005.11.017

occmed.theclinics.com

In humans, more than 3000 chemicals have been implicated in contact dermatitis [3]. Examples of physical causes include heat exposure in foundry and outdoor workers, ionizing radiation in nuclear workers and medical personnel, which can cause chronic radiation dermatitis, and friction and cold exposure in fisherman and outdoor workers. Feverfew, poison oak, ragweed, poison ivy, chrysanthemums, and sagebrush are some of the biologic agents that can cause contact dermatitis. The flower, stems, leaves, fruit, and wood are capable of causing irritation or allergic contact dermatitis. Poison ivy and oak are the commonest causes of allergic contact dermatitis followed by chrysanthemums and compositae species. Horticulturists, farmers, loggers, foresters, florists, and nursery workers are at risk of developing phytodermatitis from contact with allergens from plants. Florists can develop contact irritant dermatitis that causes daffodil itch by handling daffodil stems. In grocery workers the commonest cause of phytophotodermatitis is contact with celery, and among outdoor workers, poison ivy and oak are the main causes of work-related allergic contact dermatitis [22].

Of all nonfatal occupational illness cases in private industry reported in 1997, skin diseases and disorders accounted for 13% (57,900 cases). Of these occurrences, 6600 cases of dermatitis involved time away from work. Workers with dermatitis had a median of 3 days off from work. Service and manufacturing industries each were the cause of 29% of the cases of dermatitis with days away from work. Laborers, fabricators, operators, precision production, repair personnel, and craft workers are most commonly affected by dermatitis with time away from work [2]. In the work setting, hands are the most often affected part of the body either alone or with other parts of the body. The hands are involved in 80% to 90% of cases of occupational dermatitis [4]. External agents that commonly cause contact dermatitis are water, detergents, solvents, metal foods, rubber, cutting oils, protective equipment, and skin care products. Some researchers have reported that up to 28% of the cases are caused by detergents or water alone [5].

Occupations that have a higher occurrence of irritant contact dermatitis involve wet work, such as dishwasher, hairdresser, baker, cook, butcher, car mechanic, bartender, nurse, fisherman, food processing worker, construction worker, locksmith, and metal worker. In a population-based study, irritant contact dermatitis had an annual incidence rate of 4.5 per 10,000 workers, and allergic contact dermatitis had an incidence rate of 4.1 per 10,000 workers. The same study found that irritant contact dermatitis was linked with skin contact with detergents in 52% of the cases, disinfectants in 24% of the cases, and acidic and alkaline chemicals in 24% of the cases in the workplace [6]. In a study performed in Taiwanese electronic workers using patch testing and examination of the skin, 35.5% were found to have irritant contact dermatitis and 3.8% were found to have allergic contact dermatitis [7].

In another study in which questionnaires were given to health care workers in intensive care units, 55.6% of the workers reported occupational hand dermatitis. The rate was much higher (69.7%) in workers who washed their hands more than 35 times per shift. The same study also found that occupational hand dermatitis was not connected to race, age, duration of employment, gender, atopy, or presence of previous dermatitis. With such high rates in these intensive care unit workers, exposure to blood-borne pathogens would be a concern [8].

Anatomy of the skin

The average adult has approximately 18 square feet of skin, which consists of the outer epidermis and the deeper dermis. The outermost layer of the superficial epidermis is the outer keratin layer (stratum corneum), which is made of non-viable anucleate cells. Below this layer there is the stratum spinosum and the basal (germinative) layers. The germinative layer produces epidermal cells that move up and transform into the flat, compact, and dehydrated keratinized cells of the stratum corneum. The stratum corneum is a protective barrier of the skin that prevents internal tissues from exposure to chemicals, toxins, ultraviolet radiation, bacteria, and extreme temperatures. It is thickest on the palms of the hands and soles of the feet, so hand dermatitis mainly affects the back of the hands rather than the palms. The keratin layer allows lipophilic chemicals to be absorbed more so than hydrophilic substances. Permeability of the skin is increased if waterproof materials, such as gloves, cover the skin and if the skin has abrasions or is inflamed. The lower layers of the epidermis contain the Langerhans cells, which are dendritic antigen-presenting cells that are necessary for allergic contact dermatitis to take place. Melanocytes in the epidermis produce the pigment melanin, which protects against ultraviolet radiation. The dermis is mainly made of collagen in a ground substance, which makes the skin strong and flexible. The dermis contains blood vessels, lymphatic, nerves, and epidermal appendages [9].

Irritant contact dermatitis

Occupational irritant contact dermatitis is characterized by inflammation caused by contact of the skin with an exogenous agent in the workplace. Common skin irritants include detergent, soap, cement in construction workers, solvents, rubber gloves in hospital workers and housekeepers, fiberglass, malathion in pesticide workers, and water and water-based metal-working fluids. Workers involved with wet work, such as cleaning, metal engineering, horticulture, and construction, are commonly affected. The hand irritation mainly occurs in the dorsum of the hands and the finger web spaces, where the stratum corneum is the thinnest. Strong irritants can produce clinically noticeable changes within minutes of a single contact, whereas weak irritants may take days of exposure to produce changes. Potent irritants cause acute contact dermatitis in which erythema, swelling, and blistering occur at the site of contact of the irritant within minutes and produce pruritus and burning. As the lesions progress, crusts and scales may form. The rash is localized to the area of contact, and erythema is more prominent than vesiculation. The potency of the irritant, the duration of contact, and local condition of the skin dictate the severity of the reaction, but once an irritant is removed, the rash usually resolves completely within a few weeks.

Repeated exposure to irritants causes chronic irritant dermatitis, which causes an inflammatory reaction that may continue even if the irritant is removed. Flare-ups of the condition can be caused by re-exposure to even minor irritants. Jobs that involve wet work commonly lead to chronic irritant dermatitis, and workers with atopic eczema—especially of the hands—are at increased risk. Because of the cumulative nature of the weak exposure, a worker often does not connect the irritant with the dermatitis [10]. Chronic irritant dermatitis presents with lichenification, fissuring, and dry scaly skin on the fingers and hands. Sometimes vesicles are present. Common causes of chronic dermatitis include weak irritants, such as water and wet work, skin cleansers, solvents, cutting fluids, degreasing agents, detergents, metal-working fluids, dusts, friction, and low humidity. At-risk occupations for chronic irritant dermatitis include bartender, housekeeper, cleaner, cook, nurse, metal worker, construction worker, hairdresser, and baker. Once an affected worker is away from work, the symptoms usually decrease, but not always so.

Allergic contact dermatitis

Allergic contact dermatitis is caused by a type IV hypersensitivity reaction. As with contact irritant dermatitis, the reaction occurs at the site where the allergen contacts the skin, but secondary spread can occur if the hands are contaminated with the allergen and spread it to other areas of the body. There are different phases in the development of allergic contact dermatitis. The first phase is the sensitization phase, in which the antigen penetrates the stratum corneum of the epidermis and reaches the basal layer, where it interacts with the Langerhans cells. These cells present the antigen on their surface and move to lymph nodes close to the site of contact [11]. In the regional lymph nodes, the Langerhans cells display the antigen to T lymphocyte. This interaction produces antigen-specific T lymphocytes that enter the circulation and return to the epidermis. For hypersensitivity to develop, the individual usually must be exposed to the allergen for a certain period of time, even with potent allergens. Contact allergens tend to be low molecular weight substances that weigh less than 600 d that can form bonds with carrier proteins in the skin. Individuals vary in their susceptibility to develop hypersensitivity, and one cannot determine how susceptible a particular individual is to developing contact allergy. Hypersensitivity usually lasts indefinitely, but some individuals may lose the hypersensitivity after long periods of time [10].

When workers are re-exposed to an allergen, the elicitation phase occurs. In the elicitation phase the Langerhans cells that present the allergen cause an inflammatory reaction by causing proliferation of antigen-specific T lymphocytes and release of inflammatory mediators. When the individual is re-exposed to the allergen, the Langerhans cells, together with the antigen attached to them, cause proliferation of the antigen-specific T lymphocytes and release of inflammatory mediators, which cause the skin lesions and symptoms to develop within 12 to 48 hours of exposure. The symptoms and lesions usually resolve over a period of 3 to 4 weeks if the offending allergen is removed. If a chemical has a structure that is close to that of the substance that caused the initial sensitization, sometimes the immune system cannot distinguish between the two so that cross-sensitization occurs. This process causes the elicitation phase with the chemical that is closely related to the allergen [12]. If workers are exposed to allergens, only a small number develop sensitization in most cases. For example, only 5% to 15% of women and up to 1% of men become sensitized to nickel. An exception occurs when workers are exposed to poison ivy, in which case up to 70% of persons become sensitized. It can take 3 to 4 days for sensitization to develop after exposure to an allergen.

Workers who are continually exposed to an allergen may not develop sensitivity for months or years, which can make the diagnosis difficult. After contact, workers develop pruritis with erythema and edema followed by papules, vesicles, and bullae. After that stage, crusting and weeping may occur and there is risk of secondary infection [13]. Photoallergic contact dermatitis is a subgroup of allergic contact dermatitis in which the allergic response occurs because of ultraviolet light. Photoallergy can be caused by various substances, such as drugs (eg, tetracycline and sulfa), vegetables (eg, celery), and hydrocarbons (eg, anthracene and coal tar). A common cause of allergic contact dermatitis in landscapers, ranch workers, and outdoor workers is phytodermatitis (plant dermatitis), which is often caused by members of the Rhus family, such as poison ivy, poison oak, and poison sumac. In the acute phase the lesions are tiny vesicles and weepy encrusted lesions. The lesions are often linear at the site of contact with the plant (Fig. 1).

Other common allergens include chromate, rubber, nickel, and formaldehyde. Occupations at risk of nickel allergic contact dermatitis include textile worker, electronic worker, mechanic, hairdresser, and machinist. Textile workers, cement

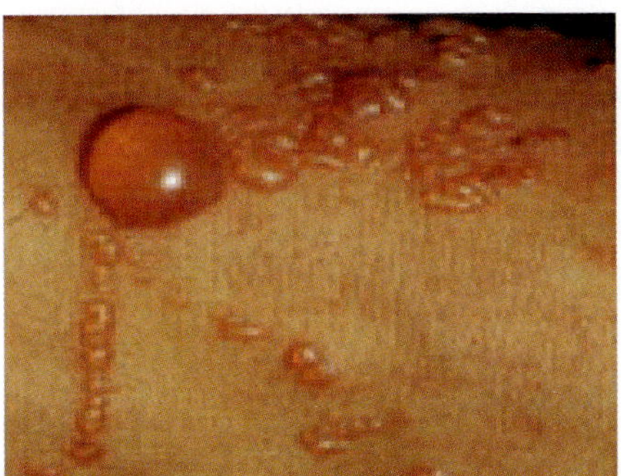

Fig. 1. Poison ivy. (*From* Habif TP. Clinical dermatology. 4th edition. St. Louis (MO): Mosby; 2004. p. 88; with permission.)

Table 1
Common causes and related occupations of allergic and irritant contact dermatitis

Allergen or irritant	Workers involved
Plants	
Poison ivy/oak	Horticulturists, outdoor workers, landscapers, farmers, landscapers
Plastic resins	
Epoxy resins	Floor layers, pipe workers, electronic workers
Acrylics	Printers, dentists, orthopedists
Metallic salts	
Nickel	Electroplaters, computer/electronic workers, ceramic workers, jewelers, dental technicians, hairdressers, tailors
Chromate	Leather tanners, cement workers, arc welders, painters
Others	
Gold, mercury, arsenic, tin, cobalt, palladium, platinum, tungsten carbide	
Rubber and rubber additives	
Topical medications	
Neosporin, benzocaine, thimersol	Medical personnel (nurses, pharmacists, doctors, dentists)
Cosmetics	
Fragrances and preservatives	Beauticians, perfume salespersons
Organic dyes	
Paraphenylenediamine	Dye workers
Pesticides	Agriculture workers
Strong alkalis and acids such as hydrofluoric acid, potassium hydroxide	Electroplaters, engravers, semiconductor workers
Heavy metals	Factory and semiconductor workers
Soaps, detergents	Nurses, waiters, dishwashers, butchers
Solvents	Dry-cleaning workers, machinists
Water	Hairdressers, dishwashers, food preparers, nurses, and other employees who wash hands frequently
Pesticide	Agriculture workers

workers, mechanics, and printers are at risk of chromate allergic contact dermatitis. Chromate dermatitis found in cement workers can take a few years to develop. Some of the common causes and related occupations of allergic and irritant contact dermatitis are listed in Table 1. (Not all the causes or occupations are listed because of the size of this article.)

Diagnosis

The cause of hand dermatitis cannot be ascertained by the pattern and types of lesions. A detailed history is paramount to ascertain the cause and select the correct allergens for patch testing, however. Sometimes incomplete recollection by a worker can hinder obtaining a complete history. Most cases of occupational contact dermatitis occur in the early years of employment, and approximately half of the cases occur in workers within 2 years of starting employment [11]. Some of the important questions to ask are listed in Box 1.

It is important to realize that material safety data sheets only list ingredients that are present in the final product at levels of more than 1%. Many agents that can cause allergic contact dermatitis in small quantities, such as preservatives, would not be listed in a material safety data sheet. Substances such as water, which can irritate with repeated exposure, are not listed [14]. In addition to taking a thorough history, the physician should perform a full physical examination and place emphasis on the type of rash, the location of the rash, and whether it is symmetrical.

Patch testing

The diagnosis of allergic contact dermatitis can be confirmed with a positive patch test. Patch testing is not useful in contact irritant dermatitis, but it is the gold standard for diagnosing allergic contact dermatitis. In the clinic setting, however, only a small percent of workers with contact dermatitis have the patch test done. The test is not without risk because it can cause hypersensitivity to the tested substance in the worker. If there is active dermatitis at the site of testing during an acute attack, the patch test should not be done because of the increased rate of false-positive reactions. Once the acute episode has resolved, however, the patch test can be done. Another problem with the patch test is that allergens available in the standardized tests focus mainly on detecting allergens common in domestic and not industrial environments. Industrial chemicals, for which there is no standardized test, can be patch tested by an experienced allergist or dermatologist. The allergist or dermatologist must be well versed in occupational issues because the right concentration of the allergen must be used and an adequate number of controls must be run. If too little allergen is applied, the test is suboptimal [13].

The sensitivity and specificity rates of the patch test are 75% to 80%. The commonly used patch testing methods are the Finn chamber and the newer True test. The Finn chamber uses a multi-well aluminum patch. Each well has a measured small quantity of allergen being tested, and the patch is taped to the skin in the upper back region. In the True test a tape with measured quantities of allergen in a thin gel film is used. After 48 hours, the patch is removed and a reading is taken. Additional readings at 72 hours and sometimes at 1 week should be undertaken; otherwise, approximately one third of positive reactions can be missed. Erythema, edema, and vesiclulation suggest a positive test result. The grading and methods of the patch test have been standardized by the International Contact Dermatitis Research Group, in which grade 0 is no reaction and grades 1 to 3 are positive grades of increasing severity based on the presence of erythema, edema, papules, vesicles, and bullae. Photoallergic dermatitis can be diagnosed using ultraviolet light and the photopatch. In certain cases, specific antibodies to

Box 1. Questions to aid in the diagnosis of dermatitis

Questions about the rash

Where did the rash begin on the body, and how did it progress (provide a description of lesions)?
When did the rash begin, and what was the relation to work, exposures, weekends, and vacation?
What are the symptoms and aggravating and relieving factors relating to the rash?
If lesions recur, what areas are involved and what treatments are effective?

Questions about the medical history

Is there a history of atopic eczema and rash before the current employment?
Is the individual taking prescribed, over-the-counter medications or using topical agents?

Questions about the workplace and previous occupational skin disease

Did skin problems occur in previous jobs and was any workers' compensation received?
How long has the employee been in the current job?
What are general work conditions, such as cold, humidity, and heat?
What control measures, such as ventilation, encapsulation, or processes, are in place?
What is the history of exposure to irritants and potential allergens and duration of exposure?
What is the history regarding material safety data sheets regarding irritants/allergens, cleansing agents used, frequency of hand washing, and use of protective creams and moisturizers?
What is the timing of exposure and its relation to the development or rash and symptoms?
What is the job description, with a detailed description of what workers actually do and whether there have been recent work changes or exposure? (A walk-through may be useful.)

Are other workers similarly affected? (Irritant contact dermatitis may affect groups of workers, whereas allergic contact dermatitis is usually sporadic.)
What types and effectiveness of personal protective equipment are used?

Questions about hobbies and other non–work-related activities

What is the detailed history of hobbies and other non-occupational activities that may expose individuals to allergens or irritants?
What types of dishwashing, laundry, and cleaning products are used, and are gloves used?

allergens in the blood can be measured using the radioallergoabsorbent test to aid in the diagnosis.

Differential diagnosis of contact dermatitis

Other skin lesions, such as impetigo, should be considered in the differential diagnosis of contact dermatitis. Gram stain and culture of the lesions rule out impetigo or secondary infection. If scabies is impetigenized, the presentation can be confused with contact dermatitis, and scraping for mites is indicated. Other conditions in the differential diagnosis include psoriasis, pomphylyx (dishydrosis), lichen simplex chronicus, and atopic dermatitis [15].

Treatment of contact dermatitis

In the treatment of contact dermatitis the first step is to avoid the exposure that produces the dermatitis once it has been identified. This avoidance is especially important for allergic contact dermatitis because even the smallest exposure to the allergen can produce dermatitis. If removal of the allergen is not possible, a worker may have to be moved to a different location or job in which there is no exposure to the allergen. Acute vesicular eruptions are treated with wet dressings for 24 to 36 hours using Burrow's solution, followed by steroid lotion. Colloidal oatmeal baths may give symptomatic relief of itching. High potency fluorinated topical glucocorticoid creams can be used once the lesions have dried out. Together with antihistamines, steroid creams improve the symptoms and hasten recovery. Secondary infection is not common, but if it occurs oral antibiotics can be used. Topical antibiotics and antihistamines should not be used because they can cause sensitization [15]. If workers have widespread lesions or lesions that involve the face or genitalia, treatment with oral corticosteroids may be indicated,

Treatment with oral corticosteroids must be continued for at 10 to 14 days. If used for short, rapidly tapered doses, a recurrence of skin lesions can occur. Some dose packs that are available are usually inadequate in doses and duration and should be avoided.

Prevention

In the workplace certain preventive measures can be implemented to prevent contact dermatitis. Pre-employment screening can detect individuals who have conditions that predispose to contact dermatitis, such as hand eczema, atopic dermatitis, and xerosis. These individuals should avoid wet work and exposure to irritants or allergens and should be advised to perform dry work. The best method for preventing contact dermatitis is eliminating or replacing substance that are irritants or allergens. If this is not possible, engineering controls, such as automation, ventilation, or encapsulating a process can be effective. If engineering controls cannot be used, administrative controls, such as job rotation, can be used. Works can be rotated between wet work and dry work to prevent prolonged exposures to wet work. Personal protective equipment is the last resort. Face shields, aprons, and plastic or synthetic gloves can be worn to prevent contact with irritants and allergens. Barrier creams and after-work creams also can be used; however, they have questionable efficacy in protecting against irritants. When used on normal skin, some moisturizers may increase skin susceptibility to irritants. Soap substitutes can provide some protection, which has been shown in some controlled clinical trials. After-work creams can reduce the incidence of contact dermatitis. Workers should be advised to use mild soaps, rinse hands thoroughly to remove chemicals, and dry the hands, especially the finger web spaces, where moisture can be trapped. Sunscreens can be used in individuals who have photo dermatitis.

Nail disorders

Ten percent of all skin problems are caused by nail disorders. The occurrence is similar in men and women and it increases with age [16]. Systemic diseases and occupational injury can cause nail disorders, and to differentiate the two causes one must consider the differential diagnosis.

The nail unit has several parts (Fig. 2). The soft tissue under the nail that provides nail growth and support is the nail bed and matrix. In the nail matrix the terminative layers divide and differentiate to produce nail plate growth. The nail plate (or nail) fits proximally into the proximal nail fold and laterally into the paronychium, which are the lateral nail folds. The cuticle (eponychium) is the keratinized border of the proximal nail fold, and the hyponychium is the tissue between the nail bed and the distal nail, which is resistant to infection. The lanula is the distal portion of the nail matrix, which is seen as the white curved opacity

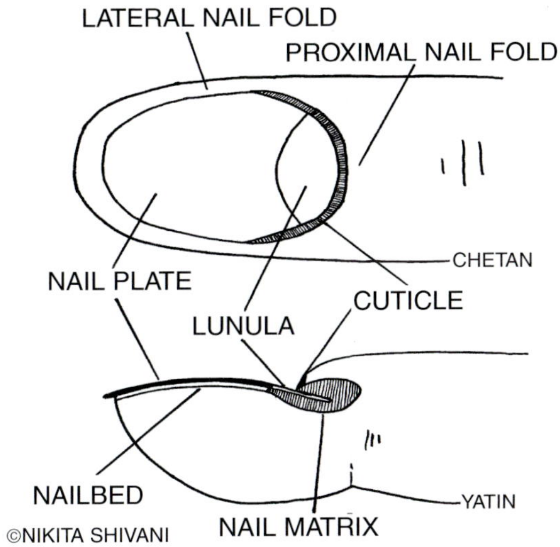

Fig. 2. Nail anatomy. (Reprinted with permission from Nikita Shivani.)

just distal to the eponychium. Where the lunula ends the nail bed begins. The nail matrix forms most of the nail plate, with some material being added to the undersurface of the nail by the nail bed.

Onycholysis (Fig. 3) is spontaneous painless separation of the nail from the nail bed. The separation starts at the hyponychium and progresses proximally. It can be work related or can be caused by nonoccupational conditions. Some of the occupational and nonoccupational causes are listed in Table 2. Nonoccupational causes include hyperthyroidism, connective tissue diseases, psoriasis, and dermatophytosis. Occupational causes include increased pressure on the nail plate from repeated minor trauma (eg, in workers with long nails that are involved in keyboarding for long periods of time). Workers involved in wet work that requires prolonged immersion in water also can develop onycholysis. Tulip workers

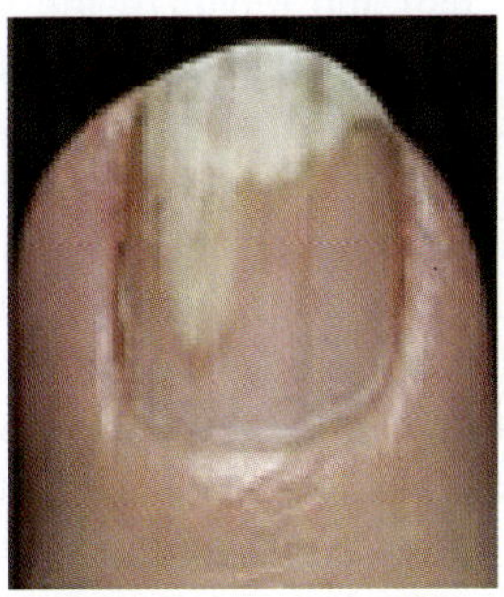

Fig. 3. Onycholysis. (*From* Habif TP. Clinical dermatology. 4th edition. St. Louis (MO): Mosby; 2004. p. 880; with permission.)

Table 2
Onycholysis

Nonoccupational causes	Occupational causes
Subungal neoplasms, warts, and growths	Gasoline
Amyloidosis	Paint removers
Habitual finger sucking	Hydroxylamine sulfate in color developers
Chronic paronychia (fungal)	Solvents
Onychomycosis	Thioglycolate
Lichen planus	Dicyanodiamide
Psoriasis	Repeated minor trauma
Hyperthyroidism and hypothyroidism	Allergic contact dermatitis from nail polish, hardeners, wraps, and artificial nails
Sarcoidosis	
Scleroderma	
Leprosy	
Photo-onycholysis: doxycycline, sulfa drugs and diuretics	
Biologic agents (bacteria/yeast/viruses)	

who separate bulbs may develop onycholysis, and it can occur in bakers and confectioners as a result of sugar. It also can be caused by allergic contact dermatitis from nail cosmetics, such nail hardeners and adhesives used in artificial nails. Other causes include fungal infections (eg, dermatophytic and yeast), bacteria (eg, *Pseudomonas*), and viruses (eg, herpes simplex) [17]. Pseudomonas often grows under the onycholytic nail and causes a greenish-black discoloration.

Subungal hematoma is a subungal collection of blood usually caused by blunt trauma, such as a heavy falling object or getting a finger caught in a door. It may be associated with a fracture of the distal phalanx, which, if present, must be addressed as part of the treatment. Depending on the size it can cause severe throbbing pain, fingertip swelling, fingertip tenderness, and eventually the loss of the nail. Usually the diagnosis is obvious, but a physician must consider other conditions, such as malignant melanoma and normal pigment bands, which are often found in the nails of African Americans. If malignant melanoma is suspected, biopsy should be taken, because melanomas often are discovered after nail trauma. Removal of the nail and repair of the nail bed laceration is usually indicated if the subungal hematoma is larger than half of the total nail area, but it has been suggested that trephination of even large subungal hematomas using a hand-held cautery or heated paper clip may be adequate treatment. If nail bed repair is needed, a digital block is necessary and the nail bed should be repaired with 6/0 or 7/0 absorbable sutures after removing the nail. After the repair, the nail should be replaced and sutured in place and left in place for 2 to 3 weeks to prevent the nail fold from closing. The patient should be advised regarding the possibility of a deformed nail despite the repair [18]. Nail bed lacerations, which can occur in workers who use sharp objects and knives, should be sutured in much the same way as lacerations associated with subungal hematomas after the nail plate is removed with blunt dissection. Significant work-related crush injury to the finger tips can destroy a part of the nail matrix so that it can no longer produce the nail plate, and a pterygium develops where the nail matrix joins the nail bed. Traumatic pterygium commonly occurs in construction workers and carpenters. If necessary, the pterygium can be removed surgically for cosmetic reasons.

Pitting is characterized by small, round, sharply defined depressions in the nail surface, and it is a common finding. Allergic and irritant contact dermatitis that affects the hands and nails can cause pitting. Psoriasis is a common nonoccupational cause of pitting. It also can occur with alopecia areata, eczema, fungal infections, pemphigus, Reiter's syndrome, and sarcoidosis.

Workers often seek help from an occupational medicine physician to diagnose and treat discolorations of the nail, and the physician must decide whether the condition is work related. To ascertain the cause of nail discoloration, a full history (including workplace exposures) and physical examination must be performed and a list of differential diagnosis made, which may include occupational and non–work-related causes. There are many different causes of discoloration of the nails, some of which are discussed herein. Organic dyes and coal tar derivatives can produce virtually any discoloration of the nails, but yellow-brown to black is the most common. Nitrosylated compounds cause a yellow discoloration of the nail. Silver intoxication seen in silver refinery workers causes blue discoloration of the lunulae, as does Wilson's disease. Pseudomonal infection of the nails causes greenish discoloration below the nail. Phenytoin has been reported to turn the nail brown. Subungal melanoma can cause brown discoloration of nails and has a bad prognosis, so it should be differentiated from benign conditions, such as pigmented bands, which are a normal finding in African Americans. Individuals who have uremia can have hand and half nail of Lindsey, in which the proximal nail is dull white like ground glass and the distal half is brown, pink, or reddish. Yellow nail syndrome occurs in patients with lymphadema, nasal sinus disease, bronchiectasis, chronic bronchitis, or lung cancer. The yellow color is caused by thickening of the nail.

Leukonychia is the presence of white bands in the nail that occur when the formation of the nail is disturbed. It can be caused by occupational or non–work-related causes. Punch operators who do a lot of keypunching can develop leukonychia because of repeated minor trauma. The transverse white bands caused by trauma follow the contour of the proximal nail fold but do not cover the whole nail width. Leukonychia punctatae are white spots in the nail caused by mild trauma, such as aggressive manicuring or tapping of the nails. The spots or bands may appear at the lunula and grow with the nail or disappear. A familial type of leukonychia has an autosomal dominant inheritance. Other causes of transverse white lines of the nails include pellagra, Hodgkin's disease, renal failure, sickle cell anemia, and nail damage from paraquat. At low levels, paraquat causes transverse white bands, but with severe exposure workers may develop onycholysis, ridging, and furrowing. Terry's nail involves white opacities of the nails in patients with cirrhosis. The white area obscures the proximal lunula but the distal nail shows the color of the nail bed. Mee's lines are white striae in the nails that can develop after chronic arsenic exposure, which can be diagnosed by analyzing hair and tissue samples for arsenic. Other conditions that cause Mee's lines are Hodgkin's disease, congestive heart failure, leprosy, malaria, chemotherapy, and carbon monoxide poisoning. The defect is in the nail itself because the nail matrix growth is disrupted by the insult. The Mee's lines move distally and the width of the lines varies. We can determine when the insult occurred by measuring the distance from the lines to the cuticle. Muehrcke lines are paired, white, transverse lines that are caused by an abnormality in the vascular bed of the nail. Unlike leukonychia, they cover the entire width of the nail plate and do not move with nail growth. These lines were first described in patients with chronic hypoalbuminemia but do occur in other conditions, such as glomerulonephritis, nephrotic syndrome, and malnutrition [19]. Trauma also has been reported as a cause of Muehrcke lines [20].

All types of eczema, including contact dermatitis, can affect the nail. Eczema can cause thick rough brittle nails, yellow discoloration, ridging, onycholysis, furrowing, subungal hematomas, and transverse leukonychia [21,22].

Disruption of the capillaries along the longitudinal dermal ridges causes splinter hemorrhages, which are usually more than 2 mm long. Subungal epidermal ridges are present longitudinally from the lunula to the hyponychium, and they fit tightly into dermal ridges. Repeated trauma or a single severe injury at work damages the capillaries in the dermal ridges and causes splinter hemorrhages. Single or a few splinter hemorrhages can be found in 20% of healthy individuals as a normal finding. With nail growth, the trapped blood moves distally with it. Non–work-related causes include systemic lupus erythematous, psoriasis, atopic dermatitis, subacute bacterial endocarditis, tichinosis, blood dyscrasias, vasculitis, and onychomycosis. Fifteen percent of patients who have endocarditis have splinter hemorrhages, and they occur more often in subacute rather than acute infection, usually in the proximal nail rather than distally [19].

Ridging of the nails can be caused by trauma. Trauma to the nail matrix, whether caused by a single acute trauma or repetitive insults, can lead to permanent changes in the nail, such as longitudinal ridges or splits that extend through the entire nail. Beau's lines are transverse ridges or depressions in the nail that are caused by temporary cessation of cell division in the proximal nail matrix. They can occur with chemotherapy, malnutrition, pemphigus, Raynaud's disease, and systemic illnesses. They can be caused by trauma and unilateral beau's lines can be caused by reflex sympathetic dystrophy.

Koilonychia is a lateral elevation and central depression of the nail that gives the nail a spoon shape (Fig. 4). Prolonged exposure to organic solvents, oils, and acids and repeated trauma can cause work-related koilonychia. Occupations such as mechanic, cabinet worker, and hairdresser are at increased risk of koilonychia. Nonoccupational causes include hemochromatosis, thyrotoxicosis, nail patella syndrome, which is autosomal dominant, Plummer Vinson syndrome, Raynaud's disease, and systemic lupus erythematosus. Almost half of the individuals with hemochromatosis can develop koilonychia. Ferritin and a complete blood count can rule out hemochromatosis and iron deficiency. Once the iron deficiency anemia is treated, the koilonychias resolves [19].

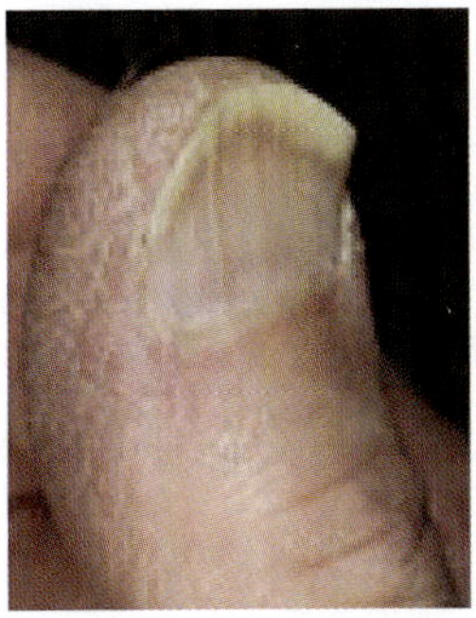

Fig. 4. Spoon nails. (*From* Habif TP. Clinical dermatology. 4th edition. St. Louis (MO): Mosby; 2004. p. 88; with permission.)

Wet workers are at increased risk of paronychial infections from yeast, bacteria, or fungi. A detailed history that includes trauma at work or exposure to wet work helps differentiate occupational and nonoccupational causes. Workers with frequent exposure of the nails to solvents may develop thin and brittle nails because the solvent partially dissolves and weakens the nail plate.

Summary

The practicing occupational medicine physician commonly treats hand dermatitis and nail disorders. An accurate diagnosis is essential. It is important to distinguish occupational and nonoccupational causes, which can be done by taking a detailed history and physical examination and, if necessary, undertaking a walk-through at the employee's workplace. The patch test can be useful in diagnosing allergic contact dermatitis but should be administered by a physician who is familiar with the test and is able to test substances that are not available in the standardized test.

References

[1] NIOSH. Occupational dermatoses: a program for physicians. Available at: http://www.cdc.gov/niosh/ocderm.html. Accessed May 19, 2005.

[2] US Bureau of Labor Statistics. Nonfatal occupational illnesses by category of illness, private industry. Available at: www.cdc.gov/niosh/pdfs/2002-120.pdf. Accessed.

[3] Cohen DE. Contact dermatitis: a quarter century perspective. J Am Acad Dermatol 2004; 51(1 Suppl):S60–3.

[4] Gawkrodger D. Patch testing in occupational dermatology. Occup Environ Med 2001;58:823–8.

[5] Fowler J. Occupational dermatology. Curr Probl Dermatol 1998;10(6):214–41.

[6] Dikel H, Kuss O, Schmidt A, et al. Importance of contact dermatitis in occupational skin disease. Am J Clin Dermatol 2002;3(4):283–9.

[7] Shiao JS, Sheu HM, Chen CJ, et al. Prevalence and risk factors of occupational hand dermatoses in electrical workers. Toxicol Ind Health 2004;20(1–5):1–7.

[8] Forrester BG, Roth VS. Hand dermatitis in intensive care units. J Occup Environ Med 1998; 40(10):881–5.
[9] Bigby M, Arndt KA, Coopman SA. Skin disorders. In: Levy BS, Wegman D, editors. Occupational health: recognizing and preventing work-related disease and injury. 4th edition. Philadelphia: Lippincott Williams & Wilkins; 2000. p. 537–51.
[10] White I. ABC of work related disorders: occupational dermatitis. BMJ 1996;313:487–9.
[11] English JSC. Current concepts of irritant contact dermatitis. Occup Environ Med 2004;61: 722–6.
[12] Habif TP. Contact dermatitis and patch testing. In: Clinical dermatology. 4th edition. St. Louis (MO): Mosby; 2004. p. 81–103.
[13] La Dou J. Occupational skdn Disorders. In: Occupational and environmental medicine. 2nd edition. Stamford (CT): Lange; 1997. p. 272–9.
[14] Herington TN, Morse LH. Injuries to the skin. In: Occupational injuries: evaluation, management, and prevention. St. Louis (MO): Mosby; 1995. p. 247–53.
[15] Ferri FF. Contact dermatitis. In: Ferri's clinical advisor. Philadelphia: Mosby; 2006. p. 246.
[16] American Academy of Dermatology. Guidelines of care for nail disorders. J Am Acad Dermatol 1996;34:529–33.
[17] E medicine. Onycholysis. Available at: www.emedicine.com /DERM/topic 299.htm. Accessed May 19, 2005.
[18] E medicine. Nail bed injuries. Available at: www emedicine.com. Accessed.
[19] Fawcett R, Linford S. Nail abnormalities: clues to systemic disease. Am Fam Physician 2004; 69:1414–24.
[20] Schwartz RA, Barnet CR. Muerhcke lines of the fingernails. Available at: www.emedicine.com/derm/topic916.htm. Accessed.
[21] Daniel CR. Diagnosis of onychomycosis and other nail disorders: a pictoral atlas. New York: Springer-Verlag; 1996. p. 40–51.
[22] Zenz C, Dickerson OB, Horvath E. Occupational dermatoses. In: Occupational medicine. 3rd edition. St. Louis (MO): Mosby; 1994. p. 93–128.

ELSEVIER
SAUNDERS

Clin Occup Environ Med
5 (2) 397–405

CLINICS IN
OCCUPATIONAL AND
ENVIRONMENTAL
MEDICINE

Rheumatic Diseases that Can be Confused with Work-Related Upper Extremity Disorders

Lisa June, MD

Private Practice, Rheumatology Associates, 4213 Maryknoll Lane, Louisville, KY 40207, USA

The rheumatic diseases have great significance for persons interested in occupational medicine because of the large number of workers affected, the significant costs associated with such disorders, and the presence of systemic arthritides in the differential diagnosis for certain occupational injuries. This article concentrates on recognizing such rheumatic conditions so that patients can be referred appropriately for further treatment and optimal outcome and so that undue burden is not put on the workplace with inappropriate workers' compensation.

Epidemiology

The prevalence of musculoskeletal disorders is so great that issues related to occupational medicine and patients who have arthritis are unavoidable: 15% to 20%, or 54 million, of the United States population have musculoskeletal disorders that range from distinct injuries to systemic diseases. Many of these musculoskeletal disorders are rheumatic disorders that can affect the upper extremities, such as osteoarthritis (21 million affected), rheumatoid arthritis (RA) (2.1 million), crystalline arthritides (2–3 million), spondyloarthropathies (400,000), systemic lupus erythematosus (SLE) (240,000), and scleroderma (50,000) [1]. Because of the aging of the baby boomers, an estimated 59 million people will have some form of arthritis by 2020 [2]. Although prevalence of these rheumatic conditions increases with age, many persons have onset during the typical working years, between ages 18 and 64. Spondyloarthropathies, for ex-

E-mail address: lisajunemd@hotmail.com

1526-0046/06/$ – see front matter
doi:10.1016/j.coem.2005.11.008

ample, virtually always have an onset at age younger than 40 [3], and RA is not unusual in young or middle-aged individuals [4].

Economic impact

The cost of musculoskeletal disorders is substantial. Approximately 30% of adult patients who have arthritis who are younger than age 64 are considered totally disabled or unable to work in their chosen occupations secondary to their musculoskeletal conditions. This status accounts for $77 billion in lost wages per year. Although two thirds of the working age population are currently employed, only 42% of working age people with musculoskeletal disorders are jobholders. Persons aged 45 to 64 account for the largest share of indirect cost secondary to lost wages. Medical treatment of the musculoskeletal diseases alone costs another $39 billion, or 0.5% of the gross national product, per year. Each year, patients with such disorders account for 315 million doctor's visits and 8 million hospitalizations. In addition to the cost of lost wages and medical care, the workplace's productivity is also affected, because an average patient with a musculoskeletal condition has 40 days of restricted activities per year [2].

Rheumatologic mimics of upper extremity occupational disorders

Inflammatory arthritis-related carpal tunnel syndrome and other entrapment neuropathies

The incidence of upper extremity disorders, so-called "cumulative movement disorders" (eg, entrapment neuropathies) has greatly increased over the last 10 years. "Cumulative trauma disorders" caused by the performance of repetitive tasks account for more than 50% of work-related medical problems in the United States [5]. Carpal tunnel syndrome (CTS) accounts for more than 30% of these disorders [6]. Patients who have RA and other inflammatory arthritides that can affect the wrist, such as crystalline disease (eg, gout, pseudogout), spondyloarthropathies, psoriatic arthritis, and SLE, often have significant tenosynovitis of the finger flexors and synovitis of the wrist, which can compress the median nerve and result in CTS (Fig. 1). The paresthesias often resolve with control of the underlying inflammatory process with appropriate medications.

CTS is the most common associated entrapment neuropathy in patients who have RA, occurring in 23% to 69% of patients [7–10]. The incidence may increase with the severity of inflammatory disease. One study showed entrapment neuropathies in up to one half of patients with severe RA with associated nodules [11]. In addition to CTS, other types of upper extremity nerve entrapment have been reported in RA, including cases that involve the posterior interosseous and ulnar nerves [12,13]. These cases are much less common in patients who have RA than CTS and are less prevalent in occupational medicine.

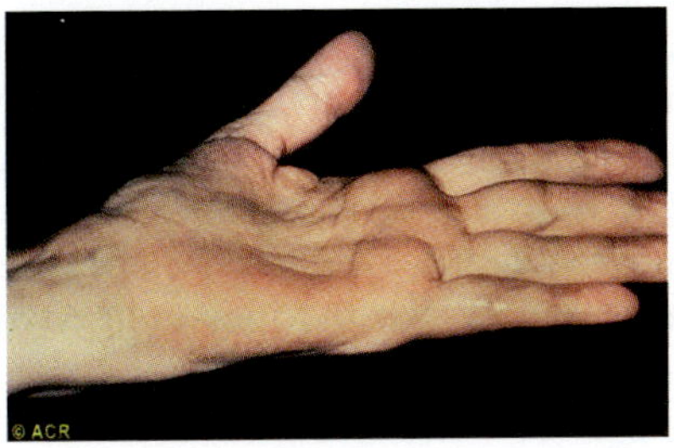

Fig. 1. Hand of rheumatoid arthritis patient with associated carpal tunnel demonstrating thenar atrophy and swelling of the volar aspect of the wrist secondary to synovitis. (*From* The American College of Rheumatology, Atlanta, GA. © 1972–2004 American College of Rheumatology Clinical Slide Collection. Used with permission.)

The presence of inflammatory arthritis and other possibly causative diseases, such as hypothyroidism in work-related CTS, has been demonstrated in several studies. One study of almost 200 patients who had what was believed to be work-related CTS were found to have other undiagnosed, although probably related, diseases, such as inflammatory arthritis [6]. Another study examined comorbid illnesses associated with 1000 patients who had CTS. RA or another inflammatory rheumatic disease was found to be present in 6.5% [14]. A review of CTS and concomitant diseases that was conducted in 2003 supported an etiologic association between RA and CTS, with an odds ration of 2.2 (confidence interval 1.4–3.4) [15].

Gout can result in CTS by two mechanisms: acute flare with the resulting swelling that impinges on the median nerve and compression of the nerve by uric acid deposits or tophi. One series that examined 2649 carpal tunnel releases found tophi as the cause of compression in 15 hands of 13 patients, for an incidence of 0.6%. The patients were predominantly male (12/13), and 8 were known to have gout and were taking medications for the same [16].

Radiographic features of tophaceous gout in the carpal tunnel have been described. One retrospective study reviewed 18 CT scans and 20 MRI of patients who had CTS with known tophi as the cause of median nerve compression. All included patients were men, with ages ranging from 35 to 76 years. The tophi were found in the floor of the carpal tunnel in 18, among the carpal bones in 17, in the radiocarpal joint in 17, and in the extensor tendons and tendon sheaths in 16. Overall, the tophi showed similar signal characteristics, described in the article to aid the radiologists in their identification [17].

When tophaceous gout is present in the carpal tunnel, the underlying complications can exceed CTS alone. One case study reported such tophaceous invasion of the tendons in a patient who had CTS that the superficialis was beyond repair, although the profundus was able to be salvaged by careful excision of the uric acid deposition [18].

Calcium pyrophosphate deposition also has been associated with CTS in various reports. All were secondary to acute inflammation or pseudogout [19–23]. One study also demonstrated hydroxyapatite crystals on the pathologic specimen in addition to calcium pyrophosphate deposition, with both crystals likely contributing to the inflammation [19].

SLE and progressive systemic sclerosis have been reported as underlying causes for CTS [24–27]. In SLE, nerve impingement is secondary to acute inflammatory arthritis. In scleroderma, CTS has been reported in the early, edematous phase of the disease and can be the presenting symptom of the collagen vascular disorder with more stereotypical findings, such as sclerosis developing later [25].

Patients who have inflammatory arthritis with an entrapment neuropathy, such as CTS, typically do not present with complaints of paresthesias alone. Joint pain, swelling, fatigue, and prolonged early morning stiffness of longer than 1 hour are common concomitant complaints for RA, psoriatic arthritis, SLE, and the spondyloarthropathies. Many patients who have crystalline disease at the wrist present with an acutely inflamed, often erythematous joint, and the complaints of pain far outweigh that of paresthesias. One exception is tophaceous gout, in which the buildup of uric acid crystals can cause nerve impingement even when the joint is not actively inflamed.

Enthesopathies

Enthesopathy is defined as inflammation at the junction of tendons, ligaments, joint capsule, or fascia to bone. Common upper extremity enthesopathies include lateral and medial epicondylitis and rotator cuff tendonitis. Enthesopathies can be associated with repetitive strain but are also commonly seen with spondyloarthropathies, which include ankylosing spondylitis, Reiter's syndrome, arthritis associated with inflammatory bowel disease, one variant of psoriatic arthritis, and a large, undifferentiated subgroup.

The various subtypes of spondyloarthropathies share certain clinical characteristics. Enthesopathies, including tendonitis and dactylitis (sausage digit), are relatively common. Many patients have an associated inflammatory low back pain with sacroiliitis. These patients often report that their low back pain is better with activity and worse after rest, unlike patients with mechanical low back pain that tends to worsen as the day goes on. Eye inflammation (eg, conjunctivitis, iritis) is a relatively common extra-articular manifestation. There is a strong association between spondyloarthropathies and HLA B27. Although this gene is present in only 9% of whites, it can be seen in up to 95% of patients with ankylosing spondylitis. The other subtypes of spondyloarthropathies have a lesser, although still strong, association with this gene.

Raynaud's syndrome

The prevalence of Raynaud's syndrome in the general population ranges from 5% to 20% in women and 4% to 14% in men [28]. In primary Raynaud's syndrome, there is no identified cause of the digital artery vasospasm. Secondary Raynaud's syndrome has a long differential diagnosis. From an occupational medicine standpoint, the use of vibrating tools, such as pneumatic drills and hammers, has been implicated [29]. Hypothenar hammer syndrome, in which trauma to the distal ulnar artery occurs, also has been associated [30]. Raynaud's syndrome is more likely to be secondary when one or more of the following features are present: onset age more than 40, male sex, ulceration of the digits, asymmetric attacks, accompanying signs or symptoms of other disease, abnormal laboratory findings, which suggest inflammatory disease, and ischemic signs proximal to the digits [28].

Rheumatologists are interested in Raynaud's syndrome because it is present frequently in rheumatic conditions such as SLE, progressive systemic sclerosis/CREST, inflammatory myopathies, Sjögren's syndrome, mixed connective tissue disease, and possibly RA. The physical finding that is most suggestive of a possible rheumatic cause of Raynaud's syndrome is an abnormal nailfold capillary examination with dilated loops and occasionally dropout areas (Fig. 2). A nailfold capillary examination may be performed at the bedside with the aid of an ophthalmoscope to serve as a magnifier. One previous meta-analysis of ten articles showed that dilated periungual capillaries were the best predictor of whether Raynaud's syndrome was associated with any underlying collagen vascular disease [31].

A simple routine laboratory evaluation, including an antinuclear antibody and erythrocyte sedimentation rate for secondary causes of Raynaud's, is rec-

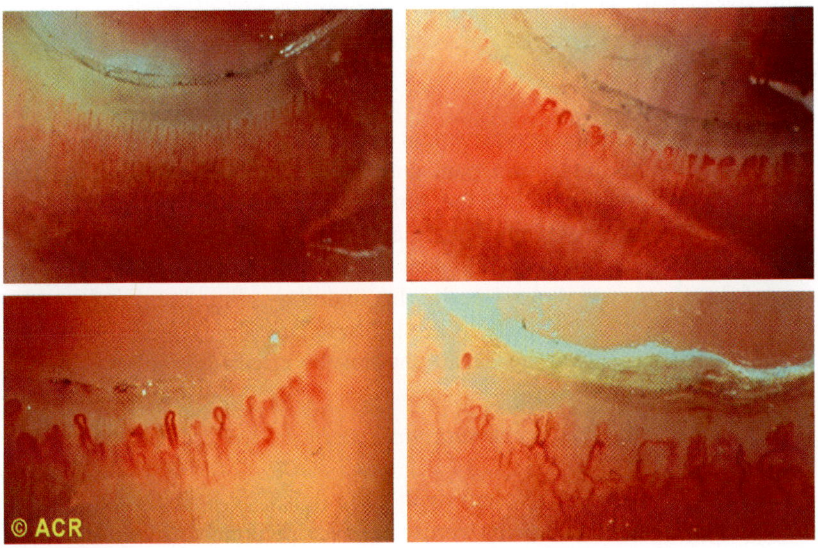

Fig. 2. Nailfold capillary examination in various patients. The upper left is normal with uniform morphology and homogeneous distribution of the small capillary loops. The upper right shows dilated loops and drop-out areas in a patient who has scleroderma. The lower right shows dilated loops in a patient who has dermatomyositis. The lower left shows giant dilated capillary loops in another patient who has dermatomyositis. (*From* The American College of Rheumatology, Atlanta, GA. © 1972–2004 American College of Rheumatology Clinical Slide Collection. Used with permission.)

ommended. If abnormal, a rheumatologic referral is reasonable for further evaluation. Extensive testing for autoimmune illnesses is not routinely recommended unless otherwise clinically indicated by abnormal nailfold capillary examination or other physical findings, such as synovitis or sclerodactyly.

Generalized pain disorders

Hypermobility syndrome

Hypermobility syndrome can be associated with widespread arthralgias without objective signs of joint swelling. Although hypermobility is relatively common, with a prevalence ranging between 10% and 30% [32–36], benign hypermobility syndrome, in which the patient also has associated joint pain, is seen in only 1% of the general population [37]. Given the prevalence of hypermobility, other causes of arthralgias should be considered before ascribing a patient's symptoms to increased flexibility. In the upper extremity, patients with hypermobile joints may be able to painlessly extend the fifth metacarpophalangeal joint more than 90°, oppose the thumb to the forearm, or extend the elbow more than 10° beyond neutral [37]. Patients who have benign hypermobility syndrome are prone to premature osteoarthritis. Physical therapy often can provide benefit for such patients [37].

Fibromyalgia

One study examined the pervasiveness of certain illnesses in patients who seek compensation for disabling arm pain and found that 73 of 102 patients with chronic upper extremity pain met the American College of Rheumatology's criteria for the classification of fibromyalgia syndrome. These patients had similar physical examinations and psychological testing as a group of patients who had fibromyalgia who were followed in the rheumatology clinic but did not attribute their symptoms to their occupations [38]. Physicians should be cautious in applying this label, because it can create the nocebo effect.

When to suspect underlying rheumatic disease in the worker with pain

Because many workers present with arthralgias, it is important to know when such joint pain is related to overuse versus a rheumatic illness. History that suggests inflammatory arthritis includes reports of swollen, erythematous, or hot joints, prolonged early morning stiffness of longer than 1 hour, and improvement with modest activity and worsening after rest. A detailed review of systems may uncover a history of psoriasis, photosensitivity, malar rash, mucositis, iritis, cytopenias, pleurisy, sicca symptoms, or Raynaud's syndrome. A few signs of inflammatory arthritis on physical examination include synovitis, warm joint effusions, erythematous joints, rheumatoid nodules, tophi, and psoriasis with nail pitting. Assessing range of motion is important because signs of hypermobility may be noted. Limitations in range of motion are also helpful in the differential diagnosis because reduced active but preserved passive range of motion suggests bursitis, tendonitis, or muscle injury, whereas decreased active and passive range of motion suggests contracture, synovitis, or mechanical abnormality of the joint [39].

When inflammatory arthritis is demonstrated on examination, appropriate laboratory evaluation may include a rheumatoid factor, antibodies to citrullinated peptides, antinuclear antibody, uric acid, erythrocyte sedimentation rate, C-reactive protein, complete blood count, and comprehensive metabolic panel. Blanket evaluations, such as arthritis panels that are not driven by the patient's history and physical examination, produce many false-positive serologic results. For example, an otherwise healthy middle-aged man with an acutely swollen, erythematous monoarthritis is much more likely to have crystalline or septic arthritis than SLE, so an antinuclear antibody test is not warranted.

All laboratories have their limitations, and this is especially evident in rheumatology. Given the high prevalence of asymptomatic hyperuricemia in the general population, an elevated uric acid level does not diagnose gout, nor does it rule out infection. Uric acid levels are normal in up to 20% of patients with acute gout, especially with polyarticular flares [40,41]. At least 20% of patients who have early RA are seronegative. Positive rheumatoid factors can be seen in 4% to 25% of the normal population, with incidence of RF positivity increasing with age [42,43]. Negative antinuclear antibody test results are helpful in ruling out SLE, but most patients with positive antinuclear antibody test results have no clinically significant connective tissue diseases. Measurements of erythrocyte sedimentation rate and C-reactive protein are often obtained to rule out inflammatory disease, but patients who have RA may have normal values even with active disease [44], and an elevated erythrocyte sedimentation rate/C-reactive protein level can be seen in the absence of disease [40]. In short, laboratory evaluation should be obtained to help clarify the clinical picture but is rarely diagnostic in itself. The history and physical examination are of much greater clinical use in eliminating unlikely causes of pain, narrowing down the differential to the most likely diagnosis for a particular patient.

Summary

Rheumatic illnesses are a common cause for musculoskeletal complaints in the general population. All ages can be affected, including people in the prime of their working years. Secondary problems, such as entrapment neuropathies, enthesopathies, and Raynaud's syndrome, can be associated with various inflammatory arthritides. A detailed history and physical examination are the most important tools in screening for potential inflammatory disease in workers with upper extremity complaints.

References

[1] Lawrence RC, Helmick CG, Arnett RC, et al. Estimates of the prevalence of arthritis and selected musculoskeletal disorders in the United States. Arthritis Rheum 1998;41:778–99.

[2] Yelin E, Callahan LF. The economic cost and social and psychological impact of musculoskeletal conditions. Arthritis Rheum 1995;38(10):1351–62.

[3] Arnett FC. Ankylosing spondylitis. In: Koopman WJ, editor. Arthritis and allied conditions. Baltimore (MD): Williams & Wilkins; 1997. p. 1197–208.

[4] Fuchs HA, Sergent JS. Rheumatoid arthritis: the clinical picture. In: Koopman WJ, editor. Arthritis and allied conditions. Baltimore: 1997. p. 1041–70.

[5] Rempel DM, Harrison RJ, Barnhart S. Work-related cumulative trauma disorders of the upper extremity. JAMA 1992;267(6):838–42.

[6] Atcheson SG, Ward JR, Lowe W. Concurrent medical disease in work-related carpal tunnel syndrome. Arch Intern Med 1998;158(14):1506–12.

[7] Herbison GJ, Teng C, Martin JH, et al. Carpal tunnel syndrome in rheumatoid arthritis. Am J Phys Med 1973;52:68–74.

[8] Barnes CG, Currey HL. Carpal tunnel syndrome in rheumatoid arthritis: a clinical and electrodiagnostic survey. Ann Rheum Dis 1967;26(3):226–33.

[9] Chamberlain MA, Corbett M. Carpal tunnel syndrome in early rheumatoid arthritis. Ann Rheum Dis 1970;29(2):149–52.

[10] Fleming A, Dodman S, Crown JM, et al. Extraarticular features of early rheumatoid disease. BMJ 1976;1:1241–3.

[11] Nakano KK. The entrapment neuropathies of rheumatoid arthritis. Orthop Clin North Am 1975; 6(3):837–60.

[12] Keret D, Porter KM. Synovial cyst and ulnar nerve entrapment: a case report. Clin Orthop 1984; 1984;Sep(188):213–6.

[13] Fernandez AM, Tiku ML. Posterior interosseous nerve entrapment in rheumatoid arthritis. Semin Arthritis Rheum 1994;24(1):57–60.

[14] Stevens JC, Beard CM, O'Fallon WM, et al. Conditions associated with carpal tunnel syndrome. Mayo Clin Proc 1992;67:541–8.

[15] Van Dijk MA, Reitsma JB, Fischer JC, et al. Indications for requesting laboratory tests for concurrent diseases in patients with carpal tunnel syndrome: a systematic review. Clin Chem 2003;49:1437–44.

[16] Rich JT, Bush DC, Lincoski CJ, et al. Carpal tunnel syndrome due to tophaceous gout. Orthopedics 2004;27(8):862–3.

[17] Chen CK, Chung CB, Yeh L, et al. Carpal tunnel syndrome caused by tophaceous gout: CT and MR imaging features in 20 patients. AJR Am J Roentgenol 2000;175(3):655–9.

[18] Mockford BJ, Kincaid RJ, Mackay I. Carpal tunnel syndrome secondary to intratendinous infiltration by tophaceous gout. Scand J Plast Reconstr Surg Hand Surg 2003;37(3):186–7.

[19] Spiegel PG, Ginsbery M, Skosey JL, et al. Acute carpal tunnel syndrome secondary to pseudogout: case report. Clin Orthop 1976;120:185–7.

[20] Rate AJ, Parkinson RW, Meadows TH, et al. Acute carpal tunnel syndrome due to pseudogout. J Hand Surg Br 1992;17(2):217–8.

[21] Chiu KY, Ng WF, Wong WB, et al. Acute carpal tunnel syndrome caused by pseudogout. J Hand Surg Am 1992;17(2):299–302.

[22] Goodwin DR, Arbel R. Pseudogout of the wrist presenting as acute median nerve compression. J Hand Surg Br 1985;10(2):261–2.

[23] Weinstein JD, Dick HM, Grantham SA. Pseudogout, hyperparathyroidism and carpal tunnel syndrome: a case report. J Bone Joint Surg Am 1968;50(8):1669–74.

[24] Sidiq M, Kirsner AB, Sheon RP. Carpal tunnel syndrome: first manifestation of systemic lupus erythematosus. JAMA 1972;222(11):1416–7.

[25] Barr WG, Blair SJ. Carpal tunnel syndrome as the initial manifestation of scleroderma. J Hand Surg Am 1988;13(3):366–8.

[26] Steen VD. Clinical manifestations of systemic sclerosis. Semin Cutan Med Surg 1998;17(1): 48–54.
[27] Sivri A, Hascelik Z, Celiker R, et al. Early detection of neurological involvement in systemic lupus erythematosus patients. Electromyogr Clin Neurophysiol 1995;35(4):195–9.
[28] Wigley FM. Clinical manifestations and diagnosis of the Raynaud phenomenon. UpToDate 2005 [CD-ROM]. Wellesley (MA): UpToDate, Inc.; 2005.
[29] Noel B. Pathophysiology and classification of the vibration white finger. Int Arch Occup Environ Health 2000;73:150–5.
[30] Spencer-Green G, Morgan GJ, Brown L, et al. Hypothenar hammer syndrome: an occupational cause of Raynaud's phenomenon. J Rheumatol 1987;14(5):1048–51.
[31] Spencer-Green G. Outcomes in primary Raynaud's phenomenon. Arch Intern Med 1998;158: 595–600.
[32] Thompson TR, Andrish JT, Bergfeld JA. A prospective study of preparticipation sports examinations of 2670 young athletes: method and results. Cleve Clin Q 1982;49(4):225–33.
[33] Al-Rawi ZS, Al-Aszawi AJ, Al-Chalabi T. Joint mobility among university students in Iraq. Br J Rheumatol 1985;24:326–31.
[34] Larsson LG, Baum J, Mudholkar GS, et al. Hypermobility: prevalence and features in a Swedish population. Br J Rheumatol 1992;32:116–9.
[35] Grahame R, Bird H. Hypermobility in New Zealand. Rheumatology 2003;42:491–2.
[36] Raskin RJ, Lawless OJ. Articular and soft tissue abnormalities in a "normal" population. J Rheumatol 1982;9:284–8.
[37] Sheon RP. Clinical manifestations and treatment of the hypermobility syndrome. In: UpToDate 2005, CD-ROM.
[38] Helfenstein M, Feldman D. The pervasiveness of the illness suffered by workers seeking compensation for disabling arm pain. J Occup Environ Med 2000;42(2):171–5.
[39] American College of Rheumatology Ad Hoc Committee on Clinical Guidelines. Guidelines for the initial evaluation of the adult patient with acute musculoskeletal symptoms. Arthritis Rheum 1996;39:1–8.
[40] Liang MH, Sturrock RD. Evaluation of musculoskeletal symptoms. In: Klippel JH, Dieppe PA, editors. Practical rheumatology. London: Times Mirror International Publishers Limited; 1995. p. 3–20.
[41] Hadler NM, Frank WA, Bress NM, et al. Acute polyarticular gout. Am J Med 1974;56: 715–9.
[42] Newkirk MM. Rheumatoid factors: what do they tell us? J Rheumatol 2002;29:2034–40.
[43] Cammarata RJ, Rodnan GP, Fennell RH. Serum anti-gamma-globulin and antinuclear factors in the aged. JAMA 1967;199:455–8.
[44] Pinals RS. Rheumatoid arthritis with a normal erythrocyte sedimentation rate. J Rheumatol 1978;5:272–4.

ELSEVIER
SAUNDERS

Clin Occup Environ Med
5 (2) 407–411

CLINICS IN
OCCUPATIONAL AND
ENVIRONMENTAL
MEDICINE

High Pressure Injection Injuries of the Hand

Roberto Gonzalez, MD, Morton L. Kasdan, MD, FACS*

Division of Plastic Surgery, University of Louisville, Louisville, KY 40290, USA

We can assume that high pressure injuries of the hand were introduced in the twentieth century as pressure machinery appeared. In the world's medical literature, Hesse [1] first reported high pressure injection injuries in 1925. It was not seen in the English literature until 1937, when Rees [2] presented a case. A 47-year-old male mechanic sustained an injury using a diesel fuel injector. The patient was managed conservatively and ultimately required amputation. This injury is considered a surgical emergency. Several variables can affect the end result, and careful assessment and aggressive treatment may improve the overall outcome [3].

Epidemiology

High pressure injection injury occurs more commonly in young male workers in the nondominant hand in approximately two thirds of the cases. The anatomic areas most frequently affected are (in order) index finger, thumb, palm, and small finger [4,5]. It is important to recognize that this injury may occur to the lower extremities, abdomen, and thorax [6]. It is important to remember that a pressure of approximately 100 psi is required to penetrate the skin [7], and most pressure guns can achieve this power and more. For example, a hydraulic pump operates at approximately 3000 psi, and fluid that leaves the pinpoint nozzle may surpass velocities of 183 m/s. Armored hydraulic pipes that carry paraffin can generate high pressures. Diesel engine injector systems compress fuel to 12,000 psi [8].

The most common substances injected are grease, paint, paint thinners, diesel fuel, oil, water, and cement, and the injury has been reported even in veterinary

* Corresponding author. PO Box 6048, Louisville, KY 40206.
E-mail address: m.kasdan@insightbb.com (M.L. Kasdan).

doi:10.1016/j.coem.2005.11.007 ***occmed.theclinics.com***

medicine while giving chicken vaccines [4–6,9,10]. Any instrument capable of generating enough pressure can cause this injury, such as the autoinjectors for medical compounds [11]. Paint is a combination of multiple chemical compounds that have a pigment (color), a vehicle or binder that functions as adherent, and solvent. After evaporating, the solvent leaves the pigment that provides the final color. The media can be an unsaturated or drying oil or polymer. Synthetic polymers are alkyd resins. Oil-based paints use soy alkyd resins as vehicles, but newer latex paints have emulsified vehicles [12]. Emulsified vehicles cause less inflammatory response than the nonemulsified alkyd resin of oil-based paints, so there is less tissue necrosis [13].

Anatomy

The site of injury is important in determining the spread of the injected material. In 1968, Kaufman [14] injected hands of cadavers with wax at 750 psi at different locations. Results indicated that injected material would continue to enter tissues until resistance is encountered. The flexor sheaths are not uniform; the C pulleys are flexible and thin, whereas the A pulleys are rigid and fibrous. Injections over the middle segments of the fingers are deflected off the fibrous sheath and spread out laterally into the superficial tissues that encircle the digit. If the puncture occurs over the proximal or distal interphalangeal joints and penetrates the sheath, then it dissects through the tendon sheath [14]. The index, long, and ring fingers have a synovial sheath that ends at the metacarpophalangeal joint level. Conversely, in the thumb and little fingers the synovial sheaths extend into the radial and ulnar bursae into the proximal palm. Depending on the digit, the proximal spread of the material can be predicted [14].

Pathophysiology and clinical course

Mason and Queen described the clinical stages of high pressure injection injuries in 1941. Multiple papers make reference to these stages, which can be summarized, in three distinct phases.

In the acute phase, the symptoms result from the injection of the foreign material. First is the swelling secondary to the presence of the material in a small space. As the inflammatory response continues, the soft tissue becomes anesthetic and white because of vascular insufficiency [15]. Several factors have been described as crucial to determining the extent of the injury: (1) Site of entry and underlying anatomy. (2) Chemical and physical characteristics of the injected material. Paint solvent is considered to be the most destructive of the injected substances because of its low viscosity, which permits extensive tracking through the soft tissues, and its corrosive nature, which produces severe tissue necrosis. Grease causes more chronic and less immediate inflammatory reaction [16,17]. (3) The pressure at the injection site (velocity). The higher the velocity, the greater the damage. An amputation rate of 100% has been reported if injuries occur at injection of more than 7000 psi [14]. (4) The duration of exposure to the injection. The greater the volume injected, the more likely an amputation [17].

In the intermediate phase, the inflammatory response continues with fibrosis and formation of foreign body granulomas [18].

In the late phase, the skin overlying the granulomas breaks down and develops ulcers and draining sinuses, which can become secondarily infected [15,18]. The development of squamous epithelioma in the sinuses has been reported [18]. Infection is usually not a primary concern because the injected materials (eg, paint, solvents) seem to be bactericidal or bacteriostatic [16]. Once necrosis ensues, however, a secondary infection may occur. The literature documents an infection rate from 11% to 60%. The bacteria isolated varies from *Staphylococcus epidermidis* to a polymicrobial flora [5,12].

Evaluation

A careful history is essential. Patients should be asked about hand dominance, occupation, time of injury, type of gun used, material injected, the amount of pressure generated, and the usual comorbidities (eg, vascular disease, diabetes). If possible, the physician should obtain the material safety data report. The initial physical examination may not reveal an obvious skin break, and it is essential to identify it because minimal symptomatology is common [15]. The time that elapses between injury and definitive therapy is a major determinant in morbidity and prognosis [19]. The skin must be examined in conjunction with the area of injury, which helps to determine the type of wound and the nature of the deficits. Observing for mottling and skin temperature changes assesses the circulatory status.

Damage to the nerves is evaluated by sense of touch and fine tactile recognition. Motor function also should be assessed. Flexion and extension at each joint are critical to assess tendon and compartment involvement. The flexor digitorum profundus, which inserts into the distal phalanx, is tested by active flexion of the distal interphalangeal joint [17]. Radiographs are useful for evaluating the extent of penetration of the injected material [5,17]. Even if the material is not radiopaque, air may be present.

Treatment

The key elements in treatment remain prompt recognition of the severe nature of the injury and aggressive early decompression and débridement [6,9,18]. Emergency department care must include tetanus prophylaxis, administration of broad-spectrum antibiotics, limb elevation, radiographs, and contacting a hand surgeon [17]. Local anesthesia and hot soaks are contraindicated because of the risk of added local swelling and ischemia [17,18].

In the operating room, débridement should be performed under regional block or general anesthesia. Exsanguination should be performed with hand elevation for 4 to 10 minutes instead of using Esmarch's wrap [17]. All affected areas must be explored. Digits should be opened by a midlateral or Brunner incision through their entire length [20]. Involvement of the thumb and little fingers should include exploration of the ulnar and radial bursa. If material is located within the palm, then the carpal tunnel and forearm should be explored [14]. If any signs of neuropathy are found, the involved nerves should be decompressed.

All nonviable tissue should be excised and copious irrigation should be used. Wounds are left open for further observation and débridement. Closure can be achieved secondarily or with skin grafting [17]. The use of steroids is controversial; they may be of benefit in certain injuries [21]. Most authors have suggested that the hand should be immobilized in the intrinsic plus position to facilitate healing, and therapy should begin as soon as tolerated [5,16].

Outcome

Even with early recognition, high pressure injection injury leads to significant impairment. Amputation incidence is high if the initial débridement is delayed more than 6 hours, especially with low-viscosity substances [16]. The reported rates for amputation varied from 16% to 55% [8,16]. The agents more associated with a poor outcome are fuel, paint thinner, and solvents [7]. These injuries can have systemic effects similar to a massive snake bite [22].

The average permanent partial impairment is approximately 15% for spray gun injuries, less than 2% for pneumatic hoses, and 6% for hydraulic fluid. Depending on the site and delay of treatment, the permanent partial impairment varies: 4% if the delay is less than 6 hours versus 17% if the delay is more than 6 hours [7]. Work loss ranges from 6 to 26 weeks, with 92% of patients returning to their prior jobs [16].

Summary

High pressure injection injuries are devastating if not properly recognized and treated. The primary care physician or nurse should refer these patients to a hand surgeon immediately because they represent a true emergency.

References

[1] Hesse E. Die chirurgische und gerichtliche medizinische bedeutung der kunstlich herrogerufenen erkrankungen. Arch Klin Chir 1925;136:277–91.

[2] Rees CE. Penetration of tissue by fuel oil under high pressure from diesel engine. JAMA 1937; 112:907–8.

[3] Jebson PJL, Sanderson M, et al. High pressure injection injuries of the hand. Wis Med J 1993;92:13–6.
[4] Schoo MJ, Scott FA. High pressure injection injuries of the hand. J Trauma 1980;20(3):229–38.
[5] Pinto MR, Turkula-Pinto LD, Cooney WP, et al. High pressure injection injuries of the hand: review of 25 patients managed by open wound technique. J Hand Surg Am 1993; 18A(1):125–32.
[6] Fialkov JA, Freiberg A. High pressure injection injuries: an overview. Emergency Medicine in Review 1991;9:367–71.
[7] Vasilevski D, Noorbergen M, Depierreux M, et al. High pressure injection injuries to the hand. Am J Med 2000;18(7):820–4.
[8] Neal NC, Burke FD. High pressure injection injuries. Injury 1991;22(6):467–70.
[9] Barr ST, Wittenborn W, Nguyen D, et al. High pressure cement injection injury of the hand: a case report. J Hand Surg Am 2002;27A(2):347–9.
[10] Burke F, Brady O. Veterinary and industrial high-pressure injection injuries. BMJ 1996;312: 1436–7.
[11] Combs J, Hise L. High pressure injection injury involving a 2-PAM chloride auto injector. Mil Med 1992;157(8):434–6.
[12] Schnall SB, Mirzayan R. High pressure injection injuries to the hand. Hand Clin 1999; 15(2):245–8.
[13] Gillespie CA, Rodehaver GT, Smith S, et al. Airless paint gun injuries: definition and management. Am J Surg 1974;128:383–91.
[14] Kaufman HD. High-pressure injection injuries: the problems, pathogenesis and management. Hand 1970;2:63–73.
[15] Luber KT, Rehm JP, Freeland AE. High pressure injection injuries of the hand. Orthopedics 2005;28(2):129–32.
[16] Hayes CW, Pan HC. High pressure injection injuries to the hand. South Med J 1982; 75(12):1491–516.
[17] Sirio CA, Smith JS, Graham WP. High pressure injection injuries of the hand: a review. Am Surg 1989;55(12):714–8.
[18] Harter BT, Harter KC. High pressure injection injuries. Hand Clinics 1986;2(3):547–52.
[19] Stark HH, Wilson JN, Boyles JH. Grease gun injuries of the hand. J Bone Joint Surg Am 1961;43A:485–91.
[20] Williams CS, Riordan DC. High velocity injection injuries of the hand. South Med J 1974; 67:295–302.
[21] Phelps DB, Hastings H, Boswick JA. Systemic corticosteroid therapy for high-pressure injection injuries of the hand. J Trauma 1977;17(3):206–10.
[22] Kasdan ML, Ryan R. High pressure injection injuries. In: Kasdan M, editor. Occupational hand and upper extremity injuries and diseases. Philadelphia: Hanley & Belfus; 1991. p. 233–7.

ELSEVIER
SAUNDERS

Clin Occup Environ Med
5 (2) 413–422

CLINICS IN
OCCUPATIONAL AND
ENVIRONMENTAL
MEDICINE

Fingertip Injuries

Johnny Chang, MD, Adam J. Vernadakis, MD,
W. Thomas McClellan, MD*

Department of Plastic and Reconstructive Surgery, Lahey Clinic Foundation, 41 Mall Road, Burlington, MA 01805, USA

The fingertip is a highly specialized part of the body that contributes to the hand's dexterity, provides a broad range of sensory capabilities, and serves a cosmetic purpose. As the most distal part of the upper extremity in exploratory and manipulative actions, the fingertip is particularly vulnerable to injury. After back injuries, hand injuries are the second most common occupational injuries that result in lost workdays, and the fingertips are the most frequently involved part of the hand. As expected, the most used fingers are the most commonly injured at work; the index finger and thumb are affected the most, whereas the ring and small fingers are affected the least. The most common mechanism of occupational finger injury that results in time off from work is laceration, but crush and avulsion injuries also occur commonly, whereas puncture, amputation, and other injuries occur less frequently [1]. Although single mechanism injuries are most common, a significant number of injuries involve more than one. Proper evaluation, diagnosis, triage, and treatment of fingertip injuries are essential for optimal outcome. Secondary reconstruction of improperly managed fingertip injuries is technically challenging and prone to complications. Correct initial management is of paramount importance for successful long-term results [2].

* Corresponding author.
E-mail address: william.t.mcclellan@lahey.org (W.T. McClellan).

doi:10.1016/j.coem.2005.11.010 *occmed.theclinics.com*

Evaluation of fingertip injuries

History

As in any medical situation, history plays a critical role in the evaluation of fingertip injuries. The mechanism of injury can quickly provide clues to the type and extent of injuries to be expected and potential treatment options. For example, sharp injuries tend to be more amenable to microsurgical repair than crush injuries. Age, hand dominance, vocation and avocation, and digits affected also play important roles in treatment choices [3]. Comorbidities, such as smoking, peripheral vascular disease, and diabetes, are prognostic factors that help to guide management. The type of contamination is important to know.

Examination

Despite discomfort to the patient, a sensory examination should be conducted before use of local anesthetic agents. It is helpful to consider the anatomy of the fingertip in doing so. Branches of the palmar digital nerves lie distal interphalangeal joint (DIP) volar to the arteries in the distal finger. The palmar digital nerve typically trifurcates or branches just distal to the joint and becomes exceedingly small beyond that point. Light touch is useful for an initial rough test, but static and moving two-point discrimination may be determined for more accurate assessment. Keep in mind that sensory deficits may be caused by transient neuropraxia rather than permanent nerve damage; serial examinations can be particularly helpful. Delayed sensory nerve repair in the hand also is generally tolerated well [4].

After sensory branches have been tested carefully, local anesthesia can be administered to allow further examination. The affected fingers can be examined systematically and evaluated by considering the anatomic components of the fingertip. If the possibility of bone pathology exists, plain films should be obtained to look for fractures. Typically, anteroposterior, lateral, and oblique films of the entire hand should be obtained; subtle pathologic conditions are often more read-

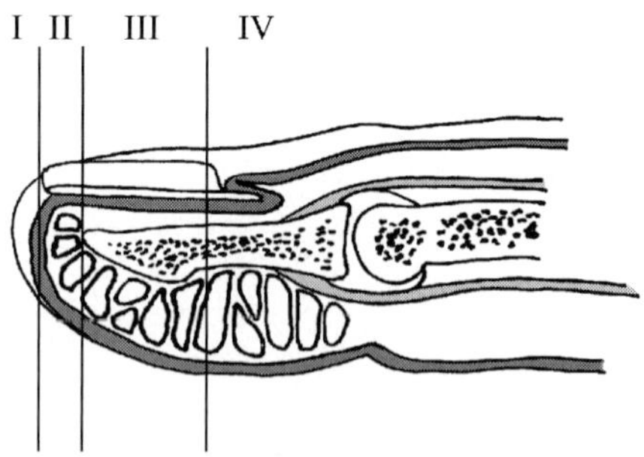

Fig. 1. Allen classification of fingertip injuries. I, skin and pulp. II, nail or nail bed. III, distal phalanx. IV, proximal to lunula.

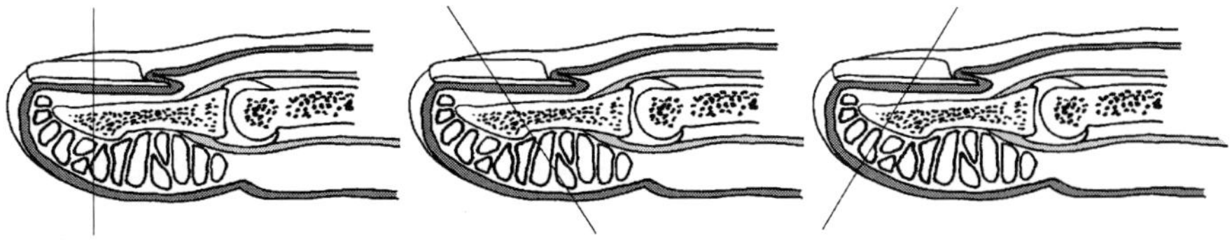

Fig. 2. Fingertip injury orientations.

ily apparent in the context of the hand as a whole. Joint integrity and tendon attachments should be evaluated via passive and active ranges of motion.

The most apparent component in an injury—the skin and pulp—should be inspected carefully to identify the amount of tissue loss, location of tissue loss, and the types of injuries involved. The nail and nail bed should be examined for subungual hematoma, laceration, and avulsion. Most importantly, vascular supply and fingertip viability should be assessed by observing blood flow and capillary refill.

Fingertip amputation classification

Various similar classification schemes have been described over the years in an attempt to categorize fingertip injuries and guide treatment. In general, these classifications are useful as frameworks for evaluating fingertip injuries and having study data. In considering fingertip injuries, it is useful to organize an examination based on some type of classification. Allen [5] proposed a simple and helpful scheme in 1980 based on the proximal extent of injury and the fingertip tissues involved (Fig. 1). These injuries also can be described by their orientations: transverse, volar oblique, or dorsal oblique (Fig. 2).

Recently, Evans and Bernardis [6] proposed the more precise pulp, nail, and bone classification (Table 1). By assigning mutually exclusive single-digit grades that describe the extent and type of injury to each of the three major fingertip components, one three-digit number can describe a fingertip injury immediately

Table 1
Pulp, nail, and bone classification of fingertip injuries

	Pulp	Nail	Bone
0	No injury	No injury	No injury
1	Laceration	Sterile matrix laceration	Tuft
2	Crush	Germinal & sterile matrix laceration	Comminuted nonarticular
3	Loss — distal transverse	Crush	Articular
4	Loss — palmar oblique partial	Proximal nail bed dislocation	Displaced basal
5	Loss — dorsal oblique	Loss — distal third	Tip exposure
6	Loss — lateral	Loss — distal two thirds	Loss — distal half
7	Loss — complete	Loss — lateral	Loss — subtotal
8		Loss — complete	Loss — complete

in more detail than is possible with Allen and similar classifications. Muneuchi and colleagues [7] later attempted to determine the pulp, nail, and bone classification numbers that delineate injuries that require conservative management from injuries that require operative management. Although such classification schemes can provide valuable guidance, the complexity of fingertip injuries requires the application of sound clinical judgment.

Management of fingertip injuries

Treatment goals

Because of the fingertip's importance and specialized functions, several fundamental treatment goals should be kept in mind when treating fingertip injuries [8]:

1. Preservation of length, especially of the thumb
2. Preservation of sensation and prevention of painful neuromas
3. Early mobilization and prevention of joint contractures
4. Quick return to patient function
5. Attention to cosmesis

Preparation

A digital block using 1% to 2% lidocaine injected into the dorsal web space on either side of a digit provides excellent coverage for up to 2 hours. If more time is needed or in cases of severe crush injuries and painful subungual hematomas, in which extended postoperative analgesia would be particularly helpful, one should use 0.5% bupivacaine. Although many texts caution against the use of epinephrine with lidocaine, recent studies have shown its use in digital blocks to be safe and helpful in maintaining clear fields without the use of tourniquets [9,10]. (The editors recommend against this practice.) Otherwise, a simple digital tourniquet can be made from gauze padding, a Penrose drain or latex glove finger, and a hemostat. After proper anesthesia and exsanguination, liberal irrigation and conservative débridement are essential for an optimal outcome [11].

Allen's type I and smaller type II injuries

Lacerations of only the skin or pulp without loss of tissue can be closed directly using fine monofilament sutures. Defects of up to 1 cm^2 with tissue loss that involves only the skin, pulp, or distal nail bed can be allowed to heal secondarily with simple occlusive or semi-occlusive dressings. Studies have supported this practice and demonstrated excellent recovery of sensation, function, and cosmesis. Recovery tends to be slow, however, and complications, such as cold intolerance and joint stiffness, are not uncommon and should be addressed with early motion and close follow-up [3]. For older patients, patients with occupations that require full use of their hands, or patients with complex medical issues, it may be prudent to shorten the joint to allow more rapid return to function.

Allen's type III and larger type II injuries that involve less than 50% of nail bed

For type II defects larger than 1 cm^2 and type III defects, which involve the distal phalanx, secondary closure is less desirable. If less than 50% of the nail bed is involved, good results with preserved sensation may be obtained through direct closure if adequate tissue remains or through several local, regional, or distant pedicled flaps. The simplest of these procedures is the V-Y plasty, or V-Y local advancement flap, which involves advancement of either a single volar V-shaped flap or bilateral flaps from either side of the finger into the defect [12]. The single volar V-Y plasty is simpler and more commonly used, and it works best in transverse or dorsal oblique injuries that preserve more of the volar tissue [13]. It is important to note that the V flap should be undermined minimally to allow advancement. Overzealous undermining of the flap may compromise its vascular supply. Excessive volar tension on the distal nail bed may result in a claw deformity, in which the distal end of the nail curves in a volar direction.

When there is inadequate remaining volar tissue for V-Y plasty, an option particularly suited for the middle and possibly index finger is the thenar flap [14,15]. The injured finger is flexed and attached to a pedicled flap raised from the thenar eminence for 10-14 days, then disconnected and closed. The skin of the thenar eminence provides an excellent functional and cosmetic match for the fingertip pulp and provides adequate tissue for single fingertip injuries with minimal donor site morbidity. Melone and colleagues [15] showed in their study of 150 cases that age is not a contraindication for thenar flaps; persistent proximal interphalangeal (PIP) joint stiffness occurred in only one of 31 patients over 50 years of age. To reduce the risk of both PIP joint stiffness and donor site morbidity, the flap should be raised as far proximally and radially on the thenar eminence as patient comfort allows. This position minimizes PIP joint flexion and relegates the donor site to less critical areas along the periphery of the palm.

For injuries that involve significant loss of soft tissue or multiple fingers, an option that works well is the cross-finger flap. A pedicled flap is raised from the dorsum of a neighboring digit and used to cover the fingertip defect. The flap is disconnected after 10 to 14 days. Meanwhile, the dorsal donor site is covered with a full-thickness skin graft. Although complications such as cold intolerance are not uncommon, patients are generally satisfied with the results of cross-finger flap reconstruction in the absence of applicable alternatives [16,17].

Finally, for injuries to multiple fingertips in which adequate donor tissue may not be available for local or regional flaps, options to consider include distant thoracic and abdominal flaps [18,19]. A patient's fingers are sutured to flaps raised from the anterior thorax or abdomen. Donor site morbidity is minimal, arm position during pedicle development is natural and comfortable, with little risk of long-term residual joint stiffness, and tissue match, although not optimal, is adequate.

Allen's type III and larger type II injuries that involve more than 50% of nail bed

For type II defects larger than 1 cm^2 and type III defects that involve the distal phalanx, if more than 50% of the nail bed is involved, it is exceedingly difficult to salvage the nail bed. Nail growth in this situation is likely to occur abnormally, with curvature toward the volar tip that results in the claw deformity. Shortening of the digit and rounding of the distal bone to allow direct closure are adequate options in cases in which other reconstructive options are not available or are not suitable based on patient history. Excision of the entire nail bed is crucial to prevent painful ingrown nail fragments and deformities. As with any shortening procedure, care also must be taken to perform neurectomies or bury nerve endings proximally in soft tissue or bone, away from the injury site, to prevent development of painful neuromas.

Allen's type IV injuries

When possible, microsurgical replantation is important to consider in type IV injuries with significant loss of fingertip length, especially when the thumb or index finger is involved. In general, replantation is more likely to be successful when the mechanism is a sharp rather than crush injury, when there is minimal delay between injury and replantation, and when the injury occurs at or proximal to the vascular trifurcation [20]. If replantation is not possible, the digit should be shortened and closed directly, as described previously. Shortening is usually contraindicated for the thumb and should be performed with caution for the index finger.

Type IV injuries also often involve the flexor and extensor tendons. When possible, the tendon insertions should be preserved or reattached. Importantly, great care should be taken to reattach the flexor digitorum profundus (FDP) tendon with proper tension closely matching its natural state [21]. Inadequate tension or complete retraction of the tendon results in a condition called lumbrical plus, in which attempts to flex the digit result in paradoxic PIP joint extension. This condition occurs because the associated lumbrical muscle, which functions to extend the PIP joint, is attached proximally to the FDP tendon. When the FDP is no longer attached to the distal phalanx, contraction instead pulls the lumbrical muscle proximally [22]. Suture of the extensor tendon to the FDP tendon results in a condition called quadriga, named after Roman charioteers who controlled the reins of four horses in concert with one hand while wielding weapons in battle with the contralateral hand. In this condition, the injured finger cannot be extended fully, and the uninjured fingers cannot be flexed fully. The injured finger reaches full flexion before any other fingers, which keeps them from flexing further because they must move in concert with the injured finger [23].

Composite grafts

Replacement of amputated digits as composite grafts without vascular anastomosis is sometimes attempted when injuries occur distal to the vascular trifurcation because of the difficulty of microsurgery on the exceedingly small distal branches. Such composite grafts tend to be more successful in children and nonsmokers with sharp or avulsion injuries [24]. Despite a general avoidance of this technique in adults, Heistein and Cook's study of 53 patients demonstrated complete graft survival in 77% of patients younger than age 18 and most adult nonsmokers without diabetes. Even with partial graft survival, composite grafts have the potential of serving as a biologic dressing and providing some additional bulk and length.

Subungual hematomas

Subungual hematomas occur frequently and are exceedingly painful because of pressure that forces the nail plate away from the nail bed. Decompression of the hematoma is always indicated, with the understanding that decompression can convert a closed distal phalangeal fracture to an open one [25]. Common methods of decompression include the creation of drainage holes in the nail plate by using a small electrocautery unit or a hot paperclip, spinning a No. 11 blade, or using an 18- or 21-gauge needle [26].

Some controversy exists over indications for nail removal to allow direct inspection of the nail bed and repair nail bed lacerations. Simon and Wolgin [27] studied 47 patients who had subungual hematomas and found nail bed lacerations in all cases associated with distal phalanx fracture and 60% of cases with more than half the nail bed involved. As a result, classic teaching recommends removal of the nail bed when the hematoma encompasses more than 50% of the nail bed or when it is associated with a distal phalanx fracture. Others argue that the nail should be removed in all cases, because any subungual hematoma implies that some nail bed laceration is supplying the hematoma. A third school of thought is that nail removal is not necessary in any case with intact nail plate and nail folds, although this belief is based on a study of children and may not apply to the adult population [28,29]. Delayed nail bed repairs are difficult and typically yield poor results. Once nail bed tissue is lost or allowed to scar, sequelae are generally permanent and irreparable. It is prudent to consider nail removal whenever there is doubt of nail bed integrity.

The nail should be removed with either a periosteal elevator or a small hemostat, taking care to avoid iatrogenic damage to the nail bed. The nail bed should be examined meticulously under loupe magnification, and lacerations should be repaired with simple interrupted fine absorbable sutures. The nail plate should be replaced as a biologic splint to maintain separation of the eponychial dorsal roof from the nail bed, and it will be displaced gradually by the distal growth of the new nail. If the original nail plate cannot be used, alternatives such as silastic or silicone sheets, adaptic, foil, nonadherent gauze, and even the suture packaging can be used, as long as care is taken to interpose the material between the eponychial fold and the nail bed.

Nail plate and nail bed injuries

Nail plate lacerations are commonly associated with an underlying distal phalanx fracture, which underscores the need for plain films of the affected hand (not just the affected digit). Improper management of nail bed injuries results in significant sequelae, including painful ingrown nails, split nails, grooving, non-adherent nail plates, and the claw deformity. If nail bed tissue loss results in significant tension on direct closure of the nail bed, longitudinal relaxing incisions can be made in the paronychial folds at the border of the nail bed [30]. Care must be taken to splint the eponychial folds open using either the native nail plate or a substitute material.

Distal phalanx fractures

Nail bed lacerations should be expected in any distal phalanx fractures. Inadequately reduced fractures can result in permanent nail deformities because of the close relationship between the nail bed and the distal phalanx. As with fractures elsewhere in the body, distal phalanx fractures should be described as open or closed, displaced or nondisplaced, and simple or comminuted.

Closed, minimally displaced fractures of the distal phalanx may require only the nail plate for maintaining reduction and can be managed with small finger splints, such as malleable, foam-backed aluminum splints. Fractures that cannot be maintained in reduction can be managed with placement of paired K wires inserted through the fracture and joint. Open fractures should be treated with copious irrigation, conservative débridement, reduction, closure, and splinting. Suprock [31] reported that with proper irrigation and débridement, prophylactic antibiotics are generally not indicated, and factors such as comorbidities and contamination should be considered in making this decision [31,32]. Postreduction plain films should be obtained.

Tendon injuries

The most common injuries to the two tendons that insert on the distal phalanx are mallet finger (baseball finger, drop finger), which results from extensor tendon injury, and jersey finger, which results from flexor tendon rupture. Mallet finger manifests as the inability to actively extend the DIP joint and occurs with forced flexion of an extended distal phalanx, such as jamming a finger on an assembly line. There can be an injury of the extensor tendon itself or avulsion of its bony insertion. When a tendinous injury occurs proximal to the DIP joint, the tendon should be repaired using a stitch that passes through the tendon core. For the most part, uncomplicated mallet finger without significant joint surface involvement should be treated conservatively with continuous extension splinting for 8 to 10 weeks followed by 2 to 3 weeks of night splinting. The physician should emphasize to patients that DIP joint extension should be maintained at all times, even when the splint is removed temporarily for cleaning [13,32,33].

Jersey finger manifests as the inability to flex the DIP joint actively. It occurs with forced extension of a flexed DIP joint. Examples include pulling on a player's jersey and power tool torquing while held in a power grip. Because retraction of the tendon or scarring of the tendon sheath can result in permanent partial or total loss of function, early operative repair is generally indicated [34].

Summary

The fingertip is a complex anatomic unit highly specialized in function and particularly prone to injury. Its complex design and the difficulty of secondary repairs demand great care in initial evaluation, diagnosis, and treatment for optimal long-term outcome significance in the future. The goals of treatment should be to preserve length, maintain sensation, mobilize early, return function expediently, and be mindful of cosmesis.

References

[1] Sorock GS, Lombardi DA, Hauser RB, et al. Acute traumatic occupational hand injuries: type, location, and severity. J Occup Environ Med 2002;44(4):345–51.

[2] Browne Jr EZ. Complications of fingertip injuries. Hand Clin 1994;10(1):125–37.

[3] Martin C, González del Pino J. Controversies in the treatment of fingertip amputations: conservative versus surgical reconstruction. Clin Orthop 1998;353:63–73.

[4] Kotwal PP, Gupta V. Neglected tendon and nerve injuries of the hand. Clin Orthop Relat Res 2005;10(431):66–71.

[5] Allen MJ. Conservative management of finger tip injuries in adults. Hand 1980;12(3):257–65.

[6] Evans DM, Bernardis C. A new classification for fingertip injuries. J Hand Surg [Br] 2000; 25(1):58–60.

[7] Muneuchi G, Tamai M, Kazuhiko I, et al. The PNB classification for treatment of fingertip injuries: the boundary between conservative treatment and surgical treatment. Ann Plast Surg 2005;54(6):604–9.

[8] Zienowicz RJ. Fingertip injuries. In: Weinzweig J, editor. Plastic surgery secrets. Philadelphia: Hanley & Belfus; 1999. p. 501–6.

[9] Andrades PR, Olguin FA, Calderon W. Digital blocks with or without epinephrine [comment]. Plast Reconstr Surg 2003;111(5):1769–70.

[10] Wilhelmi BJ, Blackwell SJ, Miller JH, et al. Do not use epinephrine in digital blocks: myth or truth? Plast Reconstr Surg 2001;107(2):393–7.

[11] Shestak KC. Fingertip injuries. In: Greco R, editor. Emergency plastic surgery. New York: Little Brown & Company; 1991. p. 89–99.

[12] Frandsen PA. V-Y plasty as treatment of finger tip amputations. Acta Orthop Scand 1978; 49(3):255–9.

[13] Jackson EA. The V-Y plasty in the treatment of fingertip amputations. Am Fam Physician 2001; 64(3):455–8.

[14] Barbato BD, Guelmi K, Romano SJ, et al. Thenar flap rehabilitated: a review of 20 cases. Ann Plast Surg 1996;37(2):135–9.

[15] Melone Jr CP, Beasley RW, Carstens Jr JH. The thenar flap: an analysis of its use in 150 cases. J Hand Surg [Am] 1982;7(3):291–7.
[16] Nishikawa H, Smith PJ. The recovery of sensation and function after cross-finger flaps for fingertip injury. J Hand Surg [Br] 1992;17(1):102–7.
[17] Kappel DA, Burech JG. The cross-finger flap: an established reconstructive procedure. Hand Clin 1985;1(4):677–83.
[18] Yamada N, Ui K, Uchinuma E. The use of a thin abdominal flap in degloving finger injuries. Br J Plast Surg 2001;54(5):434–8.
[19] Agarwal R, Agarwal S, Chandra R. The lateral pectoral flap. J Hand Surg [Br] 1999 Oct;24(5): 542–6.
[20] Yamano Y. Replantation of fingertips. J Hand Surg [Br] 1993;18(2):157–62.
[21] Lister G. Pitfalls and complications of flexor tendon surgery. Hand Clin 1985;1(1):133–46.
[22] Parkes A. The "lumbrical plus" finger. Hand 1970;2(2):164–5.
[23] Neu BR, Murray JF, MacKenzie JK. Profundus tendon blockage: quadriga in finger amputations. J Hand Surg [Am] 1985;10(6 Pt 1):878–83.
[24] Heistein JB, Cook PA. Factors affecting composite graft survival in digital tip amputations. Ann Plast Surg 2003;50(3):299–303.
[25] Helms A, Brodell RT. Surgical pearl: prompt treatment of subungual hematoma by decompression. J Am Acad Dermatol 2000;42(3):508–9.
[26] Skinner Jr PB. Management of traumatic subungual hematoma. Am Fam Physician 2005; 71(5):856.
[27] Simon RR, Wolgin M. Subungual hematoma: association with occult laceration requiring repair. Am J Emerg Med 1987;5(4):302–4.
[28] Fieg EL. Management of nail bed lacerations. Am Fam Physician 2002;65(10):1997–8.
[29] Roser SE, Gellman H. Comparison of nail bed repair versus nail trephination for subungual hematomas in children. J Hand Surg [Am] 1999;24(6):1166–70.
[30] Trumble TE. Fingertip and nailbed injuries. In: Principles of hand surgery and therapy. Philadelphia: WB Saunders; 2000. p. 192–200.
[31] Suprock MD, Hood JM, Lubahn JD. Role of antibiotics in open fractures of the finger. J Hand Surg [Am] 1990;15(5):761–4.
[32] Handoll HH, Vaghela MV. Interventions for treating mallet finger injuries. Cochrane Database Syst Rev 2004;3:570–4.
[33] Geyman JP, Fink K, Sullivan SD. Conservative versus surgical treatment of mallet finger: a pooled quantitative literature evaluation. J Am Board Fam Pract 1998;11(5):382–90.
[34] Murphy BA, Mass DP. Zone I flexor tendon injuries. Hand Clin 2005;21(2):167–71.

ELSEVIER
SAUNDERS

Clin Occup Environ Med
5 (2) 423–433

CLINICS IN
OCCUPATIONAL AND
ENVIRONMENTAL
MEDICINE

Work-Related Burns

Valerie M. Pruitt, MD, MAJ, USAF, MC

General/Trauma Surgery, Surgical Critical Care, Keesler USAF Medical Center, 81st MSGS/SGCQ, 301 Fisher Street, Room 1A132, Keesler Air Force Base, MS 39534-2519, USA

Burns sustained while performing employment duties are relatively common. Rossignol and colleagues [1] showed that 29% of burns that are severe enough to require hospitalization are work related. Burns of the upper extremity may encompass 80% of all patients admitted to a burn unit [2]. The causative agent of the burn and incidence varies by occupation. Regardless of the origin, upper extremity and especially hand burns have the potential to affect dramatically the activities of daily living, ability to perform work-related tasks, and simple social graces. The use and range of motion of the upper extremity are instrumental in allowing one to maintain independence. We rely on the upper extremity to get dressed each day, eat, shake hands for social greetings, and perform occupational duties. Although the hands constitute less than 5% of the body surface area, sequelae of burn injury can lead to minor alterations in normal anatomy with significant dysfunction and permanent disability. All upper extremity burns must be evaluated closely and repetitively, and detailed care plans must be arranged.

Epidemiology

In the Consumer Product Safety Commission's national electronic injury surveillance system, 119 hospitals participated during a 1-year period. The data collected showed that 11,759 burn injuries were treated. Of that total, 38% involved the upper extremities. The data suggested that young adults and infants are most susceptible to hand burns [3].

The opinions and assertions contained herein are the private views of the author and are not to be construed as official policy or position of the United States Government, the Department of Defense, or the Department of the Air Force.

E-mail address: Valerie.pruitt@keesler.af.mil

doi:10.1016/j.coem.2005.11.002 ***occmed.theclinics.com***

Islam and colleagues [4] examined West Virginia's state-administered workers' compensation insurance database and reported that the annual incidence rate of occupational burn was 26.4 per 10,000 workers. Among female workers, burns of the wrist and hand were the most common. For male workers, burns of the eye and adnexa were the most common followed by wrist and hand burns. Most wrist and hand burns were caused by hot liquids or objects. When compared with other occupations, welders, laborers, cooks, food service workers, and mechanics had a higher incidence of burn injury [4].

Initial evaluation and classification

Many upper extremity burns are part of a larger burn surface area. Initial assessment of the injured patient entails providing systemic support, with airway, breathing, and circulation assessed and stabilized. Particular attention to the airway is important when examination or history indicate an inhalation injury. An intravenous catheter may be necessary, and appropriate crystalloid resuscitation should be administered. One commonly used formula is 24 hours fluid volume = (4 mL lactated Ringer's solution) × (body weight in kg) × (% total body surface area burn). Half of the calculated volume is given in the first 8 hours from time of burn and the next half is given over the remaining 16 hours [5]. All involved clothing should be removed to stop any further thermal injury. All jewelry should be removed because it can cause a tourniquet effect on a hand or finger. Tetanus status should be reviewed and appropriate immunization administered. The burn must be evaluated, with documentation of depth of injury to the skin over each specific anatomic location. Each upper extremity constitutes 9% of total body surface area, with the hand being approximately 2.5% of that 9%. Accuracy of prediction of burn depth is difficult based on a single observation. A burn is a dynamic process and may change over the course of the first days. Less than 50% of the time, the depth and body surface area measurements remain unchanged with repeat examination [6,7].

Thickness of the skin of the hand and a patient's age and gender must be considered while accessing the depth of a burn. Young patients have thin skin over their entire body, and at approximately age 5 it equals adult thickness. In the older population, dermal atrophy begins at approximately age 50 and leads to thinner skin throughout the body [6]. The skin of the hand itself differs from palmer to dorsal surface. Palmer skin is thicker, hairless, without pigment, and relatively nonmobile because of fibrous septae that anchor it to the underlying fascia. The dorsal hand skin is thin, haired, pigmented, and mobile. There is also minimal soft tissue between the dermis and extensor tendons.

The history and clinical examination determine the depth of the burn because no satisfactory objective test is readily available and easy to use. The depth depends on the thickness of the skin, heat dissipating capability of the skin, duration of contact with the burn source, and actual heat of the burn source [6]. Once the individual is stabilized, the burned upper extremity must be elevated.

Nonocclusive dressings are recommended. Repeat examinations are warranted to assess for any evidence of impaired circulation and possible need for escharotomy, which is of particular importance for circumferential burns. The hand must be splinted in the intrinsic plus position [8].

Burns are classified into four basic groups as discussed. Superficial partial-thickness burns involve the epidermis to a depth of the dermal papillae [9]. The burn appears shiny pink to bright red and wet. It blanches with pressure because the papillary vascular plexus is intact and vasodilated. Blisters may be present. Light touch and temperature changes cause pain because sensation to pinprick is preserved. The burn usually heals in 10 to 14 days spontaneously with no scarring [10]. Deep partial-thickness burns involve the epidermis and dermis but epidermal appendages (eg, hair follicles, sweat and sebaceous glands) are spared. These burns appear waxy white or pale pink and edematous. They feel soft and elastic and blisters are present [9]. Pressure is usually the only recognizable sensation. Healing can take up to 6 weeks [11] and is initiated from viable cells in deep skin adnexae with scarring [10]. Full-thickness burns destroy the epidermis, the dermis, and the epidermal appendages. These burns appear pale white to brown/black, with the eschar dry and leathery to the touch [9]. The area is insensate, so pain is minimal if present. The wound heals slowly by epithelial ingrowth from the margins [10], which leaves a scar with a definite risk of contracture [12]. Fourth-degree burns involve deep structures, such as tendons, muscle, bone, or joint space. They are difficult to manage and often require amputation or flap coverage.

Box 1. Burns that should be referred to a burn unit

- Partial-thickness burns more than 10% total body surface area
- Burns that involve the face, hands, feet, genitalia, perineum, or major joints
- Full-thickness burns in any age group
- Electrical burns, including lightning injury
- Chemical burns
- Inhalation injury
- Burn injury in patients with pre-existing medical disorders that could complicate management, prolong recovery, or affect mortality
- Burn injury in patients who require special social, emotional, or long-term rehabilitative intervention

Data from Committee on Trauma, American College of Surgeons. Resources for optimal care of the injured patient. 1999. Chicago: American College of Surgeons; 1998.

Of special note, scald full-thickness burns appear red instead of the more typical white. This appearance is from hemoglobin that has been fixed within the skin when the burn was sustained [9].

The American College of Surgeons committee on trauma recommends that burns listed in Box 1 be referred to a burn unit.

Thermal burns

Thermal burns can be caused by hot liquids, flames, hot surfaces, and electricity. Immediate immersion in cool water can decrease the depth of the burn and provide analgesia. Scalds have varying depths of burn within the same area depending on the length of time the hot liquid was in contact with the skin. Flash burns by nature may look concerning but are usually superficial unless the ignited clothing was extinguished by beating it with a hand. Flame burns can be some of the most serious hand burns and are generally full thickness [13]. Regardless of the heat source of the burned upper extremity, the most important factors in treatment are escharotomy/fasciotomy if indicated, dressings that help minimize infection and allow range of motion, appropriate splinting, early excision and grafting, and hand therapy.

Circulation of the burned upper extremity must be evaluated from the shoulder to the fingertips. Brachial, radial, and ulnar pulses are examined. Notation of rapid capillary refill, pink/warm digits, and Doppler pulsatile flow in the palmer arch and digital vessels confirms adequate circulation. For extensive, deep, partial- and full-thickness burns, the circulation should be re-evaluated continuously. Always look for signs of a compartment syndrome.

Full-thickness burned skin is nonpliable. The dermis, which contains the elastin fibers, is destroyed. The burned skin acts as a restrictive barrier, and as the area becomes edematous it can cause a tourniquet effect if circumferential. After a burn, the edema continues to progress and becomes maximal at 36 hours after injury [14]. This potential tourniquet effect can lead to poor circulation around the wound and distal structures. Any indications of poor circulation warrant an escharotomy. In a well-defined full-thickness burn that is circumferential on admission, an escharotomy may be performed as a preventive measure before circulatory alterations are noted. The incision does not affect future management because the skin must be excised. Escharotomy is especially important to consider if a lengthy transport for the individual is required to the definitive medical treatment center.

Escharotomy is a full-thickness incision through the eschar to expose the subcutaneous fat. The goal is to maintain perfusion and preserve nerve function. The procedure may be performed at the bedside if necessary. Local anesthesia or intravenous sedation is administered. The incision is made through the burned skin into the subcutaneous fat. The incision extends the entire length of the circumferential wound onto partial-thickness burned or unburned skin proximally and distally. With the upper extremity in the anatomic position, the incisions on the forearm are on the anterior ulnar and radial sides and continue parallel distally. The elbow should be crossed if indicated, with the ulnar incision anterior to the medial epicondyle to avoid the ulnar nerve. The wrist should be incised onto the thenar and hypothenar eminences. The hand incisions are placed dorsally between the metacarpal bones. Finger escharotomies are placed on the midlateral line on the ulnar side of the digit. The incision should be placed to avoid the neurovascular bundle and extend from the web space to the distal phalanx. A second incision on the radial side of the digit may be required if adequate circulation is not achieved with a unilateral incision.

Fasciotomy is sometimes required for full-thickness burns that involve the muscle or electrical injuries. A fasciotomy is an incision through skin, subcutaneous tissue, and the fascia to relieve the pressure within the muscular compartment. A fasciotomy is performed for elevated compartment pressure (ie, compartment syndrome) [14]. This procedure should be performed in the operating room.

Dressings and topical creams

Dressings should protect the wound from desiccation and infection. They should be simple to allow easy dressing changes, encourage patient compliance, and enable continued use of the extremity for range-of-motion purposes. Various topical creams can be used on burn wounds. Single, double, or triple antibiotic ointments are acceptable for superficial thickness burns that will heal without intervention and smaller burns when a serious infection is not a concern. For deeper burns or more extensive burns, the options include silver sulphadiazine, mafenide, and 0.5% silver nitrate.

Silver sulfadiazine is one of the most widely used creams. It is easy to apply and readily available. Treatment with silver sulfadiazine does have the side effect of potential leukopenia during the first week. This condition is transient, resolves with discontinuation of the cream, and does not recur with repeat application [15,16]. Mafenide has antibacterial activity that is particularly effective against pseudomonas and enterococcus [16]. It penetrates burn wound eschars. Mafenide may cause a metabolic acidosis and increase respiratory minute ventilation when applied to large surface areas [15]. It can be painful with application. 0.5% silver nitrate provides good antimicrobial coverage [16]. It is cumbersome to apply because it stains black anything with which it comes into contact. Electrolyte wasting may occur with its use.

Some newer dressings that are especially designed for hand burns may be of benefit over the standard gauze in extensive hand burns. The dressings are made into a glove and include Biobrane (Dow B Hickman, Sugarland, Texas) and GoreTex (WL Gore and Associates, Flagstaff, Arizona). Biobrane is available as a glove that is applied after the wound has been cleansed. It takes approximately 1 day to adhere. No further dressings are needed, and the individual may participate in aggressive therapy. It is not intended for deep burns, and the wounds under the membrane continue to require close observation for signs of potential infection [17]. GoreTex gloves are applied over a thin layer of silver sulfadiazine and provide an impermeable barrier to water yet semi-permeable barrier to water vapor. The glove allows range-of-motion therapy. The dressing must be changed once daily, and the glove can be washed and reused [17].

In summary, for thermal burns the treatment depends on the depth of burn. Superficial partial-thickness burns require local wound care and early therapy for range of motion. Analgesic medications may be needed depending on the extent of burn and individual patient characteristics. Deep partial-thickness burns should be evaluated by a specialist. Certain circumstances and locations may be managed with local wound care. The timeline for surgical intervention varies but usually falls within a 2- to 3-week period [2]. Full-thickness burns require surgical intervention in most instances. Circumferential burns are highly susceptible to circulation alterations, and escharotomy may be warranted early in the individuals care before transport.

Electrical burns

Electrical burns have a different pathology from that seen with thermal burns. The electrical injury can be categorized as high voltage (>1000 V) and low voltage (<1000 V). The actual amount of current that passes through tissue is the amperage, but this measurement is not independent, so volts are used for classification [18]. Electrical injuries have a point of contact with an entrance site and transmit through the body to a grounded site. They present a difficult diagnostic dilemma. The cutaneous wound does not reflect the degree of injury to deeper structures. The hand and upper extremities are the most frequent sites of entry [19].

Initial first-line management does not differ from thermal burns, except electrocardiograph monitoring should be initiated to access for any electrically induced arrhythmias. Accurate assessment of the electrical wound on the upper extremity changes with time. The initial electrical current affects tissue types differently secondary to their respective resistance properties [20]. Necrosis of tissue can occur from devascularization caused by injury to blood vessels. The necrosis can progress for 4 to 5 days and is often most severe near the entrance and exit site and along bone [18]. This deeper injury to muscle can cause myoglobinuria and hemoglobinuria with nephrotoxic effects [21]. The need for fasciotomy of the upper extremity is more common with high-voltage burns. The muscles within the fascial compartment can be injured, which leads to increased swelling and compartment syndrome.

A thorough neurologic examination should be performed early in the post-electrical injury and repeated persistently. Delayed degeneration of small sized blood vessels within the spinal cord days after injury can lead to resultant permanent localized paresis to quadriplegia [20]. Electrical burns often require extensive débridement of damaged tissues as an emergency. Amputation rates are reported to occur in 26% to 65% of cases [18].

Chemical burns

Chemicals are used daily in industry. Chemical products that can cause a cutaneous burn number more than 25,000 [22]. The upper extremities and especially the hands are susceptible because many of the chemicals are found in cleaning agents. The major determinant of the extent of injury is the duration of contact with the skin and the agent. Treatment is initially based on limiting the chemical contact to stop the burn process.

Once a chemical burn is suspected, all affected clothing must be removed and immediate water lavage at the scene must be initiated if possible. For acid burns, up to 2 hours of water lavage is recommended [23]; alkali burns may require up to 12 hours [22]. Low-pressure shower lavage is preferred to tub immersion secondary to the chemical runoff in the water. Delay in irrigation can lead to a more extensive injury. A delay of just a few minutes for initiation of irrigation after a chemical contact may allow the epidermis to be destroyed. Blisters and necrotic tissue are debrided because they may contain residual chemical agents [22].

Some chemicals require specific therapies. Oxidizing agents, such as sodium hypochlorite, chromic acid, and potassium permanganate, can coagulate protein and cause severe irritation. Milk, egg whites, or milk of magnesia may be used initially before copious irrigation [22,23]. Reducing agents, such as hydrochloric acid, alkyl mercury agents, and nitric acid, should be neutralized with soap, soda lime, or magnesium hydroxide before lavage [22,23].

White phosphorus burns can be seen after explosions. Phosphorous is used to make fireworks and military weapons and is used in the illegal manufacture of methamphetamines. The phosphorus particles are oxidized by air as they shower the skin. The particles must be removed manually. Initial treatment involves irrigating once, quickly, with a dilute 1% to 3% solution of copper sulfate and then proceeding with water lavage. The copper sulfate allows identification and débridement of the phosphorous by staining it black [22].

In industry, phenols are used for plastics, organic polymers, cleaning agents, and cosmetics. Phenol is also used for chemical face peels and nerve ablation injections. Phenol is not water soluble [23]. Therapy consists of wiping the skin with undiluted polyethylene glycol 300 or 400 immediately [23,24]. Phenol is quickly absorbed by the skin and can lead to nephropathy [23].

Elemental sodium, potassium, and lithium are found in burning metal fragments. Use of water for irrigation is contraindicated because it causes these substances to ignite spontaneously and intensify the burn. To extinguish the burning metal, sand or a class D fire extinguisher should be used. The burn is covered with mineral oil or a cooking oil to isolate the metal from water. The metal fragments are removed and only then is copious lavage applied. After appropriate initial decontamination and water lavage of chemical injuries, burns are assessed for severity of depth. Treatment principles are similar to those for thermal injuries.

Hydrofluoric acid burns

Hydrofluoric acid is used widely in industry and research facilities. Occupational uses are ubiquitous and include glassware and ceramic industries, semiconductor industries, and treatment of textiles [25–27]. The manufacturing of insecticides, fertilizers, solvents, dyes, plastics, refrigerant fluids, and high octane fuels also involve hydrofluoric acid [25]. Anhydrous hydrofluoric acid is the purified form and has a concentration of more than 99%. Aqueous hydrofluoric acid is the more dilute form and is a colorless liquid [25].

Hydrofluoric acid burns can be deceiving based on clinical inspection. With dilute solutions and small parts of the body surface involved, the burn can be minor. Tepperman [28] reported a case of mortality 10 hours after a 2.5% body surface area burn with 70% hydrofluoric acid. The reason for this chemical being so lethal is secondary to electrolyte imbalances. Hydrofluoric acid causes a mild caustic burn to the skin it contacts, but the surface destruction is less than equimolar solutions of hydrochloric and sulfuric acids [25]. Hydrofluoric acid readily crosses lipid membranes, which allows it to diffuse in the subcutaneous tissues and release the freely dissociable fluoride ion [25]. This ion produces severe toxicity by complexing primarily with calcium and magnesium to form insoluble salts [27,29], which interferes with calcium metabolism in the soft and bony tissues and results in cell destruction and severe pain [27]. Systemic toxicity is manifested mainly by severe hypocalcemia and, less dramatically, hypomagnesemia. If not recognized and treated immediately, electrolyte imbalance can lead to cardiac arrhythmias and asystole.

Major hydrofluoric acid burns are defined in Box 2 and are associated with possible electrolyte imbalances that result in severe systemic abnormalities.

Digits and subungual tissue are the most frequent injury sites. The clinical presentation varies, depending on the concentration of the hydrofluoric acid, duration contact, and route of exposure (ie, contact with skin or ocular, inhalation, or ingestion) [25]. In 1943, the National Institute of Health separated exposures to hydrofluoric acid into three categories. Solutions with less than 20% concentration may not produce symptoms for 24 hours. Twenty percent to 50% concentrations produce burns that are apparent usually within 1 to 8 hours. More than 50% concentrations produce immediate tissue destruction and pain [25].

First-line therapy involves immediate, copious irrigation of the exposed area. Remove any clothing/work articles that may have had acid contact. The length of time for optimal hydrotherapy is debated but seems to be approximately 20 minutes [25]. Persons who assist with the care of a new hydrofluoric acid burn should use self-protection (eg, nonabsorbent gloves, eye protection, and plastic aprons) to avoid contamination.

After irrigation, the burn must be assessed. If the burn meets any of the criteria from Box 1, immediate transfer to an emergency department is warranted. For minor burns, topical treatment is the next line of therapy after water irrigation. Calcium gel, 2.5%, is the most widely used agent [30]. If the commercial product is not available it can be prepared extemporaneously by mixing 3.5 g calcium

Box 2. Hydrofluoric acid burns with a high risk of developing lethal electrolyte imbalances

1% body surface area burn with anhydrous hydrofluoric acid
5% body surface area burn with >70% concentrated hydrofluoric acid
7% body surface area burn with 50%–70% concentrated hydrofluoric acid
10% body surface area burn with 20%–50% concentrated hydrofluoric acid
20% body surface area burn with <20% concentrated hydrofluoric acid
Prolonged exposure or long delay for treatment in minor hydrofluoric acid burns
Ingestion of hydrofluoric acid at concentrations >5%
Inhalation of hydrofluoric acid at concentrations >5%

From Dunser MW. Critical care management of major hydrofluoric acid burns: a case report, review of the literature, and recommendations for therapy. Burns 2004;30:392; with permission.

gluconate powder with a 5-oz tube of water-soluble surgical lubricant. The gel should be massaged into the skin for at least 30 minutes [25] up to several hours [31]. Pain relief is the clinical goal, which is secondary to inactivation of the free fluoride ion with the calcium. The therapy should be recommenced if pain returns. Uncontrollable or nonrelenting pain is a clinical marker of potentially deeper, more serious burns. Local anesthesia should not be used because it may mask the pain perception. A surgical glove can be used as a dressing over the gel in hand burns [27,32,33]. Chemical exposure around finger beds can cause subungual pain. The nail bed must be treated and may require nail removal [26,27].

Infiltration of the area with calcium gluconate is recommended for exposures to hydrofluoric acid concentrations more than 20% [34] or if one of the following two criteria are met: (1) throbbing, severe pain or (2) burns with a central, hard gray area with surrounding erythema [35]. The subcutaneous tissue beneath the burn is injected using a 27- or 30-gauge needle from peripheral sites, instilling a dose of 0.5 mL of 10% calcium gluconate per cm^2 [36]. After placement of the needle, the calcium solution is slowly injected while continuously withdrawing the needle. A 5% calcium gluconate concentration also can be used in an attempt to avoid irritation to the tissues and prevent possible keloids from the higher concentrations [34]. Infiltration is not recommended for the digits to avoid producing edema and increasing compartment pressures [34]. Calcium chloride cannot be substituted for calcium gluconate [29].

For more extensive burns, intra-arterial calcium infusions are used to inactivate fluoride ions regionally from hydrofluoric acid. This approach is especially useful in digit and hand burns, in which subcutaneous injection should be avoided [37]. Intravenous regional calcium gluconate recently was demonstrated to be as effective as intra-arterial infusions [38,39]. In some circumstances that involve high-concentration exposures, prompt excision of the area is warranted [25].

Summary

Work-related upper extremity burns often occur. The cause directs the course of action. Thermal burns should be assessed for system alterations, and depth of burn should be determined. Deep partial-thickness burns and more severe burns require a specialist evaluation. Chemical burns must be irrigated and the agent identified. Some chemical burns, such as those that involve phenols and metal fragments, require specific topical applications before water lavage. Hydrofluoric acid burns can cause life-threatening electrolyte abnormalities with a small, highly concentrated acid burn. The goal with any extremity burn is to provide the patient with a multidisciplinary team approach to achieve a functional, useable extremity.

References

[1] Rossignol AM, Locke JA, Boyle CM, et al. Epidemiology of work-related burn injuries in Massachusetts requiring hospitalization. J Trauma 1986;26:1097–101.
[2] Luce EA. The acute and subacute management of the burned hand. Clin Plast Surg 2000;27(1): 49–63.
[3] Pruitt BA. Epidemiology and general considerations. In: Salisbury RD, editor. Burns of the upper extremity. Philadelphia: WB Saunders; 1976. p. 11–5.
[4] Islam SS, Nambiar AM, Doyle EJ, et al. Epidemiology of work-related burn injuries: experience of a state-managed workers' compensation system. J Trauma 2000;49:1045–51.
[5] Armstrong JH. Resuscitation of the burn patient. In: Shatz DV, Kirton OC, McKenney MG, et al, editors. Manual of trauma and emergency surgery. Philadelphia: WB Saunders; 2000. p. 200–9.
[6] Heimbach D, Engrav L, Grube B, et al. Burn depth: a review. World J Surg 1995;16:10–5.
[7] Hlava P, Moserova J, Konigova R. Validity of clinical assessment of the depth of a thermal injury. Acta Chir Plast 1983;25:202.
[8] Tredget EE. Management of the acutely burned upper extremity. Hand Clin 2000;16(2):187–203.
[9] Howell JW. Management of the acutely burned hand for the nonspecialized clinician. Phys Therapy 1989;69(12):1077–90.
[10] Sykes PJ. Severe burns of the hand: a practical guide to their management. J Hand Surg Br 1991;16B(1):6–12.
[11] Yakuboff KP, Kurtzman LC, Stern PJ. Acute management of thermal and electrical burns of the upper extremity. Orthop Clin North Am 1992;23(1):161–9.
[12] Morgan ED, Bedsoe SC, Barker J. Ambulatory management of burns. Am Fam Physician 2000;62(9):2015–32.
[13] Harrison DH, Parkhouse N. Experience with upper extremity burns. Hand Clin 1990;6(2): 191–209.

[14] Wong L, Spence RJ. Escharotomy and fasciotomy of the burned upper extremity. Hand Clin 2000;16(2):165–74.
[15] Monafo WW. Initial management of burns. N Engl J Med 1996;335(21):1581–6.
[16] Wolf SE, Herndon DN. Burns and radiation injuries. In: Moore EE, Feliciano DV, Mattox KL, editors. Trauma. 5th edition. New York: McGraw-Hill; 2004. p. 1088–9.
[17] Logsetty S, Heimbach DM. Modern techniques for wound coverage of the thermally injured upper extremity. Hand Clin 2000;16(2):205–14.
[18] Achauer B, Applebaum R, Vanderkam VM. Electrical burn injury to the upper extremity. J Plast Surg 1994;47:331–40.
[19] Salisbury RE, Dingeldein GP. The burned hand and upper extremity. In: Green DP, editor. Operative hand surgery. 2nd edition. New York: Churchill-Livingstone; 1988. p. 2135–64.
[20] Ko SH, Chun W, Kim HC. Delayed spinal cord injury following electrical burns: a 7-year experience. Burns 2004;30:691–5.
[21] Wright PE. Special hand disorders. In: Canale ST, editor. Campbell's operative orthopaedics. St. Louis: Mosby; 1998. p. 3501–16.
[22] Reilly DA, Garner WL. Management of chemical injuries to the upper extremity. Hand Clin 2000;16(2):215–24.
[23] Bentivegna PE, Deane LM. Chemical burns of the upper extremity. Hand Clin 1990;6(2):253–9.
[24] Stewart CE. Chemical skin burns. Am Fam Pract 1985;31(6):149–57.
[25] Kirkpatrick JJR, Enion OS, Burd DAR. Hydrofluoric acid burns: a review. Burns 1995;21(7): 483–93.
[26] Flood S. Hydrofluoric acid burns. Am Fam Pract 1988;37(3):175–82.
[27] Bertolini JC. Hydrofluoric acid: a review of toxicity. J Emerg Med 1992;10:163–8.
[28] Tepperman PB. Fatality due to acute systemic fluoride poisoning following a hydrofluoric acid skin burn. J Occup Med 1980;22:691–2.
[29] Sheridan RL, Ryan CM, Quinby WC, et al. Emergency management of major hydrofluoric acid exposures. Burns 1995;21(1):62–4.
[30] Bracken WM, Cuppage F, McLaury RL, et al. Comparative effectiveness of topical treatments for hydrofluoric acid burns. J Occup Med 1985;27:733–9.
[31] Browne TD. The treatment of hydrofluoric acid burns. J Soc Occup Med 1974;24:80–9.
[32] Roberts JR, Merigan KS. Acute hydrofluoric acid exposure. Am J Emerg Med 1989;7:125–6.
[33] Bullock C. Hydrofluoric acid burns cooled with calcium carbonate slurry. Emerg Med News 1989;July:17.
[34] Trevino MA, Herrmann GH, Sprout WL. Treatment of severe hydrofluoric acid exposures. J Occup Med 1983;25(12):861–3.
[35] Paterson JD. Control of the fluorine hazard. Br J Ind Med 1956;16:301–3.
[36] Dibbell DG, Iverson RE, Jones W, et al. Hydrofluoric acid burns of the hand. J Bone Joint Surg Am 1970;52A:931–6.
[37] Dunser MW, Ohlbauer M, Rieder J, et al. Critical care management of major hydrofluoric acid burns: a case report, review of the literature, and recommendations for therapy. Burns 2004;30:391–8.
[38] Graudins A, Burns MJ, Aaron CK. Regional intravenous infusion of calcium gluconate for hydrofluoric acid burns of the upper extremity. Ann Emerg Med 1997;30:604–7.
[39] Henry JA, Hla KK. Intravenous regional calcium gluconate perfusion for hydrofluoric acid burns. Clin Toxicol 1992;30:203–7.

ELSEVIER
SAUNDERS

Clin Occup Environ Med
5 (2) 435–443

CLINICS IN
OCCUPATIONAL AND
ENVIRONMENTAL
MEDICINE

Factitious Disorders

Dean S. Louis, MD[a,*], Christopher Doro, MD[a], Radford J. Hayden, PA-C[a,b]

[a]*Division of Hand Elbow and Microsurgery, Department of Orthopaedic Surgery, University of Michigan Medical Center, 2098 South Main Street, Ann Arbor, MI 48103, USA*
[b]*College of Health Professions, Physician Assistant Studies, University of Detroit Mercy, PO Box 19900, Detroit, MI 48219-0900, USA*

Most patients who present for medical care have a bona fide concern about their health status. They have experienced symptoms such as pain or a change in function (ie, weight loss, fatigue, loss of function, loss of appetite) that have prompted the consultation. In the usual course, a diagnosis is rendered, and treatment is undertaken. Most of the time a happy outcome can be expected. There are times, however, when a person presents to a physician and has made a conscious but nonverbalized decision to be ill and become a patient. Such individuals are the subject of this article. They have factitious disorders and are seen with various recognizable presentations [1,2].

History

The psychiatric literature is full of reports of various forms of self-mutilation, including delicate self-cutting [3], auto-amputation of various body parts [4], and even attempted surgery upon oneself. Individuals who behave in such fashion are not in touch with reality and are not trying to hide anything. In contrast to this noncovert injurious behavior, there is a contrasting group of patients who try to hide the origins of their presenting infirmity. Although past psychological thought in this area referred to subconscious motivations to explain such patients'

* Corresponding author.
E-mail address: dslouis@med.umich.edu (D.S. Louis).

doi:10.1016/j.coem.2005.11.016 ***occmed.theclinics.com***

denial of knowledge of the cause, current thought has changed. In its 1994 manual, the American Psychiatric Association considers malingering and factitious disorders to be conscious attempts (efforts) by individuals so involved [5].

Definitions

Malingering

Malingering is the intentional reporting of nonexistent signs or symptoms for secondary gain. The gain may be for emotional reasons, to avoid a task, or for monetary or other gain, such as drugs. These individuals are feigning illness [6–8].

Factitious disorders

A factitious disorder is a self-created problem (ie, a nonhealing wound) that is totally created by the person involved. A person so afflicted is causing disease. Unlike a malingerer, who pretends to have a disease, people with factitious illness have and are causing disease [9–12].

Differential considerations

Many conditions may mimic factitious disorders. Malingering has been mentioned, but the fine line of the presence or absence of disease separates these two enities clearly [6,7]. For dysfunctional syndromes, various painful and painless dysfunction syndromes may be confused with factitious illness [13,14]. Reflex sympathetic dystrophy is covered elsewhere in this issue. It is currently considered under the category of complex regional pain syndrome (CRPS), type I. The major distinction between CRPS and factitious disorders is the presence and relative absence of pain in the two conditions, respectively. The hallmark of CRPS is pain, and it is the dominant presenting symptom [14]. Factitious illnesses generally present with a dysfunctional posture, but pain is not the major presenting issue.

A large problem is caused when the diagnosis of a factitious disorder is not made (or considered) and another label is applied (eg, CRPS). If a patient with a factitious disorder is given a label (CRPS) and offered treatment (eg, a stellate ganglion block), then the entire situation becomes mired with the inappropriate treatment for the wrong diagnosis. How confusing can this be to patients, who seek illness behavior and have their self-inflicted problems sanctified by a doctor's inappropriate diagnosis [15]? There are recognizable patterns of dysfunction. Current teaching must extend to the point that all physicians are aware of these subtle nuances. The wrong diagnosis, followed by the wrong treatment, may have devastating consequences. This is perhaps most well known as the nocebo effect, which essentially occurs when a person who manifests illness behavior is given a label such as CRPS, which reinforces their behavior [16–19].

Acknowledged patterns of factitious illness

Several patterns of behavior result in characteristic postures of the upper extremity that are so recognizable as to be almost pathognomonic of the condition.

Factitious lymphedema

The edematous limb that results from this behavior is characteristic. There is a circumferential line just proximal to the area where the edema is. The limb distal to this point is markedly edematous. As is usual in these circumstances, the patient denies knowledge of a cause for the problem. In his classic article in 1975, Richard Smith [20] talked about making early "rounds" and finding a tourniquet about the involved arm in which there was distal lymphedema. Figs. 1 and 2 graphically display the typical indentations found on the forearm and leg, respectively, of patients who caused the observed lymphedema. Other authors also have recognized this condition [1,2,21].

Factitious ulcers

Any wound that does not heal—surgical or otherwise—should be considered the possible result of wound manipulation [10]. The extent of such manipulation may range from a small cutaneous ulcer (Fig. 3) to multiple ulcers (Fig. 4). We have seen extensive areas on the dorsum of the forearm that remained in an excoriated state because of self-manipulation.

The clenched fist and other dysfunctional postures

Patients sometimes present with their fingers tightly clenched into their palm or palms. In the classic presentation, the thumb and index finger are spared, whereas the ulnar three digits are tightly flexed (Fig. 5) [22]. The variations of this form of posturing are endless, including adduction of the thumb only with the fingers spared, extension of the thumb alone, scissoring of the fingers (Fig. 6), extension posturing of one digit (Fig. 7), and even the combination of adduction of the thumb and flexion of the index finger (Fig. 8).

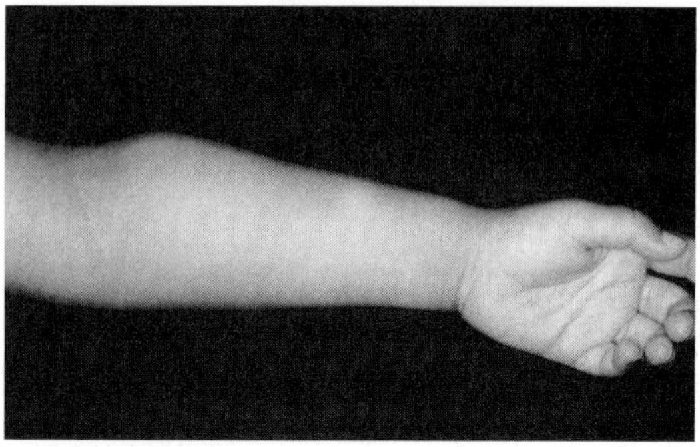

Fig. 1. The woman whose forearm and hand are depicted presented with swelling of the forearm and hand. The area in which the tourniquet was applied at the elbow is obvious. (© Dr. Dean S. Louis, MD, Ann Arbor, MI.)

The SHAFT syndrome

In 1978, Wallace and Fitzmorris [23] reported on their experience with an entity that they described with the acronym SHAFT. These patients were described as Sad, Hostile, Anxious, Frustrating, and Tenacious. They usually had a history of multiple operations by various other surgeons and reported bad results from all. They usually presented with seductive entreaties such as "You are my

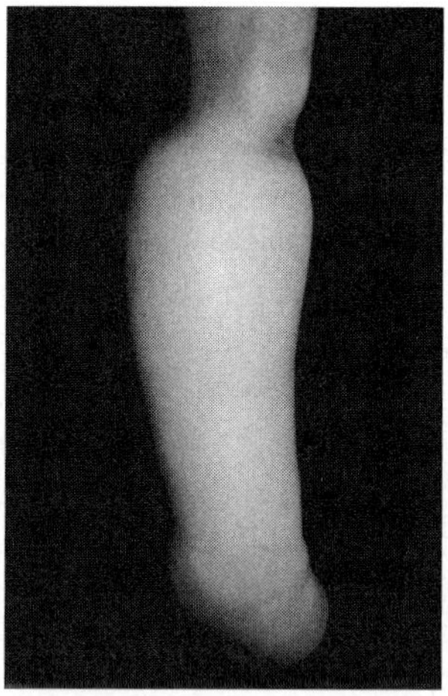

Fig. 2. This is the right lower extremity of a 15-year-old girl. She presented with an edematous limb. When she was placed in a hip spica that elevated her leg, the swelling rapidly receded. She prevailed upon her parents to have the cast taken off. The area in which the tourniquet was applied is obvious. She ultimately underwent an above-knee amputation. After that, similar problems developed in her remaining limbs. (© Dr. Dean S. Louis, MD, Ann Arbor, MI.)

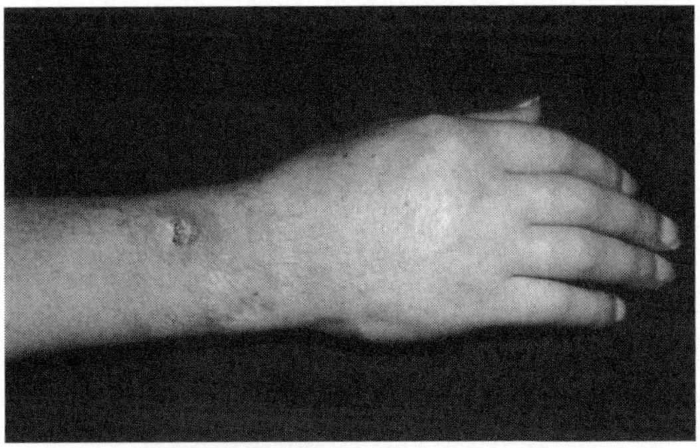

Fig. 3. This figure depicts an ulcer that would not heal in a man who said he had sustained an injury at work. The crater of the ulcer was painted with fluorescein dye, and a light but bulky dressing was applied. The next morning an ultraviolet light focused on his other hand showed fluorescence of the finger nails as a result of wound manipulation. (© Dr. Dean S. Louis, MD, Ann Arbor, MI.)

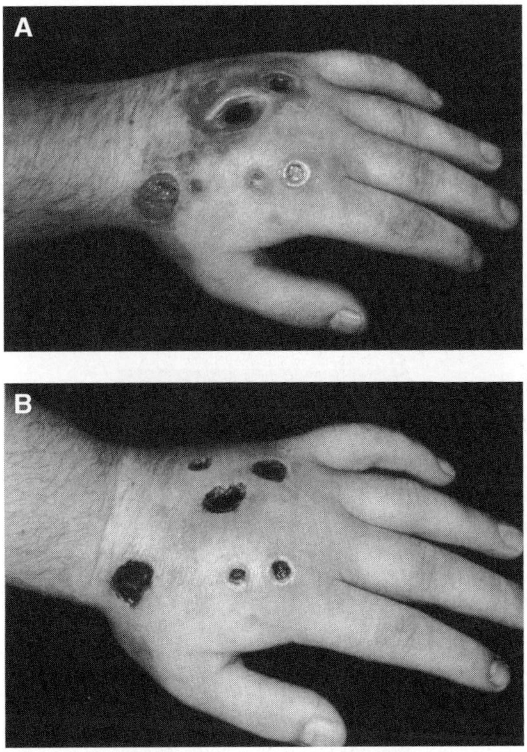

Fig. 4. (*A,B*) This is the left hand of a young man who had sustained a trivial trauma at work that did not break the skin. He denied any knowledge of the cause of the lesions. It was assumed that these were cigarette burns, and he was placed in a cast. Two weeks after the cast was applied it was removed. All of the previous wounds had healed. Two weeks after this picture was taken, he returned with the lesions weeping again. Psychiatric care was recommended. (© Dr. Dean S. Louis, MD, Ann Arbor, MI.)

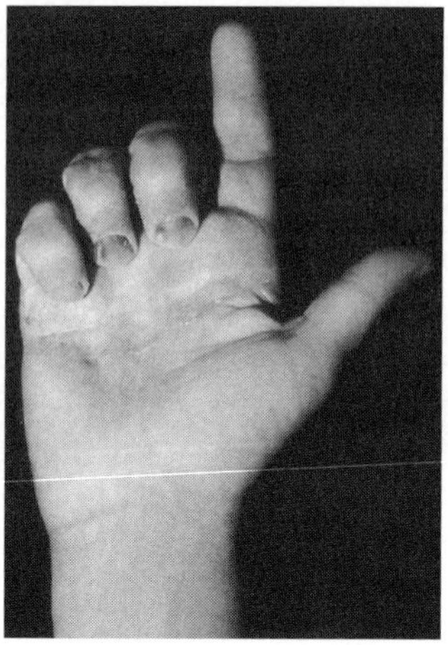

Fig. 5. This is the right hand of a young woman who initially presented with lymphedema and then converted to this posture. At long-term follow-up, this condition had been maintained for 8 years. (© Dr. Dean S. Louis, MD, Ann Arbor, MI.)

last hope" and "Everyone says you are the best." Postoperatively, another tune plays: "You did not tell me it would be this bad" or "I should not have let you do this to me." Recognition of patient history in this regard is critical because it is a lose-lose situation. Nothing but grief comes from patients so encumbered, and surgery is not an answer.

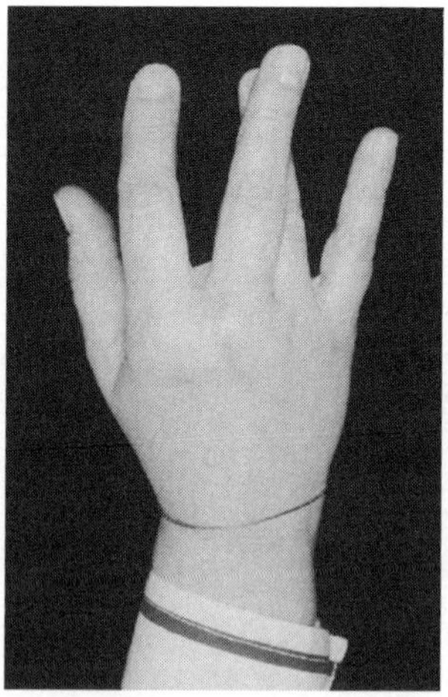

Fig. 6. This is the right hand of a woman who mysteriously developed overlapping of her fingers. Electromyography demonstrated an electrical pattern in the interosseous muscles consistent with sustained voluntary contractures. (© Dr. Dean S. Louis, MD, Ann Arbor, MI.)

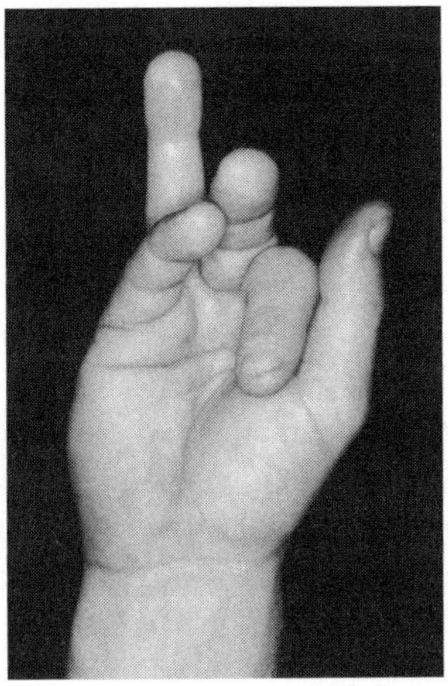

Fig. 7. This is the right hand of a Viet Nam veteran who was making a claim for Agent Orange exposure, which was granted. He underwent biofeedback, and the posture resolved. He was seen again 15 years later, and had resumed the posture seen. He was never gainfully employed. (© Dr. Dean S. Louis, MD, Ann Arbor, MI.)

Differential diagnosis

The patterns described herein are easily recognizable once one has had sufficient experience. That seems to be a great problem because many physicians are unwilling to accept such diagnoses, although there is abundant literature about these afflictions. It may be that these problems are not addressed in medical school and residency. At the time of this writing, 1908 references were available

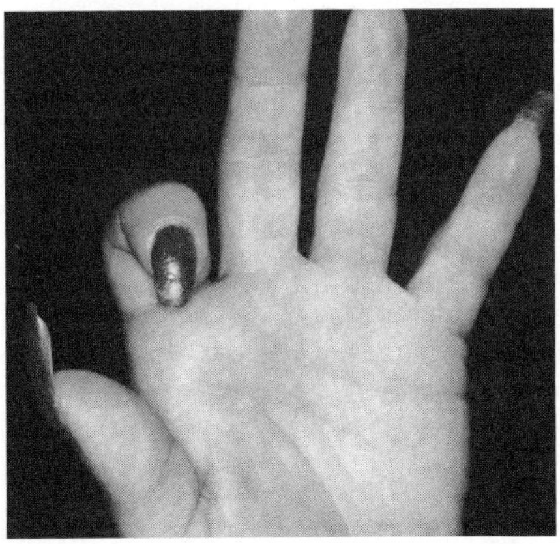

Fig. 8. This is the left hand of a woman who denied any significant antecedent history. Her thumb adducted and her index finger flexed mysteriously. When asked to attempt to straighten out, extend, and abduct the fingers, there was a palpable co-contraction of her flexor and extensor muscles. (© Dr. Dean S. Louis, MD, Ann Arbor, MI.)

by a quick computer search. Unfortunately, we have seen patients who have undergone amputations for problems that were clearly factitious but were misdiagnosed (see Fig. 2).

Summary

Factitious disorders are real clinical entities. An awareness of the patterns of presentation and of the important differential conditions should lead to appropriate subsequent management, which includes psychiatric consultation [12]. There is an abundant literature regarding these conditions. Feldman and Ford [24] addressed these issues at length in their book "Patient or Pretender." They have included extensive case histories that illustrate to what extent patients will go to simulate illness.

References

[1] Louis DS. Recognizable dysfunction syndromes. Hand Clin 1993;9:213–20.
[2] Louis DS, Lamp MK, Greene TL. The upper extremity and psychiatric illness. J Hand Surg [Am] 1985;10:687–93.
[3] Pho PN. The syndrome of delicate self cutting. Br J Med Psychol 1969;42:195–206.
[4] Bensiers JM, Paauw DS. Apotemnophilia masquerading as medical morbidity. Del Med J 2003; 96(7):674–6.
[5] American Psychiatric Association. Diagnostic and statistical manual of mental disorders. 4th edition. Washington, DC: American Psychiatric Association; 2000.
[6] LoPiccolo CJ, Goodkin K, Baldewicz TT. Current issues in the diagnosis and management of malingering. Ann Med 1999;31:166–74.
[7] Hall HV, Pritchard DA. Detecting malingering and deception. Boca Raton (FL): St. Lucie Press; 1996.
[8] Barsky AJ. Forgetting, fabricating, and telescoping. Arch Intern Med 2002;162:981–4.
[9] Hardie TJ, Reed A. Pseudologic fantastica, factitious disorder, and impostership: a deception syndrome. Med Sci Law 1998;38:198–201.
[10] Phelps DB, Buchler U, Boswick JA. The diagnosis of factitious ulcer of the hand: a case report. J Hand Surg [Am] 1977;2:105–8.
[11] Al-Qattan MM. Factitious disorders of the upper limb in Saudi Arabia. J Hand Surg [Br] 2001; 26:414–21.
[12] Grunert BK, Sanger JR, Matloub HS, et al. Classification system for factitious syndromes in the hand with implications for treatment. J Hand Surg [Am] 1991;16:1027–30.
[13] Dobyns JH. Pain dysfunction syndrome. In: Gelberman R, editor. Operative nerve repair. Philadelphia: JB Lippincott; 1991. p. 1489–94.
[14] Cooney WP, Schuind F, editors. Upper extremity pain dysfunction: somatic and sympathetic disorders. Hand Clin 1997;13(3):319–526.
[15] Stutts JT, Kasdan ML, Hickey SE, et al. Reflex sympathetic dystrophy misdiagnosis in patients with dysfunctional postures of the upper extremity. J Hand Surg Am 2000;25:1152–6.
[16] Benson H. The nocebo effect: history and physiology. Prev Med 1997;26:612–5.
[17] Kasdan ML, Lewis K, Bruner A, et al. The nocebo effect: do no harm. J South Orthop Assoc 1999;8:108–13.
[18] Hahn RA. The nocebo phenomenon: concept, evidence, and implications for public health. Prev Med 1997;26:607–11.

[19] Schweiger A, Parducci A. Nocebo: the psychologic induction of pain. Pavlov J Biol Sci 1981;16:140–5.
[20] Smith RJ. Factitious lymphedema of the hand. J Bone Joint Surg Am 1975;57:89–94.
[21] Reading G. Secretan's syndrome: hard edema of the dorsum of the hand. Plast Reconstr Surg 1980;65:182–7.
[22] Simmons BP, Vasile RG. The clenched fist syndrome. J Hand Surg [Am] 1980;5:420–7.
[23] Wallace PF, Fitzmorris CF. The S-H-A-F-T syndrome in the upper extremity. J Hand Surg [Am] 1978;3:492–8.
[24] Feldman MD, Ford CV. Patient or pretender. New York: John Wiley & Sons; 1994.

ELSEVIER
SAUNDERS

Clin Occup Environ Med
5 (2) 445–454

CLINICS IN
OCCUPATIONAL AND
ENVIRONMENTAL
MEDICINE

Complex Regional Pain Syndrome Type I in the Upper Extremity

Christopher Doro, MD[a,*], Radford J. Hayden, PA-C[a,b], Dean S. Louis, MD[a]

[a]*Department of Orthopaedic Surgery, University of Michigan Medical Center, 2098 South Main Street, Ann Arbor, MI 48103, USA*
[b]*College of Health Professions, Physician Assistant Studies, University of Detroit Mercy, PO Box 19900, Detroit, MI 48219-0900, USA*

Complex regional pain syndrome (CRPS) refers to a group of neuropathic pain disorders that usually follow a traumatic event. Patients with this diagnosis generally suffer from pain, sensory changes, edema, sweating, and temperature disturbance in the affected limb. Although the exact prevalence of the condition is unclear, a rapid increase in the incidence of reported cases of CRPS has occurred [1]. This increase has been partly caused by the diagnostic criteria put forth in 1994, which lacked specificity [2], and the increased awareness of this condition by personal trial lawyers. A general awareness of this condition is still relatively poor, because an average of 30 months pass and 4.8 different physicians are seen before patients who have CRPS are referred to a pain center for adequate therapy [3]. This article reviews the current literature on CRPS as it pertains to the upper extremity.

Evolution of current nomenclature

The signs and symptoms of what is currently called CRPS were first described in soldiers during the Civil War by Mitchell in 1864. He stated "The irritation of a nerve at the point of wound, might give rise to changes in the circulation and nutrition of parts in its distribution, and that these alterations might be themselves

* Corresponding author.
E-mail address: cdoro@umich.edu (C. Doro).

1526-0046/06/$ – see front matter
doi:10.1016/j.coem.2005.11.006

of a pain producing nature" [4]. He later named this condition "causalgia" [5]. Since its first description, what we currently refer to as CRPS has had multiple names. In 1900, Sudeck [6] described similar symptoms after fractures and is given credit for the first description of this syndrome. Sudeck's syndrome traditionally has referred to spotty or cystic bony atrophy seen with CRPS. The sympathetic nervous system was believed to be involved in CRPS as early as 1916 [7]. Leriche [8] also was of the opinion that sensory fibers that supply peripheral parts of the body may pass through the sympathetic ganglion to reach the cord. Livingston adapted this theory and propagated the idea that the sympathetic nerve fibers were part of a vicious circle in which pain afferents create an abnormal state of activity in the spinal cord gray matter, which results in pain and vasomotor changes [9]. The term "reflex sympathetic dystrophy" (RSD) is credited to Evans [10]. In his article he presented cases in which sympathetic blockage or sympathectomy provided relief and supported a sympathetic etiology. Many alternate terms, in addition to the aforementioned, have been used for CRPS: algodystrophy, posttraumatic dystrophy, minor causalgia, sympathalgia, shoulder-hand syndrome, and postinfarctional sclerodactylia. Because of these ambiguities, in 1993 the International Association for the Study of Pain re-evaluated the terminology and defined CRPS. CPRS type I is used to describe the clinical features traditionally called RSD, whereas type II is used for a similar syndrome that occurs after a known nerve injury, traditionally referred to as causalgia. These are typically named nerves and the affected area is not limited to the territory of the injured nerve [11]. The term RSD has become a misnomer, because no reflex or consistent link to the sympathetic nervous system has been discovered, and dystrophy is not a dependable finding in these patients [12]. These topics are addressed later in this article. Because the term RSD is imprecise and assuming, the term CRPS is used herein.

Pathophysiology

A hyperactive sympathetic nervous system was originally believed to play a primary role in the CRPS disease process. This theory was promoted by reports of reduction in symptoms after sympathetic interruption [10,13–15]. Most of these older studies were retrospective case series. In more recent double-blind random trials, no difference has been noted between sympathetic blockage and placebo [16–18]. Additional evidence questions a hyperactive sympathetic nervous system. Two studies have shown a decrease in serum norepinephrine and epinephrine in the affected limb versus the normal limb [19,20]. Newer concepts focus on the increase in adrenergic receptor sensitivity for circulating catecholamines. Research has demonstrated that patients who have CRPS have an exaggerated vasoconstrictive and pain response to norepinephrine when compared with controls or the contralateral limb [21,22]. Animal studies have demonstrated an increased pain response to alpha-2 adrenergic receptor agonists after sympathectomy [23]. All of these studies suggest upregulation of adrenergic receptors in nociceptive fibers, which was shown in rats with immunoassay [24]. This would allow sympathetic activation of afferent pain fibers. With physiologic activation of the sympathetic nervous system in patients with CRPS, multiple studies have shown that an increase can be detected in the vasoconstrictor and pain response [25,26]. Newer theories speculate that circulating catecholamines may activate sensitized tissue and produce the clinical picture observed in CRPS [27]. This finding still does not account for why sympathetic blocking agents have not been shown to be effective. Some authors believe that this is a result of blocks lacking specificity in their action [28]. Additional studies are needed to prove definitively the sympathetic nervous system's role in CRPS.

Sudeck's postulation was that an exaggerated inflammatory response was responsible for the symptoms seen in what we currently call CRPS [6]. This theory has been gaining support recently. Consistent with this hypothesis is the observation that treatment with corticosteroids has been shown to provide some relief [29]. Indium scanning has been performed in patients with labeled IgG and compared with the contralateral upper extremity [30]. Most of the affected hands showed an increased extravasation of macromolecules independent of arterial flow, which was seen in 14 of the 17 patients with acute CRPS (<5 months). Only one of the six patients with chronic disease was positive, however, which clearly demonstrates a regional inflammatory process. Histologic studies have demonstrated some changes at the cellular level [31]. Muscle specimens showed increased lipofuscin pigment (degenerative product produced during lipid peroxidation of the cell membrane that increases normally with age), atrophic fibers, and thickened basal membranes of the capillaries. The nerves were largely normal, and only a loss of C-fibers was seen in four of eight patients. These findings do not support an immune-mediated inflammation. Studies performed on CRPS blood samples also are not consistent with immune-mediated inflammation. No differences have been found in lymphocyte populations [32] or pro- and anti-inflammatory cytokines [33] between patients who have CRPS and controls. These findings have given rise to a theory of neurogenically mediated inflammation. Nociceptive C-fibers have an efferent neurosecretory role, and when stimulated, they release neuropeptides into their innervated territory, which cause vasodilation and protein extravasation [34]. When nerve fibers are transcutaneously stimulated in patients who have CRPS, increased vasodilation and protein extravasation are seen when compared with healthy controls [35]. Increased serum levels of calcitonin gene-related peptide (neuropeptide mainly responsible for vasodilation) were elevated in CRPS serum samples [36]. Finally, intradermal substance P provokes an increased protein extravasation in the affected and unaffected limb of patients who have CRPS [37]. The pain, hyperesthesia, skin temperature, increased sweating [38], hair growth [39], and bony changes [40] that are seen clinically in CRPS may be mediated at least in part by neuropeptides and neurogenic inflammation. An inflammatory process at some level is involved in the pathophysiology of CRPS; however, it is unclear if neurogenic inflammation plays a primary role or is an epiphenomenon associated with the disease process.

It is generally accepted that the central nervous system plays a role in the disease process of CRPS [41–44]. The most obvious example of this is thermoregulatory dysfunction. In cases of CRPS, increased skin temperature has been documented in affected limbs from diminished vasoconstrictor response, which is from intense sympathetic inhibition [45]. This finding is consistent with findings mentioned previously that show lower levels of norepinephrine and catecholamines in affected limbs. This sympathetic inhibition is so intense that it is able to override normal thermoregulatory vasoconstrictor reflexes, which must indicate a central disturbance [45]. Other evidence for central disturbances is the observation of increased physiologic tremor seen in 57% of patients who have CRPS [46]. Finally, the abnormal unilateral changes in sudomotor activity also may have a central explanation [45,47].

Genetic considerations have not yet proved useful in identifying causes of CRPS. The innate cytokine profile was not altered in patients who have CRPS, which argues against a genetic predisposition [48]. Two studies have shown increased frequencies of HLA-DR2 [49] and DQ1 [50] in patients with CRPS type I, however, which suggests a genetic component. The significance of the increased frequency of two different alleles is unknown.

Patients who have CRPS have been reported to have an increased incidence of psychological distress, with anxiety and depression being the most common manifestations [51,52]. Multiple studies have examined the psychological profiles in patients who have CRPS and have not shown any abnormalities specific to CRPS or any type evidence of predisposing psychological factors [53,54]. Contributing to this information, two studies have compared patients who have CRPS with other chronic pain patients and have shown no psychological dysfunction unique to CRPS [55,56]. Ciccone and colleagues [56] stated "The burden of proof would appear to be upon those who advocate the non-organic hypothesis to provide credible evidence of psychological involvement in the etiology of RSD." It seems that psychological symptoms are a result and not a cause of CRPS. A recent study suggested that the increased systemic concentrations of norepinephrine and epinephrine in patients who have CRPS may be related to psychological symptoms [57].

Epidemiology

CRPS has been reported after surgery, nerve injury, fracture, gunshot wounds, spinal cord injury, stroke, and myocardial infarct [43]. The reported incidence of CRPS after a fracture in general is reported to be 1% to 2% [58]. Higher incidences have been found after distal radius fractures (1%–37%) [59,60]. Zyluk [61] suggested that there is a higher incidence in highly comminuted fractures and in fractures treated with closed reduction and casting (versus percutaneuos pinning). In 10% to 26% of CRPS cases, no precipitating factors can be found [58]. A higher incidence of CRPS is reported in women (76%) and in patients in the age range of 40 to 49 [58]. No correlation to diabetes, smoking, or alcohol has ever been found [61]. The incidence of recurrent CRPS type I is 1.8% per year, and 50% are spontaneous recurrences [62].

Clinical features

There is a vast range of symptoms seen in CRPS type I. In general, signs and symptoms are characterized by sensory, autonomic, inflammatory, trophic, and motor disturbances. Pain is the most common finding and is reported in 74% to 93% of patients [42,58,63]. Pain is typically described as burning or is disproportionate to the inciting event. Allodynia has been reported in 26% to 79% of cases, with other sensory changes accompanying it, such as hyperalgesia (22%–63%) and hyperesthesia (65%–76%) [42,58,63]. Autonomic and inflammatory signs and symptoms frequency have been reported in affected limbs: color difference (86%–92%), temperature asymmetry (78%–92%), edema (69%–80%), and hyperhydrosis (47%–52%) [58,63]. Trophic changes may be present and are more common in chronic disease, such as skin changes, nail changes, and diffuse bony osteoporosis [58,63]. Finally, motor changes have been reported: weakness (75%), dystonia (14%), and tremor (23%–57%) [58,63].

The International Association for the Study of Pain diagnostic criteria for CRPS type I from 1993 are as follows: (1) there is a presence of an initiating noxious event (not required for diagnosis), (2) spontaneous pain or allodynia/hyperalgesia occurs, is not limited to the territory of a single nerve, and is disproportionate to the inciting event, (3) there is evidence of edema, skin blood flow, or abnormal sudomotor activity in the affected limb since the inciting event, and (4) this diagnosis is excluded by the existence of conditions that would otherwise account for the degree of dysfunction and pain [11]. These criteria were designed to standardize CRPS diagnostic criteria and limit the confusion in the literature caused by other terms. The criteria were based on decisions from an expert panel and were not validated clinically, however. More recent studies have shown the limitations of the criteria. The sensitivity of the criteria was high (0.98); however, the specificity was low (0.36), and nearly 40% of persons who have diabetes met the criteria requirements for CRPS [2]. This finding could lead to inconsistent diagnosis of CRPS, which has been suggested in the literature [2,64] and could confound the entire body of literature on CRPS. More recently, authors have put forth modifications of the guidelines and separated symptoms and signs into sensory, sudomotor/edema, vasomotor, and motor/trophic categories to improve the specificity of the criteria [63]. The International Association for the Study of Pain did meet recently, and some changes were made to the criteria for CRPS; however, these reports are not yet published [65]. Zyluk [66] has proposed a scoring system for the upper extremity to compare patients who have CRPS more accurately.

The current criteria for CRPS type I are based on clinical findings. No single gold standard test is available to provide the diagnosis. Radiographs, bone scintigraphy, and MRI have been used to evaluate CRPS [67]. In particular, bone scanning has been shown to be sensitive and specific in the subacute period [68]. After 26 weeks, however, this test becomes much less sensitive and specific, and currently most authors do not recommend routine use of bone scanning [69,70]. Sympathetic testing also has been used to evaluate CRPS, such as thermography [71] and quantitative sudomotor axon reflex testing [47]. Although these tests do show quantitative differences, their clinical role is unclear.

Treatment

A plethora of heterogeneous treatments has been suggested in treatment of CRPS, from spinal cord stimulation to nonsteroidal anti-inflammatory drugs. Relatively few randomized, double-blind trials have definitely shown efficacy of one form of treatment over another, however [72,73].

Past regional treatment regimens were predominantly aimed at the sympathetic nervous system and reported good outcomes [10,13,15]. They were based on poorly constructed studies, however. After critical review of the literature, less than one third of patients obtained full pain relief from blocks with agents such as guanethidine [72,73]. Most patients require some type of pharmacotherapy regimen. These treatments are aimed at pain management or associated problems, such as depression, anxiety, and insomnia. Among these medications used are tricyclic antidepressants, anticonvulsants, nonsteroidal anti-inflammatory drugs, corticosteroids, narcotics, clonidine, nifedipine, calcitonin, bisphosphonates, topical anti-inflammatory agents, and alpha-adrenergic antagonists. Few of these agents have any evidence more than level 4, which demonstrates clinical effectiveness for CRPS type I [65]. Oral corticosteroids are an exception and have been shown in a randomized trial to provide some long-term relief [29]. Recently in a randomized, double-blind study, methylprednisolone and lidocaine were administered via Bier block and were not found to improve symptoms [74].

The role of surgical management is limited in CRPS type I. In contrast, some recent data have shown improvement from surgical release in CRPS type II [75]. In general, despite earlier reports [14], it is currently accepted that any destructive surgery on the peripheral or central nervous system should be avoided [43]. Surgery represents a repeated painful stimulus that could exacerbate or stimulate a new attack. Amputation should be approached with great trepidation. Dielissen and colleagues [76] showed that after amputation, pain relief was rare and unpredictable, often with recurrence in the residual limb. Two of 28 patients wore a prosthesis. The inclusion criteria for patients in this study are open to question.

Treatment has shifted paradigms, from one focused on pathophysiology to one focused on restoration of function [77]. A stepwise progression of therapy should be used to achieve functional restoration. Treatment should start as early as possible, and each step should be accomplished within 2 to 3 weeks. The summary of the consensus guidelines are as follows: the first step involves motivation and desensitization followed by flexibility exercises, edema control, and isometric strengthening. The third step involves stress loading and general aerobic conditioning. The last step involves ergonomics, normalization of use, and vocational rehabilitation. If patients fail to progress at any level, then blocks, psychotherapy, or pharmacotherapy can be considered. This algorithm should be individualized and flexible to accommodate each patient.

Summary

CRPS type I remains a troubling condition for afflicted patients. The confusion surrounding nomenclature for this condition reflects the evolving pathophysiologic concepts [78]. Despite the large volume of literature in recent years, the role of inflammation and the central and sympathetic nervous system still need clarification. Treatment should be based on a multidisciplinary experienced team approach that is focused on functional restoration. Undoubtedly, future clinical trials will provide more insight to optimal treatment of CRPS.

References

[1] Harden RN. Complex regional pain syndrome. Br J Anaesth 2001;87(1):99–106.
[2] Bruehl S, Harden RN, Galer BS, et al. External validation of IASP diagnostic criteria for complex regional pain syndrome and proposed research diagnostic criteria: International Association for the Study of Pain. Pain 1999;81(1–2):147–54.
[3] Allen G, Galer BS, Schwartz L. Epidemiology of complex regional pain syndrome: a retrospective chart review of 134 patients. Pain 1999;80(3):539–44.
[4] Mitchell SW, Morehouse CR, Keen WW. Gunshot wounds and other injuries of the nerves. Philadelphia: JB Lippincott; 1864. p. 105.
[5] Mitchell SW. Injuries of nerves and their consequences. Philadelphia: JB Lippincott; 1872.
[6] Sudeck P. Über die akute entzundliche Knochenatrophie. Arch Klin Chir 1900;62:147–56.
[7] Leriche R. De la causalgie, envisagee comme une nevrite du sympathique et l'excision des plexus nerveux periarterials. Presse Med 1916;24:178–80.
[8] Leriche R. The surgery of pain. Baltimore: Williams and Wilkins; 1939.
[9] Livingston WK. Pain mechanisms: a physiologic interpretation of causalgia and its related states. New York: Macmillan; 1947. p. 226–7.
[10] Evans JA. Reflex sympathetic dystrophy. Surg Clin North Am 1946;26:780–90.
[11] Stanton-Hicks M, Janig W, Hassenbusch S, et al. Reflex sympathetic dystrophy: changing concepts and taxonomy. Pain 1995;63(1):127–33.
[12] Wong GY, Wilson PR. Classification of complex regional pain syndromes: new concepts. Hand Clin 1997;13(3):319–25.
[13] Wang JK, Johnson KA, Ilstrup DM. Sympathetic blocks for reflex sympathetic dystrophy. Pain 1985;23(1):13–7.
[14] Olcott C, Eltherington LG, Wilcosky BR, et al. Reflex sympathetic dystrophy–the surgeon's role in management. J Vasc Surg 1991;14(4):488–92.
[15] Glynn CJ, Basedow RW, Walsh JA. Pain relief following post-ganglionic sympathetic blockade with IV guanethidine. Br J Anaesth 1981;53(12):1297–302.
[16] Blanchard J, Ramamurthy S, Walsh N, et al. Intravenous regional sympatholysis: a double-blind comparison of guanethidine, reserpine, and normal saline. J Pain Symptom Manage 1990; 5(6):357–61.

[17] Jadad AR, Carroll D, Glynn CJ, et al. Intravenous regional sympathetic blockade for pain relief in reflex sympathetic dystrophy: a systematic review and a randomized, double-blind crossover study. J Pain Symptom Manage 1995;10(1):13–20.
[18] Ramamurthy S, Hoffman J. Intravenous regional guanethidine in the treatment of reflex sympathetic dystrophy/causalgia: a randomized, double-blind study. Guanethidine Study Group. Anesth Analg 1995;81(4):718–23.
[19] Harden RN, Duc TA, Williams TR, et al. Norepinephrine and epinephrine levels in affected versus unaffected limbs in sympathetically maintained pain. Clin J Pain 1994;10(4):324–30.
[20] Drummond PD, Finch PM, Smythe GA. Reflex sympathetic dystrophy: the significance of differing plasma catecholamine concentrations in affected and unaffected limbs. Brain 1991; 114(Pt 5):2025–36.
[21] Arnold JM, Teasell RW, MacLeod AP, et al. Increased venous alpha-adrenoceptor responsiveness in patients with reflex sympathetic dystrophy. Ann Intern Med 1993;118(8):619–21.
[22] Ali Z, Raja SN, Wesselmann U, et al. Intradermal injection of norepinephrine evokes pain in patients with sympathetically maintained pain. Pain 2000;88(2):161–8.
[23] Moon DE, Lee DH, Han HC, et al. Adrenergic sensitivity of the sensory receptors modulating mechanical allodynia in a rat neuropathic pain model. Pain 1999;80(3):589–95.
[24] Birder LA, Perl ER. Expression of alpha2-adrenergic receptors in rat primary afferent neurons after peripheral nerve injury or inflammation. J Physiol 1999;515(Pt 2):533–42.
[25] Drummond PD, Finch PM, Skipworth S, et al. Pain increases during sympathetic arousal in patients with complex regional pain syndrome. Neurology 2001;57(7):1296–303.
[26] Baron R, Schattschneider J, Binder A, et al. Relation between sympathetic vasoconstrictor activity and pain and hyperalgesia in complex regional pain syndromes: a case-control study. Lancet 2002;359(9318):1655–60.
[27] Perl ER. Causalgia, pathological pain, and adrenergic receptors. Proc Natl Acad Sci U S A 1999;96(14):7664–7.
[28] Baron R, Levine JD, Fields HL. Causalgia and reflex sympathetic dystrophy: does the sympathetic nervous system contribute to the generation of pain? Muscle Nerve 1999;22(6):678–95.
[29] Christensen K, Jensen EM, Noer I. The reflex dystrophy syndrome response to treatment with systemic corticosteroids. Acta Chir Scand 1982;148(8):653–5.
[30] Oyen WJ, Arntz IE, Claessens RM, et al. Reflex sympathetic dystrophy of the hand: an excessive inflammatory response? Pain 1993;55(2):151–7.
[31] van der Laan L, ter Laak HJ, Gabreels-Festen A, et al. Complex regional pain syndrome type I (RSD): pathology of skeletal muscle and peripheral nerve. Neurology 1998;51(1):20–5.
[32] Ribbers GM, Oosterhuis WP, van Limbeek J, et al. Reflex sympathetic dystrophy: is the immune system involved? Arch Phys Med Rehabil 1998;79(12):1549–52.
[33] van de Beek WJ, Remarque EJ, Westendorp RG, et al. Innate cytokine profile in patients with complex regional pain syndrome is normal. Pain 2001;91(3):259–61.
[34] Holzer P. Neurogenic vasodilatation and plasma leakage in the skin. Gen Pharmacol 1998; 30(1):5–11.
[35] Weber M, Birklein F, Neundorfer B, et al. Facilitated neurogenic inflammation in complex regional pain syndrome. Pain 2001;91(3):251–7.
[36] Birklein F, Schmelz M, Schifter S, et al. The important role of neuropeptides in complex regional pain syndrome. Neurology 2001;57(12):2179–84.
[37] Leis S, Weber M, Isselmann A, et al. Substance-P-induced protein extravasation is bilaterally increased in complex regional pain syndrome. Exp Neurol 2003;183(1):197–204.
[38] Kumazawa K, Sobue G, Mitsuma T, et al. Modulatory effects of calcitonin gene-related peptide and substance P on human cholinergic sweat secretion. Clin Auton Res 1994;4(6):319–22.
[39] Paus R, Peters EM, Eichmuller S, et al. Neural mechanisms of hair growth control. J Investig Dermatol Symp Proc 1997;2(1):61–8.
[40] Bjurholm A. Neuroendocrine peptides in bone. Int Orthop 1991;15(4):325–9.
[41] Sieweke N, Birklein F, Riedl B, et al. Patterns of hyperalgesia in complex regional pain syndrome. Pain 1999;80(1–2):171–7.

[42] Birklein F, Riedl B, Sieweke N, et al. Neurological findings in complex regional pain syndromes: analysis of 145 cases. Acta Neurol Scand 2000;101(4):262–9.
[43] Wasner G, Schattschneider J, Binder A, et al. Complex regional pain syndrome: diagnostic, mechanisms. CNS involvement and therapy. Spinal Cord 2003;41(2):61–75.
[44] Stanton-Hicks M. Complex regional pain syndrome. Anesthesiol Clin North Am 2003; 21(4):733–44.
[45] Wasner G, Heckmann K, Maier C, et al. Vascular abnormalities in acute reflex sympathetic dystrophy (CRPS I): complete inhibition of sympathetic nerve activity with recovery. Arch Neurol 1999;56(5):613–20.
[46] Deuschl G, Blumberg H, Lucking CH. Tremor in reflex sympathetic dystrophy. Arch Neurol 1991;48(12):1247–52.
[47] Birklein F, Sittl R, Spitzer A, et al. Sudomotor function in sympathetic reflex dystrophy. Pain 1997;69(1–2):49–54.
[48] van de Beek WJ, Remarque EJ, Westendorp RG, et al. Innate cytokine profile in patients with complex regional pain syndrome is normal. Pain 2001;91(3):259–61.
[49] Mailis A, Wade J. Profile of Caucasian women with possible genetic predisposition to reflex sympathetic dystrophy: a pilot study. Clin J Pain 1994;10(3):210–7.
[50] Kemler MA, van de Vusse AC, van den Berg-Loonen EM, et al. HLA-DQ1 associated with reflex sympathetic dystrophy. Neurology 1999;53(6):1350–1.
[51] Bruehl S, Husfeldt B, Lubenow TR, et al. Psychological differences between reflex sympathetic dystrophy and non-RSD chronic pain patients. Pain 1996;67(1):107–14.
[52] Geertzen JH, de Bruijn-Kofman AT, de Bruijn HP, et al. Stressful life events and psychological dysfunction in complex regional pain syndrome type I. Clin J Pain 1998;14(2):143–7.
[53] Bruehl S, Carlson CR. Predisposing psychological factors in the development of reflex sympathetic dystrophy: a review of the empirical evidence. Clin J Pain 1992;8(4):287–99.
[54] van der Laan L, van Spaendonck K, Horstink MW, et al. The Symptom Checklist-90 Revised questionnaire: no psychological profiles in complex regional pain syndrome-dystonia. J Pain Symptom Manage 1999;17(5):357–62.
[55] DeGood DE, Cundiff GW, Adams LE, et al. A psychosocial and behavioral comparison of reflex sympathetic dystrophy, low back pain, and headache patients. Pain 1993;54(3):317–22.
[56] Ciccone DS, Bandilla EB, Wu W. Psychological dysfunction in patients with reflex sympathetic dystrophy. Pain 1997;71(3):323–33.
[57] Harden RN, Rudin NJ, Bruehl S, et al. Increased systemic catecholamines in complex regional pain syndrome and relationship to psychological factors: a pilot study. Anesth Analg 2004; 99:1478–85.
[58] Veldman PH, Reynen HM, Arntz IE, et al. Signs and symptoms of reflex sympathetic dystrophy: prospective study of 829 patients. Lancet 1993;342:1012–6.
[59] Dijkstra PU, Groothoff JW, ten Duis HJ, et al. Incidence of complex regional pain syndrome type I after fractures of the distal radius. Eur J Pain 2003;7(5):457–62.
[60] van der Laan L, Goris RJ. Reflex sympathetic dystrophy: an exaggerated regional inflammatory response? Hand Clin 1997;13(3):373–85.
[61] Zyluk A. Complex regional pain syndrome type I: risk factors, prevention and risk of recurrence. J Hand Surg Br 2004;29(4):334–7.
[62] Veldman PH, Goris RJ. Multiple reflex sympathetic dystrophy: which patients are at risk for developing a recurrence of reflex sympathetic dystrophy in the same or another limb. Pain 1996; 64(3):463–6.
[63] Harden RN, Bruehl S, Galer BS, et al. Complex regional pain syndrome: are the IASP diagnostic criteria valid and sufficiently comprehensive? Pain 1999;83(2):211–9.
[64] Reinders MF, Geertzen JH, Dijkstra PU. Complex regional pain syndrome type I: use of the International Association for the Study of Pain diagnostic criteria defined in 1994. Clin J Pain 2002;18(4):207–15.
[65] Harden RN. Pharmacotherapy of complex regional pain syndrome. Am J Phys Med Rehabil 2005;84(3 Suppl):S17–28.

[66] Zyluk A. A new clinical severity scoring system for reflex sympathetic dystrophy of the upper limb. J Hand Surg Br 2003;28(3):238–41.
[67] Marshall AT, Crisp AJ. Reflex sympathetic dystrophy. Rheumatology (Oxford) 2000;39(7): 692–5.
[68] Holder LE, Mackinnonn SE. The use of three-phase radionucleotide bone scanning in the diagnosis of reflex sympathetic dystrophy. J Hand Surg Am 1984;9A:556–63.
[69] Lee GW, Weeks PM. The role of bone scintigraphy in diagnosing reflex sympathetic dystrophy. J Hand Surg Am 1995;20(3):458–63.
[70] Harden RN. Complex regional pain syndrome. Br J Anaesth 2001;87(1):99–106.
[71] Bruehl S, Lubenow TR, Nath H, et al. Validation of thermography in the diagnosis of reflex sympathetic dystrophy. Clin J Pain 1996;12:316–25.
[72] Kingery WS. A critical review of controlled clinical trials for peripheral neuropathic pain and complex regional pain syndromes. Pain 1997;73(2):123–39.
[73] Cepeda MS, Lau J, Carr DB. Defining the therapeutic role of local anesthetic sympathetic blockade in complex regional pain syndrome: a narrative and systematic review. Clin J Pain 2002;18(4):216–33.
[74] Taskaynatan MA, Ozgul A, Tan AK, et al. Bier block with methylprednisolone and lidocaine in CRPS type I: a randomized, double-blinded, placebo-controlled study. Reg Anesth Pain Med 2004;29(5):408–12.
[75] Placzek JD, Boyer MI, Gelberman RH, et al. Nerve decompression for complex regional pain syndrome type II following upper extremity surgery. J Hand Surg Am 2005;30(1):69–74.
[76] Dielissen PW, Claassen AT, Veldman PH, et al. Amputation for reflex sympathetic dystrophy. J Bone Joint Surg Br 1995;77(2):270–3.
[77] Stanton-Hicks M, Baron R, Boas R, et al. Complex regional pain syndromes: guidelines for therapy. Clin J Pain 1998;14(2):155–66.
[78] Ochoa JL. Truths, errors, and lies around "reflex sympathetic dystrophy" and "complex regional pain syndrome." J Neurol 1999;246:875–9.

ELSEVIER
SAUNDERS

Clin Occup Environ Med
5 (2) 455–469

CLINICS IN
OCCUPATIONAL AND
ENVIRONMENTAL
MEDICINE

Fibromyalgia and Myofascial Pain Syndromes and the Workers' Compensation Environment: An Update

Radford J. Hayden, PA-C[a,b,*], Dean S. Louis, MD[a], Christopher Doro, MD[a]

[a]*Division of Hand, Elbow and Microsurgery, Department of Orthopaedic Surgery, University of Michigan Medical Center, 2098 South Main Street, Ann Arbor, MI 48103, USA*
[b]*College of Health Professions, Physician Assistant Studies, University of Detroit Mercy, PO Box 19900, Detroit, MI 48219-0900, USA*

Background

In 1990, Wolfe et al developed the criteria for the classification of fibromyalgia (FM) that included patients with widespread pain in combination with tenderness at 11 or more of 18 specific tender points [1]. Myofascial pain syndrome (MFPS) is described as a trigger point characterized by a zone of tenderness in a taut band of muscle that, when stimulated by palpation or needle injection, causes localized contraction of myofibrils as opposed to contraction of the entire muscle belly [2,3]. These pain syndromes may follow trauma and are associated with acute and chronic musculoskeletal stress.

Significant controversy continues to exist as to whether FM and MFPS are true diagnoses that reflect specific pathology or are merely terms used to describe clinical conditions that provide patients with the reassurance that their symptoms are real and provide clinicians with therapeutic direction. Pearce [4] dismissed these terms as distinct disease entities based on the dearth and lack of demonstrable pathology. He suggested that the pain complaints are more general and related to neural dysfunction with nociceptive and neurogenic origins. Ehrlich [5]

* Corresponding author. Division of Hand, Elbow and Microsurgery, Department of Orthopaedic Surgery, University of Michigan Medical Center, 2098 South Main Street, Ann Arbor, MI 48103.
E-mail address: rhayden@med.umich.edu (R.J. Hayden).

doi:10.1016/j.coem.2005.11.001 ***occmed.theclinics.com***

referred to FM as a "virtual disease" and pointed out that the main criteria for the diagnosis of FM and MFPS are "tender points," which he states represent "circular reasoning" and are suspect because they are self-reported. He recommended abandoning FM as a diagnosis and treating the real physical and psychological symptoms that characterize chronic pain.

Persons who support these terms as being specifically diagnostic point to the fact that many other medical maladies are diagnosed based on similar vague and subjective complaints. White [6] listed polymyalgia rheumatica, migraine headache, and trigeminal neuralgia as examples. Nielson[7] agreed that there is a lack of empirical evidence for specific pathophysiology but finds the terms useful because they have produced meaningful scientific knowledge regarding the perception and modulation of pain and provided patients some assurance that despite being in pain it does not necessarily mean disability or incapacity. Goldenberg [8] supported the use of these terms as a way of reassuring the patient and physician that other patients exist with similar complaints in the absence of significant disease, which affords the establishment of a caring and nonconfrontational relationship between patient and clinician.

How the use of these terms affects workers' compensation patients is unclear. In addition to FM and MFPS, other terms such as "cumulative trauma disorder," "cervical brachial syndrome," "repetitive strain injury" and "chronic fatigue syndrome" are used to explain chronic pain in the working population. Gildenberg and DeVaul [9] reported on four categories that best describe patients who have chronic pain: (1) overwhelmed, (2) need to suffer, (3) assigned, and (4) psychogenic. The overwhelmed patient develops chronic pain responses in overwhelming circumstances and responds to major illnesses and crisis by escape and withdrawal behaviors. These behaviors are usually rewarded by time off or disability payments, which reinforces the behavior. In the psychogenic group, psychiatric disorders such as depression, anxiety, conversion reactions, unresolved grief, and psychosis are common. Of these four categories of chronic pain patients, the "overwhelmed" individual in the work environment and perhaps less frequently the "psychogenic" individual would be likely candidates to obtain secondary gains through workers' compensation.

Epidemiology and prevalence

The prevalence of FM in the general population is estimated to be approximately 2% and increases with age, approximating 7% in women between 60 and 80 years of age [10]. Eighty percent of patients who have FM are women, with a mean patient age between 30 and 60 years. At the time of the original classification of FM, white persons accounted for 93% of the patients, followed by Hispanics at 5% and African Americans at 1%. Arnold and colleagues [11] reported on familial aggregation of FM. Studying patients aged 40 to 55 years with a diagnosis of FM who had at least one first-degree relative aged 18 years or older, they concluded that FM and reduced pain thresholds aggregate in families with FM significantly associated with major mood disorders [11].

Little information isolates FM as a primary diagnosis in workers' compensations patients. Helliwell and colleagues [12] developed epidemiologic criteria for soft tissue disorders of the arm, including workers' compensation illnesses, such as carpal tunnel syndrome and lateral epicondylitis. They concluded that nonspecific arm pain remained a diagnosis by exclusion and that it may be associated with or be a lesser form of FM. They did not specify age, sex, or type of work performed. A review of the National Institute for Occupational Safety and Health Manual on Musculoskeletal Disorders in the Workplace revealed that most studies conducted in the upper extremity are problem specific, such as for epicondylitis and carpal tunnel syndrome. No available data on nonspecific upper limb pain were found [13]. Sarmer and colleagues [14] investigated the prevalence of carpal tunnel syndrome in patients with known FM and concluded that 10% of the patients who have FM actually had carpal tunnel syndrome by electrodiagnostic evaluation.

The economic costs of FM in the work environment were studied by Robinson and colleagues [15]. Administrative claims from a Fortune 100 manufacturer were used to quantify direct and indirect costs associated with FM. Four thousand six hundred ninety-nine patients with at least one claim between 1996 and 1998 were contrasted with a 10% random sample of the overall beneficiary population. They found that the total costs for FM claimants were approximately $5905 versus $2485 for the typical beneficiary. The prevalence of disability was twice as high among FM employees than overall employees. For every dollar spent on FM-specific claims, employers spent another $57 to $143 on additional direct and indirect costs. They also concluded that hidden costs of disability and comorbidities greatly increased the true burden of FM [15]. Additional studies have evaluated health costs and their determinance in women who have FM and confirmed that comorbidity and disability were statistically significant contributors to the direct cost of health care and noted a 20% increase with each additional comorbid condition [16,17].

Etiology research update

A significant amount of research attention has been devoted to explaining the pathophysiologic basis for patients' complaints of diffuse pain, trigger point discomfort, and fatigue. Frank and colleagues [18] reported on mutations of the serotonin receptor genes HTR3A and HTR3B in patients who suffered from FM and suggested that variants of these genes may contribute to altered nociception and play a significant role in abnormal pain perception. Sprott and colleagues [19] evaluated muscle tissue by electronmicroscopy and found increased DNA fragmentation and disorganization of the myofibrils and actin filaments. The number of mitochondria was less than would be seen in normal controls, and morphologically these intracellular structures were enlarged. Dan and colleagues [20] reported on an association between polymorphism of the dopamine D4 receptor exon III gene and its relationship to unusual personality profiles commonly seen in patients who have FM who score unusually low on personality inventories.

Hormonal influences have been investigated. An evaluation of the hypothalamic-pituitary-gonadal axis and low cortisol concentrations have been identified in women who have FM [21]. It remains unclear as to whether low cortisol levels are the result of depression, fatigue, and sleep disturbances or the cause of these complaints. Bennett [22] evaluated the hypothalamic-pituitary-adrenal axis and the deficiency of growth hormone in a subset of patients diagnosed with FM, and he suggested that growth hormone replacement therapy may be a viable treatment option. Hope [23] noted severe myalgia in female patients after discontinuing hormone replacement therapy. Akkus and colleagues [24] evaluated elevated levels of substance P from the cerebrospinal fluid of patients who have FM. Substance P mediates the neurotransmission of pain from the periphery to central nervous system and is modulated by ovarian steroids. Their study suggested that ovarian steroids influence the serotonin system and its role in pain perception. Blanco and colleagues [25] studied alpha I antitrypsin, a potent anti-inflammatory chemical, and in two patients with severe hereditary alpha I antitrypsin deficiency who were treated by infusions of purified human alpha I antitrypsin their FM symptoms were controlled efficiently. Serum hyaluronic acid levels were studied to determine their value as serologic markers for FM, and in separate studies no correlation was identified [26,27].

In 2001, Brown and colleagues [28] linked extracapsular silicone release from silicone breast implant ruptures to FM; however, these findings were refuted by Bowlin [29] in 2002 and by Lipworth and colleagues in 2003 [30]. Smoking and its affects on patients who have FM also were studied, and although smokers reported significantly more discomfort, paresthesias, and overall functional difficulties, there was no significant difference between smokers and nonsmokers regarding their complaints of fatigue and trigger points [31]. Chest expansion, maximal inspiratory pressure, and maximal expiratory pressures are all reduced in patients who have FM, which led the authors to conclude that measuring chest expansion may be a useful clinical parameter in diagnosis [32].

Electrodiagnostic studies were evaluated by Miller and colleagues [33] to evaluate muscle force, perceived effort, and voluntary activation with sensitive twitch interpolation in patients diagnosed with FM. They concluded that poor motivation, reflex pain inhibition, and muscle contractile failure were not important in the pathogenesis of fatigue in patients; however, subjective responses to exercise were commonly excessive. Chung and colleagues [34] used electrodiagnostic studies to evaluate the increased sympathetic activity in myofascial pain areas. They concluded that sympathetic outflow increases in painful areas and electrical activity could be helpful in diagnosing the discreet areas of trigger tenderness noted in FM and MFPS.

MRI has been used to investigate patients who have chronic pain syndromes. In 2000, Sprott and colleagues [35] used 31P MR spectroscopy to evaluate fibromyalgic muscle tissue. Specifically they were evaluating inorganic phosphate, phosphocreatine, and ATP and phosphodiesters. Compared with controls, there were increases in the levels of phosphodiesters in patients with a diagnosis of FM, but they were unable to correlate this finding with weakness and fatigue in these patients. In 2003, Cook and colleagues [36] assessed psychological responses to painful stimuli, responses to painful and nonpainful stimuli, and nonpainful warm stimuli. Using conventional and functional imaging techniques, they concluded that patients who had FM were significantly more sensitive to experimental heat pain than controls, and patients who had FM exhibited greater activity than the control subjects in the prefrontal, supplemental motor, insular, and anterior cingulate cortices. They also concluded that this was objective physiologic evidence to explain fibromyalgic pain. Montoya and colleagues [37] used MRI in patients to evaluate the effects of social support provided by the presence of a significant other during painful stimulation. They compared patients with a diagnosis of FM and migraine headaches and noticed an enhanced sensitivity in the patients who had FM when they were stimulated in the presence of their significant others versus stimulation when alone. They concluded that pain processing is significantly influenced by the presence of a social support system, which indicates a significant behavioral component. Brain imaging studies, such as positron emissions training and functional MRI evaluations, consistently reflect areas of hyperactivity within the important neural pain appreciation centers. The conclusion has been that patients who have FM have a heightened pain sensitivity status centrally mediated [38,39], with significant future research implications. It seems that more study is needed.

The influence of comorbidities

The role of comorbidities in patients who have FM and MFPS cannot be overstated. Box 1 represents the most up-to-date list of associated diagnoses that is continually updated as more research is conducted on patients who have FM and MFPS. As the debate continues as to whether FM is a distinct entity or a biopsychosocial syndrome [40], continued overlap with other obfuscating terminology, such as repetitive strain injury, occupational overuse syndrome, and cumulative trauma disorder, remains an issue. Martinez-Lavin [41] discussed the overlap of FM with other medical conditions, including polymyalgia rheumatica, Sjögren's syndrome, Lyme disease, and systemic lupus erythematosus, and pointed out the need to wait for these latter diagnoses to fully declare themselves before categorizing a patient as having FM. She cautioned against labeling patients as "simulators" or "hypochondriacs."

Conte and colleagues [42] evaluated parental psychological adjustment in patients with juvenile primary fibromyalgic syndrome and found that these adolescents demonstrated significant increases in the levels of depression and anxiety and higher pain sensitivity compared with control groups. Abnormal child psychological adjustment placed these children at risk for developing significant pain syndromes in the future. Additional studies on affective disorders in families

Box 1. Identified comorbidities in patients who have fibromyalgia

- Depression
- Anxiety
- Borderline personality disorder
- Cognitive impairment
- Fatigue
- Sleep disorders
- Irritable bowel syndrome
- Headache (migraine)
- Temporal mandibular syndrome
- Paresthesia
- Generalized weakness
- Dry mouth
- Morning stiffness
- Raynaud's-like symptoms
- Sickle cell anemia

confirm the correlation of affective and anxiety disorders and enhanced pain sensitivity in association with FM and MFPS and other somatic illnesses [43–45]. Comorbid depression and anxiety were studied by Thieme and colleagues [46], who found that 32.3% of the patients who have FM revealed an anxiety disorder and 34.8% revealed a mood disorder. Finset and colleagues [47] reported that depressed mood impedes pain treatment in patients with diagnosed FM.

The misinterpretation of perceived or experienced pain also has been evaluated. Sayar and colleagues [48] described patients who suffer from alexithymia, a condition of misinterpretation of emotional arousals as symptoms of physical illness. These individuals focus on and amplify somatic sensations and interpret them as distress. Gracely and colleagues[49] described "pain catastrophizing" behaviors that result in increased magnitude of neuroactivation in central nervous system areas concerned with the perception of pain, emotion, and motor activity resulting in exaggerated responses. Goubert and colleagues [50] used the Tampa Scale for kinesiophobia to evaluate patients who have FM and noted that high pain fear resulted in overall reduction of range of motion during standard physical examination, less activity during daily life, and being prone to discontinue activities associated with pain, especially activities that are expected to increase pain. They also concluded that pain-specific fear has been shown to be a better predictor of disability than medical status variables or pain itself.

Sleep disturbances are a well-described comorbidity in FM and MFPS. Landis and colleagues [51] correlated sleep quality and fatigue using an actigraf, which is an instrument worn on the nondominant wrist that is used to measure the daily sleep/wake patterns based on the assumption that wakefulness is associated with arm movements and sleep is not. They concluded that the actigraf was a good objective indicator of poor sleep patterns and noted that patients who have FM showed increased levels of activity at night compared with healthy controls.

Update on treatment of fibromyalgia and myofascial pain syndromes

Effective therapy for poorly defined medical illness is the bane of all clinicians. In cases of FM and MFPS, treatment has been directed at alleviating discomfort at specific trigger points, ameliorating patients' generalized complaints using medications, and using physical therapy and alternative medicines to improve a general sense of well-being. Box 2 lists the suggested treatment options for FM and MFPS.

One of the most common treatments is directed at specific trigger points. Known as trigger point infiltration therapy, the injections consist of lidocaine, cortisone, or a combination thereof, but "dry needling" has been found to be as effective. Meyer [52] indicated that the corticosteroids are not appropriate for patients who have FM and MFPS. Majlesi and Unalan [53] reported that high powered pain threshold static ultrasound techniques before stretching muscles that contain specific trigger points were more successful than conventional ultrasound techniques in relieving discomfort.

The treatment of the comorbidities—especially directed to anxiety and depression—is also a mainstay of treatment in FM. Pregabalin was studied by

Box 2. Reported treatments for fibromyalgia and myofascial pain syndrome

- Trigger point injections with anesthesia
- Dry needling technique (no anesthesia)
- Antidepressants
- Cannabis
- Pregabalin
- Laser trigger point injection treatment
- Magnetic stimulation
- High power ultrasound
- Physical therapy (various modalities)
- Balneotherapy (spa mineral baths; Dead Sea bathing)
- T'ai Chi
- Ribonse supplementation
- No use of cosmetics
- Dietary changes
- Religiosity

Crofford and colleagues [54]. In 529 patients, a dose of 300 to 450 mg/d resulted in significant improvement in complaints of pain, sleep disturbances, and fatigue. Antidepressants, including venlafaxine, milnacipran, and duloxetine, which to some degree are all serotonin and norepinephrine reuptake inhibitors, have been studied and shown to be effective in alleviating patient complaints of depressive affect and improving overall generalized discomfort [55–57]. Lithium has been suggested as an alternative treatment because it causes a brief rise in parathyroid hormone, which suggests a calcium-parathyroid axis dysfunction as a cause of FM [58]. Cannabinoids may be effective in patients who have FM migraine headaches and irritable bowel syndrome, which suggests a clinical endocannabinoid difficiency [59], and amitriptyline has been used in conjunction with low-power laser treatments directed at trigger points with relief of tender point discomfort, muscle spasm, and morning stiffness [60]. Antiviral medications, such as valacyclovir, and injections of botulinum toxin have not been found to be effective therapy in cases of FM or MFPS [61,62].

Physical therapy using various modalities—from exercises to heat treatments, ultrasound treatments, massage, and pool-based therapies—has proved beneficial [63–66]. The long-term efficacy is somewhat controversial. One study showed that improvements in patients who were affected with FM were short lived and that improvements in self-efficacy and physical fitness were not associated with improvement in clinical manifestations [67]. Spa treatment, including balneotherapy (mineral/sulfur bath exposure), has been found to be beneficial [68]. The simple carbohydrate ribose given as a supplement to patients who have FM to counteract any muscle adenine nucleotide metabolism aberrations was reported by Gebhart and Jorgenson [69]. Yildiz and colleagues [70] reported on the beneficial effects of hyperbaric oxygen therapy, and Winocur and colleagues [71] concluded that hypnorelaxation is an effective mode of treatment for myofascial pain disorder. Body movement treatment, such as T'ai Chi, has been reported to be beneficial to patients who have FM [72]; however, body awareness therapy, such as Quigong, either alone or in combination with mindfulness meditation has not found to be useful in these patients [73,74]. Researchers have suggested that patients who use fewer cosmetic products may suffer less with FM [75]. Finally, significant alterations in diet [76] and the effects of religiosity on the diurnal cortisol levels in patients who have FM have been studied [77] and found to be helpful in controlling symptomatology.

Nielson and Jensen [78] studied 198 individuals who have FM to examine the association between treatment variables and coping strategies and treatment outcomes, such as pain severity, activity levels, and the ability to engage in activities of daily living. They reported that positive treatment outcomes were related to (1) an increased sense of control of pain, (2) a belief that one is not necessarily disabled by FM, (3) a belief that pain is not necessarily a sign of damage, (4) decreased guarding, (5) increased use of exercise, (6) seeking support from others, (7) activity pacing, and (8) use of coping self-statements. Their study was limited to patients who had diagnosed FM and not compared with a controlled group [78].

The issue of disability and the work place: authors' preferred method

Although not traditionally considered occupationally related diagnoses, it is not inconceivable to put FM and MFPS in the same category as cumulative trauma disorders, repetitive strain injuries, cervical brachial syndromes, and similar condition when considering the issue of exacerbation of a previously existing condition and assigning culpability to the workplace. Kivimaki and colleagues [79] prospectively studied new-onset FM and its influence caused by stress in the workplace and concluded that a high work load, low decision latitude, and the experience of being bullied at work were associated with a two- to fourfold risk of new FM. Turk and colleagues [80] recommend a thorough psychological evaluation of patients who have FM to assist in determining their disability because of their high levels of emotional distress and reduced quality of life. This approach seems appropriate in light of the fact that comorbidities and increased physician use have been identified in patients who have FM [81]. Keeping in mind Kasdan and colleagues' admonition to avoid the "nocebo effect" (avoidance of creating negative expectations about symptoms that can have devastating consequences on patient recovery, which is the opposite of the placebo effect), the question remains as to whether there are ways to determine objectively the amount of disability in patients who have FM and MPS and ferret out malingerers [82].

Khostanteen and colleagues [83] studied whether individuals could simulate FM. They found that using the American College of Rheumatology's criteria for FM, examiners could distinguish patients who had chronic FM, normal individuals, and motivated simulators with 80% accuracy. Their study did, however, show that only 11 of 18 simulators (61%) were correctly identified. Gervais and colleagues [84] found that effort testing in patients who have FM to determine incomplete effort and potential exaggeration of cognitive deficits was critical in determining disability, and other researchers have suggested that additional work, including the development of more objective evaluative tools [85], and changing the focus from tender point specificity to overall impairment are needed [86].

Various health status instruments have been used to evaluate the severity of FM, including the FM impact questionnaire, the clinical assessment questionnaire, the arthritis impact measurement scales, the modified health assessment questionnaire, and the sickness impact profile [87]. Almost all of these assessments rely to a significant degree on self-reporting, and it is difficult—if not impossible—to validate the results. None of these instruments has been applied to patients who have FM in the workers' compensations setting, disability milieu, or after trauma. Zelle and colleagues [88] studied the influence of workers' compensation on functional recovery of patients suffering from trauma 10 to 28 years after the incident. Patients with workers' compensation insurance payments had significantly inferior long-term outcomes than patients who were not being compensated in this manner. It has been suggested that employers and human resources managers make an effort to accommodate patients with a diagnosis of FM and MFPS to reduce illness-related disability [89].

Finally, Hadler and Ehrlich [90] discussed the "conundrum of disability determination." FM, chronic fatigue syndrome, functional somatic syndromes, and medically unexplained symptoms are conditions with no readily demonstrable pathology. Hadler stated that "FM is the medicalization of misery" [91]. Despite the lack of traditional components of classic medical diagnoses such as defined pathology, objective physical examination and laboratory testing, and reasonably reliable and consistent treatment, these diagnoses have reached a point of successful adjudication of financial awards. How does one determine who bears the burden of financial responsibility and the degree of disability? Hadler and Ehrlich offered solutions to the problem, including indemnity coverage as a "rider" on a disability policy specific for these functional somatic syndromes and more enlightened and responsible interplay between a patient's personal physician and an insurance company's evaluating physician, in an attempt to reach a reasonable settlement.

On the hand service at the University of Michigan, the approach is as objective as possible. Terms such as FM, MFPS, chronic fatigue syndrome, and cumulative trauma disorders are used to reassess a patient and establish a true diagnosis that can be treated appropriately. We avoid "labeling" and determine work status, the degree of disability and futureablity of gainful employment based on objective evidence of disease in conjunction with a patient's employer to determine the constitutional ability to perform the tasks being asked of the patient. We are vigilant for malingering and are not uncomfortable putting into the medical record notations on patients who exhibit exaggerated responses and inhibition of function not consistent with identifiable pathology. In our communications, we sometimes wonder what the results of surveillance might be in these patients.

In patients who do not seem to be feigning illness, the basic approach is rest. They are offered casting or splinting that they would wear continuously and remove only for personal hygiene reasons. They are given work restrictions that range from no work at all to no use of the involved extremity. The overall attitude presented to them is strongly positive because we constantly reinforce that this approach will make them feel better and that we expect to start a brief occupational therapy program in approximately 4 weeks and return them to their full unrestricted work shortly thereafter. Narcotics are avoided. If patients claim that a pre-existing condition has been exacerbated by their job, preinjury pathology must be well documented or they are returned to their referring physicians and no input regarding this claim—except the notation of a lack of established preinjury pathology—is noted in our communications.

Summary

FM and MFPS are terms used to describe a constellation of complaints that includes generalized ache and specific tender trigger points often accompanied by fatigue and sleep disturbances. In 1990, criteria for the diagnosis of FM was presented by the American College of Rheumatology and included complaints of pain and 11 of possible 18 trigger points. It is seen most frequently in white women between 30 and 60 years of age and represents approximately 2% of the general population; it increases to approximately 7% in women between 60 and 80 years of age. Familial aggregation has been reported. There is little information in the literature regarding FM and MFPS in the workplace. Nonspecific arm pain and such diagnoses as epicondylitis and carpal tunnel syndrome have been associated in patients who have FM. Economic costs of patients who have FM in the work environment were studied, and researchers found that costs were approximately twice as much as in a typical beneficiary, as was the prevalence of disability compared with other employees.

No specific cause has been identified. Abnormal pain perception and significant association with comorbidities, including anxiety, depression, fatigue, and sleep disturbances, are well documented. Effective treatment is primarily directed to symptomatic treatment of discomfort and management of the comorbidities. Trigger injection therapy, antidepressant medications, physical therapy, and many alternative treatments, including balneotherapy, hypnorelaxation, and T'ai Chi, have been used with some success.

The issue of disability continues to be a source of controversy primarily because of the subjective basis for the diagnosis and lack of objective evaluation tools. It has been suggested that patients who have FM in the workplace be allotted some latitude in the type of work that they do to help their symptom control and reduce costs and length of disability. Better communication between personal physicians and insurance company physicians and the development of a "rider" on a total disability policy have been proposed as possible solutions for these patients.

References

[1] Wolfe F, Smythe HA, Yunus MB, et al. The American College of Rheumatology 1990 criteria for the classification of fibromyalgia: report of the multicenter criteria committee. Arthritis Rheum 1990;33(2):160–72.

[2] Gerwin RD. Neurobiology of the myofascial trigger point. Clin Rheumatol 1994;8:747–62.

[3] Gerwin RD. Myofascial pain syndromes in the upper extremity. J Hand Ther 1997;10(2):130–6.

[4] Pearce JMS. Myofascial pain, fibromyalgia or fibrositis? Eur Neurol 2004;52:67–72.

[5] Ehrlich GE. Fibromyalgia, a virtual disease. Clin Rheumatol 2003;22:8–11.

[6] White KP. Fibromyalgia: the answer is blowin' in the wind. J Rheumatol 2004;31(4):636–9.

[7] Nielson WR. Fibromyalgia: beyond the rhetoric. J Rheumatol 2004;31(4):827–8.

[8] Goldenberg DL. Fibromyalgia: to diagnose or not. J Rheumatol 2004;31(4):633–5.

[9] Gildenburg PL, DeVaul RA. The chronic pain patient. In: Pain and headache. New York: Karger; 1985. p. 1–148.

[10] Wolfe F, Ross K, Anderson J, et al. The prevalence and characteristics of fibromyalgia in the general population. Arthritis Rheum 1995;38:19–28.

[11] Arnold LM, Hudson JI, Hess EV, et al. Family study of fibromyalgia. Arthritis Rheum 2004; 50(3):944–52.

[12] Helliwell PS, Bennett RM, Littlejohn G, et al. Towards epidemiological criteria for soft tissue disorders of the arm. Occup Med 2003;53:313–9.

[13] National Institute for Occupational Safety and Health. Musculoskeletal disorders in workplace factors: a critical review of epidemiologic evidence for work-related musculoskeletal disorders of the neck, upper extremity, and low back. Washington, DC: US Department of Health and Human Services; 1997.
[14] Sarmer S, Yavuzer G, Kucukdeveci A, et al. Prevalence of carpal tunnel syndrome in patients with fibromyalgia. Rheumatol Int 2002;22(2):68–70.
[15] Robinson RL, Birnbaum HG, Morely MA, et al. Economic cost and epidemiologic characteristics of patients with fibromyalgia claims. J Rheumatol 2003;30:1318–25.
[16] Penrod JR, Bernatsky S, Adam V, et al. Health services costs and their determinance in women with fibromyalgia. J Rheumatol 2004;31(7):1391–8.
[17] Robinson RL, Birnbaum HG, Morely MA, et al. Depression and fibromyalgia: treatment and cost when diagnosed separately or concurrently. J Rheumatol 2004;31(8):1621–9.
[18] Frank B, Niesler B, Bondy B, et al. Mutational analysis of serotonin receptor genes: HTR3A and HTR3B in fibromyalgia patients. Clin Rheumatol 2004;23:338–44.
[19] Sprott H, Salemi S, Gay RE, et al. Increased DNA fragmentation and ultra structural changes in fibromyalgic muscle fibers [extended report]. Ann Rheum Dis 2004;63:245–7.
[20] Dan B, Hagit C, Lily N, et al. An association between fibromyalgia and the dopamine D4 receptor exon III repeat polymorphism and relationship to novelty seeking personality traits. Mol Psychiatry 2004;9(8):730–1.
[21] Gur A, Cevik R, Sarac AJ, et al. Hypothalamic-pituitary-gonadal axis and cortisol in young women with primary fibromyalgia: the potential role of depression, fatigue and sleep disturbance in the occurrence of hypocortisolism. Ann Rheum Dis 2004;63(11):1504–6.
[22] Bennett RM. Adult growth hormone deficiency in patients with fibromyalgia. Curr Rheumatol Rep 2002;4(4):306–12.
[23] Hope S. Myalgia after stopping hormone replacement therapy. J Br Menopause Soc 2004; 10(3):126.
[24] Akkus S, Delibas N, Tamer MN. Do sex hormones play a role in fibromyalgia? Rheumatology 2000;39(10):1161–3.
[25] Blanco IE, deSerres FJ, Ferandez-Bustillo E, et al. Alpha I–antitrypsin and fibromyalgia: new data in favour of the inflammatory hypothesis of fibromyalgia. Med Hypotheses 2005;64: 759–69.
[26] Wigley RD, Page B, Chambers EM. Hyaluronic acid serum levels in fibromyalgia, nonspecific arm disorder, and controls. J Rheumatol 2001;28(11):2563.
[27] Werle E, Jakel HP, Muller A, et al. Serum hyaluronic acid levels are elevated in arthritis patients, but normal and not associated with clinical data in patients with fibromyalgia syndrome. Clin Lab 2005;51(1–2):11–9.
[28] Brown SL, Pennello G, Berg WA, et al. Silicone gel breast implant rupture, extracapsular silicone, and health status in a population of women. J Rheumatol 2001;28(5):996–1003.
[29] Bowlin SJ. Silicone gel breast implants. J Rheumatol 2002;29(11):2468–9.
[30] Lipworth L, Tarone RE, McLaughlin JK. Breast implants and fibromyalgia: a review of the epidemiologic evidence. Ann Plast Surg 2004;52(3):284–7.
[31] Yunus MB, Arslan S, Aldag JC. Relationship between fibromyalgia features and smoking. Scand J Rheumatol 2002;31(5):301–5.
[32] Ozgocmen S, Cimen OB, Ardicoglu O. Relationship between chest expansion and respiratory muscle strength in patients with primary fibromyalgia. Clin Rheumatol 2002;21:19–22.
[33] Miller TA, Allen GM, Gandevia SC. Muscle force, perceived effort, and voluntary activation of the elbow flexors assessed with sensitive twitch interpolation in fibromyalgia. J Rheumatol 1996;23(9):1621–7.
[34] Chung JW, Ohrbach R, McCall Jr WD. Effect of increased sympathetic activity on electrical activity from myofascial painful areas. Am J Phys Med Rehabil 2004;83(11):842–50.
[35] Sprott H, Rzanny R, Reichenbach JR, et al. 31-P magnetic resonance spectroscopy in fibromyalgic muscle. Rheumatology 2000;39(10):1121–5.
[36] Cook DB, Lange G, Ciccone DS, et al. Functional imaging of pain in patients with primary fibromyalgia. J Rheumatol 2004;31(2):364–78.

[37] Montoya P, Larbig W, Braun C, et al. Influence of social support and emotional context on pain processing and magnetic brain responses in fibromyalgia. Arthritis Rheum 2004;50(12): 4035–44.
[38] Martinez-Lavin M. Fibromyalgia as a sympathetically maintained pain syndrome. Curr Pain Headache Rep 2004;8(5):385–9.
[39] Staud R. Evidence of involvement of central neural mechanisms in generating fibromyalgia pain. Curr Rheumatol Rep 2002;4(4):299–305.
[40] Gur H. Fibromyalgia: a distinct entity or a biopsychosocial syndrome. Isr Med J 2003; 5(12):885.
[41] Martinez-Lavin M. Overlap of fibromyalgia with other medical conditions. Curr Pain Headache Rep 2001;5(4):347–50.
[42] Conte PM, Walco GA, Kimura Y. Temperament and stress response in children with juvenile primary fibromyalgia syndrome. Arthritis Rheum 2003;48(10):2923–30.
[43] Hudson JI, Arnold LM, Keck Jr PE, et al. A family study of fibromyalgia and affective spectrum disorder. Biol Psychiatry 2004;56(11):884–91.
[44] Bradley LA. Psychiatric comorbidity in fibromyalgia. Curr Pain Headache Rep 2005;9(2): 79–86.
[45] Raphael KG, Janal MN, Nayak S, et al. Familial aggregation of depression in fibromyalgia: a community-based test of alternate hypotheses. Pain 2004;110(1–2):449–60.
[46] Thieme K, Turk D, Flor H. Comorbid depression and anxiety in fibromyalgia syndrome: relationship to somatic and psychosocial variables. Psychosom Med 2004;66:837–44.
[47] Finset A, Wigers SH, Gotestam KG. Depressed mood impedes pain treatment response in patients with fibromyalgia. J Rheumatol 2004;31(5):976–80.
[48] Sayar K, Gulec H, Topbas M. Alexithymia and anger in patients with fibromyalgia. Clin Rheumatol 2004;23(5):441–8.
[49] Gracely RH, Geisser ME, Giesecke T, et al. Pain catastrophizing and neural responses to pain among persons with fibromyalgia. Brain 2004;127(4):835–63.
[50] Goubert L, Crombez G, Van Damme S, et al. Confirmatory factor analysis of the tampa scale for kinesiophobia: invariant two-factor model across low back pain patients and fibromyalgia patients. Clin J Pain 2004;20(2):103–10.
[51] Landis CA, Frey CA, Lentz MJ, et al. Self-reported sleep quality and fatigue correlates with actigraphy in midlife women with fibromyalgia. Nurs Res 2003;52(3):140–7.
[52] Meyer H. Myofascial pain syndrome and its suggested role in the pathogenesis and treatment of fibromyalgia syndrome. Curr Pain Headache Rep 2002;6(4):274–83.
[53] Majlesi J, Unalan H. High power pain threshold ultrasound technique in the treatment of active myofascial trigger points: a randomized, double blind case controlled study. Arch Phys Med 2004;85(5):833–6.
[54] Crofford LJ, Rowbotham MC, Mease PJ, et al, and the Pregabalin 1008–105 study group. Pregabalin for the treatment of fibromyalgia syndrome: results of a randomized, double-blind, placebo-controlled trial. Arthritis Rheum 2005;52(4):1264–73.
[55] Sayar K, Aksu G, Ak I, et al. Venlafaxine treatment of fibromyalgia. Ann Pharmacother 2003; 37(11):1561–5.
[56] Arnold LM, Lu Y, Crofford LJ, et al. For the duloxetine fibromyalgia trial group: a double-blind, multicenter trial comparing duloxetine with placebo in the treatment of fibromyalgia patients with or without major depressive disorder. Arthritis Rheum 2004;50(9):2974–84.
[57] Samborski W, Lezanska-Szpera M, Rybakowski JK. Effects of antidepressant mirtazapine on fibromyalgia symptoms. Annales Academiae Bialostocensis 2004;49:265–9.
[58] Fontrier T. Lithium for fibromyalgia. Anesth Analg 2004;98(5):1505.
[59] Russo EB. Clinical endocannabinoid deficiency (CECD): can this concept explain therapeutic benefits of cannabis in migraine, fibromyalgia, irritable bowel syndrome and other treatment-resistant conditions? Neuroendocrinol Lett 2004;25(1–2):31–9.
[60] Gur A, Karakoc M, Nas K, et al. Effects of low power laser and low dose amitriptyline therapy on clinical symptoms and quality of life in fibromyalgia: a single-blind, placebo-controlled trial. Rheumatol Int 2002;22(5):188–93.

[61] Kendall SA, Schaadt MLC, Graff LB, et al. No effect of antiviral (valacyclovir) treatment in fibromyalgia: a double-blind, randomized study. J Rheumatol 2004;31(4):783–4.
[62] Paulson GW, Gill W. Botulinum toxin is unsatisfactory therapy for fibromyalgia. Mov Disord 1996;11(4):459.
[63] Mior S. Exercise in the treatment of chronic pain. Clin J Pain 2001;17(4):377–85.
[64] Altan L, Bingol U, Aykac M, et al. Investigation of the effects of pool-based exercise on fibromyalgia syndrome. Rheumatol Int 2004;24(5):272–7.
[65] Smith M, Gokula M, Weismantel A. Does physical therapy improve symptoms of fibromyalgia? J Fam Pract 2003;52(9):717–9.
[66] Redondo JR, Justo CM, Moraleda FV, et al. Long-term efficacy of therapy in patients with fibromyalgia: a physical exercise-based program and a cognitive-behavioral approach. Arthritis Rheum 2004;51(2):184–92.
[67] Karagulle Z, Donmez A. Balneotherapy for fibromyalgia at the Dead Sea. Rheumatol Int 2002;21(5):210–1.
[68] Zijlstra TR, van de Laar MAFJ, Bernelot Moens HJ, et al. Spa treatment for primary fibromyalgia syndrome: a combination of thalassotherapy, exercise and patient education improves symptoms and quality of life. Rheumatology 2005;44(4):539–46.
[69] Gebhart B, Jorgenson JA. Benefit of ribose in a patient with fibromyalgia. Pharmacotherapy 2004;24(11):1646–8.
[70] Yildiz S, Kiralp MZ, Akin A, et al. A new treatment modality for fibromyalgia syndrome: hyperbaric oxygen therapy. J Int Med Res 2004;32(3):263–7.
[71] Winocur E, Gavish A, Emodi-Perlman AE, et al. Hypnorelaxation as treatment for myofascial pain disorder: a comparative study. Oral Surg Oral Med Oral Pathol Oral Radiol Endod 2002; 93(4):429–34.
[72] Taggart HM, Arsianian CL, Bae S, et al. Effects of T'ai Chi exercise on fibromyalgia symptoms and health-related quality of life. Orthop Nurs 2003;22(5):353–60.
[73] Mannerkorpi K, Arndorw M. Efficacy and feasibility of a combination of body awareness therapy and qigong in patients with fibromyalgia: a pilot study. J Rehabil Med 2004;36(6): 279–81.
[74] Astin JA, Berman BM, Bausell B, et al. The efficacy of mindfulness meditation plus qigong movement therapy in the treatment of fibromyalgia: a randomized controlled trial. J Rheumatol 2003;30(10):2257–62.
[75] Sverdrup B. Use less cosmetics-suffer less from fibromyalgia? J Womens Health 2004;13(2): 187–94.
[76] Logan AC. Complementary and alternative medicine use and fibromyalgia. Arthritis Rheum 2002;47(4):456–8.
[77] Dedert EA, Studts JL, Weissbecker I, et al. Religiosity may help preserve the cortisol rhythm in women with stress-related illness. Int J Psychiatry Med 2004;34(1):61–77.
[78] Nielson WR, Jensen MP. Relationship between changes in coping and treatment outcome in patients with fibromyalgia syndrome. Pain 2004;109(3):233–41.
[79] Kivimaki M, Leino-Arjas P, Virtanen M, et al. Work stress and incidence of newly diagnosed fibromyalgia prospective cohort study. J Psychosom Res 2004;57(5):417–22.
[80] Turk DC, Monarch ES, Williams AD. Psychological evaluation of patients diagnosed with fibromyalgia syndrome: a comprehensive approach. Rheum Dis Clin North Am 2002;28(2):219–33.
[81] Bernatsky S, Dobkin PL, De Civita M, et al. Comorbidity and physician use in fibromyalgia. Swiss Med Wkly 2005;135(5–6):76–81.
[82] Kasdan ML, Lewis K, Bruner A, et al. The nocebo effect: do no harm. J South Orthop Assoc 1999;8(2):108–13.
[83] Khostanteen I, Tunks ER, Goldsmith CH, et al. Fibromyalgia: can one distinguish it from simulation? An observer-blind controlled study. J Rheumatol 2000;27(11):2671–6.
[84] Gervais RO, Russell AS, Green P, et al. Effort testing in patients with fibromyalgia and disability incentives. J Rheumatol 2001;28:1892–9.
[85] Smythe H. Fibromyalgia: can one distinguish it from malingering? More work needed; more tools supplied. J Rheumatol 2000;27(11):2536–40.

[86] Wolfe F. Sayin' "stand and deliver, for you are a bold deceiver": faking fibromyalgia. J Rheumatol 2000;27(11):2534–5.
[87] Wolfe F. The fibromyalgia syndrome: a consensus report on fibromyalgia and disability. J Rheumatol 1996;23(3):534–9.
[88] Zelle BA, Panzica M, Vogt MT, et al. Influence of workers' compensation eligibility upon functional recovery 10 to 28 years after polytrauma. Am J Surg 2005;190:30–6.
[89] Assefi NP, Coy TV, Uslan D, et al. Financial, occupational, and personal consequences of disability in patients with chronic fatigue syndrome and fibromyalgia compared to other fatiguing conditions. J Rheumatol 2003;30(4):804–8.
[90] Hadler NM, Ehrlich GE. Fibromyalgia and the conundrum of disability determination. J Occup Environ Med 2003;45(10):1030–3.
[91] Hadler NM. Fibromyalgia and the medicalization of misery. J Rheumatol 2003;30:1668–70.

ELSEVIER
SAUNDERS

Clin Occup Environ Med
5 (2) 471–482

CLINICS IN
OCCUPATIONAL AND
ENVIRONMENTAL
MEDICINE

Occupational and Physical Therapy for Work-Related Upper Extremity Disorders: How We Can Influence Outcomes

Dennis F. Driver, PT, DPT, MS, OCS, MTC

Concentra Health Services, 6360 West Sam Houston Parkway, Suite 200, Houston, TX 77041, USA

More than 5 million American workers experience some type of work-related injury or illness every year. Workers' compensation medical and indemnity benefits totaled more than $53.4 billion in 2002, which was an increase of 7.2% over the $49.8 billion paid in 2001 [1]. Work-related upper extremity disorders represent a disproportionate amount of these costs when compared with other occupational injuries and illnesses [2,3]. Work-related upper extremity disorders have a greater potential for delayed functional recovery, which complicates the medical care and financial cost of the individual cases relative to non–work-related claims [4].

Occupational and physical therapists play an integral role in the treatment and return to work of injured workers. Currently, up to one third of the total workers' compensation medical costs are derived from physical medicine services, including the use of hot and cold packs, therapeutic exercises, and massage. Managing the cost of physical medicine services, including the use of passive modalities, is a necessary step in total cost control for workers' compensation [5]. A therapist's ability to help manage a case and influence outcomes is vital toward reducing overall case cost and improving the health of an injured worker. With this in mind, therapists must be aware of the confounding medical and psychosocial factors of upper extremity disorders and the influence that they can have on the recovery of workers. Therapists must understand that psychosocial factors must be identified and managed, along with any mechanical injury sustained in a workplace environment.

E-mail address: Dennis_Driver@Concentra.com

doi:10.1016/j.coem.2005.11.011 **occmed.theclinics.com**

Driven by the legalities of workers' compensation requirements, rehabilitation can involve a daunting cast of players, including employee, employer, company health staff, representatives of federal and state agencies, and lawyers, not to mention a quagmire of regulations, policies, and procedural mandates. Only through a total team approach that involves all members of the treatment team (eg, physician, therapist, employee, employer, insurance carrier, and, potentially, case manager) can outcomes be improved and case costs decreased. Therapists must be careful to assess all aspects of a case, provide recommendations and a plan of care that enables a worker, and not cause unnecessary delays in case closure. These delays can and will increase the duration of a case, with a resulting economic impact on the employee, employer, and overall economy that is immeasurable.

This article provides an overview of outcomes factors associated with case closure of upper extremity disorders and standard therapy treatment interventions and the associated implications in promoting case closure.

Outcomes

When a worker sustains an occupational upper extremity injury, the primary goal is to return the individual to the previous level of function in as rapid, effective, and cost efficient a manner as possible. In an ideal world nothing should limit a worker's recovery, nor should the worker use the event for unmerited additional personal gain. Unfortunately, recovery is a complicated process influenced not only by medical factors but also by social, economic, legal, and psychosocial factors [6]. Patients who receive workers' compensation are at risk of having higher pain ratings, lower satisfaction reports, and longer average time for full return to work than clients who do not receive compensation for similar type diagnosis [7,8]. They also are not as likely to have a successful response to treatment as persons who do not receive compensation [9,10].

Although most studies have focused on workers' compensation status as the prime variable in a patient's potential to have a delayed recovery, the level of physical demand associated with the work tasks to which a patient must return also can impede rapid return to work. One investigation found that return to work demand level had a direct effect on the time to return to full duty, regardless of workers' compensation status [11]. Work demand level may have an effect on functional recovery time and delay the return to full work status, which subsequently may affect a patient's perception of success of a particular medical intervention. Consequently, a therapist must have a clear understanding of a patient's job at the onset of treatment and, whenever necessary, should obtain additional information about job tasks directly from a patient's company. If a patient is being treated while on restricted duty or while off work, he or she must be given a clear understanding and expectation regarding how and when he or she will return to work.

It has been suggested that early medical intervention and diagnostics can enhance outcome and reduce long-term incapacitation and disability [12,13]. The use of early therapy intervention also has been associated with decreasing case duration in patients who receive workers' compensation. Several authors have suggested elimination of splints/braces and initiating early range of motion with active exercise for injured workers [14]. A therapist's treatment should play a critical role in promoting early mobility, focusing on functional activities, and initiating aerobic exercise while limiting the use of passive modalities. Patients who cooperate with the appropriate rehabilitation program are likely to have a shorter return-to-work interval than those who do not [15,16]. Researchers have speculated that patients who are most highly motivated to return to work are the same patients who comply with early therapy programs and actively participate in their rehabilitation.

Psychosocial aspects

Although it is generally acknowledged that adverse psychosocial issues can impede recovery in a patient with a lumbar spine affliction, the acknowledgment that psychosocial factors have a similar negative impact on upper extremity disorders is less well studied and accepted by clinicians. The psychosocial aspects of traumatic injuries differ significantly from those of nonspecific musculoskeletal involvement. An injury to an individual's hand affects more than just that person's ability to work. Several factors come into play as a result of trauma, including self-identity, body concept, physical activity, future employment, and a significant alteration in the ability to fulfill usual social and familiar roles and obligations [17]. Early referral to a multidisciplinary program to help evaluate the need for physical and psychological rehabilitation is often appropriate for such patients who do not make the expected progress in therapy.

Illness behavior (ie, a maladaptive response to an injury or illness that is out of proportion to the physiologic insult) must be recognized and managed appropriately early in the course of care [18]. The treating therapist is often in a better position than the physician to recognize illness behavior and other psychosocial contributors early in the course of the illness, because the therapist spends longer periods with a patient during therapy and is seen more frequently. When a therapist identifies significant psychosocial issues or evidence of distress, it is imperative to alert the treating physician so that an appropriate management plan can be developed. Injured workers who experience physical illness or injury are at increased vulnerability for developing psychological problems, including depression and anxiety.

These difficulties can lead to a decrease in resources to deal with the demands of recovery from physical illness and injury. Although most clients adjust well to the psychosocial demands of their condition, approximately 20% to 25% of clients who undergo medical care experience clinically significant psychological symptoms that interfere with their recovery [19]. The sooner the psychological problems are identified and treated, the better the outcome, and if a therapist identifies symptoms of depression or anxiety in a patient, the situation should be discussed with the physician so that appropriate management is initiated. Regular aerobic exercise has been demonstrated to be beneficial as a treatment for depression and anxiety; it is particularly important that a therapist incorporate aerobic conditioning into the session and set up a home program of regular aerobic exercise.

The question of why a worker reports an injury has been investigated and debated intensely. A strong psychosocial underlay seems to influence a worker's decision to seek treatment for musculoskeletal injury or disease. Research has shown that physical activities performed at work, the physical conditions under which the work is conducted, and the actual work environment are related to the occurrence of injury reporting [20]. The data also suggest that low control on the job, monotonous work, time pressure, lack of social support by colleagues, conflicts with supervisor or colleagues, and overall pay satisfaction are associated risk factors in the injury reporting and recovery process [21–23].

Patients who receive compensation for an injury or illness can be more difficult to treat and manage, are more likely to have a prolonged case duration, and are more likely to become disabled than patients with similar conditions who are not receiving compensation. The workers' compensation system provides compensation for being disabled and incapacitated and, in many cases, provides little financial motivation to an injured employee to make a full effort toward rehabilitation [24]. Compensation may allow a high-risk employee to use an injury improperly as a solution to life's problems. Consequently, high-risk patients may have either a conscious or unconscious need to hold on to symptoms and may want to avoid establishing a therapeutic alliance with their health care providers. It is helpful to remember that a normal response to injury or illness is regression; being consistent and firm and setting reasonable limits is essential. With this in mind, therapists need to be conscious regarding the adherence a worker has toward the rehabilitation program. Although adherence seems to be vital to the success of rehabilitation programs, recent reviews of adherence are less than encouraging. There seems to be a wide range of rehabilitation program adherence in various studies, ranging from 40% to 91% in a sports injury–specific population and 4% to 92% in a general medical patient population [25,26] These findings indicate that therapists should take note when patients cancel or miss appointments and be able to clinically assess adherence to home exercise programs.

Although experts have speculated that patients who are most highly motivated to return to work are the same patients who comply with early therapy programs and actively participate in their rehabilitation, it is also likely that patients become more motivated if a therapist works to establish a therapeutic rapport during the initial sessions. When dealing with clients, a therapist's communication style is important in outcome management. There is evidence for the importance of the practitioner-client relationship from the client's perspective. Clients describe good therapists as persons who show an interest in them, are friendly and empathetic, and listen to their concerns. "Good" therapists are also described as individuals who take a more personal approach, and "bad" therapists are deemed to be more impersonal [27,28]. It is important for the practitioner-client relationship that a practitioner strive to understand the situation from a client's point of view. One primary goal is to enlist clients as collaborators in their own rehabilitation process.

Manual therapy

The use of manual therapy by the therapy profession has become a primary treatment of choice for orthopedic injuries within the past decade. Although there are numerous philosophical schools of thought regarding techniques in manual therapy, there is an equal debate regarding what simply constitutes a manual therapy intervention. The American Academy of Orthopedic Manual Physical Therapists has defined manual therapy as a clinical approach using skilled, specific, hands-on techniques that include, but are not limited to, manipulation and mobilization, which are used by a physical therapist to diagnose and treat soft tissues and joint structures for the purpose of modulating pain, increasing range of motion, reducing or eliminating soft tissue inflammation, inducing relaxation, improving contractile and noncontractile tissue repair extensibility or stability, facilitating movement, and improving function [29].

Although there has been much discussion in the therapy professions regarding the ability to diagnose pathologic conditions, the professions are better situated to identify and treat movement dysfunctions and leave the diagnosis of disease to medical-based colleagues. Dysfunction is best defined as a state of altered mechanics with either an increase of decrease from the expected normal or the presence of an aberrant motion [30]. Classic manual therapy interventions were used to restore joint motion and function and aid in pain reduction. The recent increase in manual therapy use has expanded the classic philosophy of improving joint range of motion combined with neuropsychological effects of the relief of pain, reduction in muscle tone, improvement in fascial and neural mobility, and improvement in neuromuscular activity. The treatment approaches have shifted from the belief in correcting positional faults to restoring joint mechanics to improve neural afferent discharge and muscle recruitment and decrease reflex muscle splinting. Researchers suggest that treatment directed at the joint not only has a direct effect on muscle activity but also reduces nociceptor discharge from the joint and improves muscle recruitment [31–33].

Although there is no proof that one specific manual therapy technique is preferable, the body of research and published case studies involving upper extremity disorders indicates that a hands-on manual therapy approach is a more preferable intervention than a modality/pain relieving approach in regards to patient recovery and outcomes [34–48]. Several randomized, controlled studies have based outcomes measures not only on symptom reduction but also on function grip strength and pain-free lifting ability [49]. One study involved randomization of patients who had lateral epicondyalgia into three cohorts (1) ultrasound and exercise group, (2) mobilization and exercise group, and (3) no treatment. The clients were seen for ten sessions over 3 weeks for the initial modalities or mobilization interventions. After the initial 3 weeks, a graduated exercise program was started. At the time of discharge, outcome measurement, including pain assessed on a visual analog scale, grip strength, and pain-free wrist extension lifting measurements, was noted. The group that received manual therapy demonstrated greater improvement in all parameters. The improvements in the objective strength test may lead to support of a modulatory effect on the neuromuscular recovery of tissue that allows for faster progress with an exercise program.

Strengthening

The initiation and timing of strengthening activities are widely controversial in rehabilitation intervention programs. Of primary concern is that with sore and damaged muscle tissue, any type of resistive overload could cause further structural damage. Physical inactivity initiates muscle atrophy, with protein synthesis falling within hours. Prolonged inactivity initially demonstrates loss in the type I slow twitch muscle fibers, which affects the endurance ability of a worker. Damage that occurs during or immediately after exercise has been attributed to protein degradation. An inflammatory process begins approximately 2 hours after injury and can last up to 5 days [50]. Tissue damage and postactivity delayed-onset muscle soreness has been attributed to a chemical reaction in the muscle. After an unusual or new strenuous activity, damage occurs that is characterized by changes in the sarcoplasmic reticulum and disruption to the cell membranes. This disruption of muscle cell membranes allows proteins, such as creatine kinase and histamines, to leak into the extracellular environment and potentially stimulate nociceptors [51,52].

One potential hypothesis that has been developed suggests that strenuous eccentric exercise would not increase muscle damage after repeated bouts of high-force eccentric exercise [53]. In one clinical study, changes in plasma proteins were measured after performing maximal eccentric activity to the biceps to detect muscle damage. Pre- and postactivity levels of plasma creatine kinase and glutamic-oxaloacetic transaminase were recorded and evaluated. Based on the findings of these recordings, strenuous exercise performed with predamaged or irritated muscles did not exacerbate damage or affect the repair process. This finding indicates that despite mechanical and chemical changes present in contractile tissue, initiation of exercise does not prolong the recovery time for the damaged muscle. Therapists should be cautioned when working with sore muscles not to expect maximal force generation from injured workers.

Recent investigations have concluded that most tendonopathies are more likely to be degenerative than inflammatory in nature [54]. Antidotal evidence indicates that up to 35% of the healthy population aged 35 years or older has some type of degenerative tendon changes [55]. The absence of any inflammatory infiltrate indicates that there is minimal stimulus for a normal biologic healing process. Several investigators have indicated that eccentric loading is an important component to the initiation of remodeling of tendon pathologies [56,57].

Although strengthening exercise results in microscopic muscle damage, a repeated bout of the same activity produces only modest changes in damage, which may explain why industrial workers complain of delayed muscle onset soreness after job activity changes. After performing days, weeks, or years of the same activity, when a worker takes on a new job duty either temporarily or permanently, a "job training and conditioning" effect causes some muscular soreness. With prolonged specific job activity, muscle demonstrates a unique ability to resist damage and, if any damage does occur, it is repaired at a faster rate.

Neural involvement: mechanical

The involvement of neural tissue in entrapment syndromes in the upper extremity is well documented in the medical and therapy literature. In chronic disorders the peripheral nerve involvement may become the primary pain generator. It has been estimated that in chronic lateral epicondyalgia disorders, the dorsal interossi nerve and cubital tunnel may be involved in up to 80% of all cases. Studies also have estimated that 92% of all carpal tunnel syndromes may involve a double crush syndrome in the median nerve distribution [58,59]. Consequently, an assessment of the neck should be included on all initial assessments of entrapment syndromes of the arm.

Over the past decade there has been an increase in interest in neural provocation and tension test in the therapy domain. A methodologic approach to neural tissue provocation tests for the upper quarter has been documented. This approach offers guidelines for evaluation that allow testing techniques to be tailored to the severity of a neuropathic pain disorder. The suggested evaluation approach incorporates provocation positioning that is directed toward the median, radial, and ulnar nerve trunks from a proximal to distal direction and vice versa [60].

Neural involvement: organic

Although there is a component of neural entrapment and irritation in the workers' compensation population, therapists must have the essential skills to screen for organic disease processes and the confidence to refer a client to appropriate medical professionals for additional diagnostic screening and management. When investigating carpal tunnel claims, a therapist must be aware that this disorder is one of the most common causes of occupational disability in this country. Research has found that less than half of all cases are identified as work related [61]. It has been suggested that age-related, hormone-related disorders or hormone supplementation or ceasing hormone supplementation programs may be significant risk factors for neurogenic disorders [62]. More significant are controllable risk factors that afflicted workers can help control in the prevention and treatment of organic neurogenic disorders. Behavioral risk factors that have been found to have a strong correlation include obesity, smoking/tobacco use, faulty stress management techniques, and infrequent physical activity [63].

Therapists can play a beneficial role in the overall health of an injured worker and serve as a fitness consultant. Patients are much more likely to experience musculoskeletal aches and pains at work, particularly with sedentary work, if they get no regular exercise outside of work. Studies suggest that a general wellness program that includes healthy diet, proper hydration, and general aerobic exercise is beneficial to median nerve function and may be associated with a reduction in other nerve-based hand and upper extremity symptoms [64–67]. Any patient referred for therapy with a work-related upper extremity disorder should be assessed for and instructed in a home fitness program that incorporates general aerobic and resistance training. A therapist must consider the potential need for dietary counseling for proper nutrition and weight loss. A referral to a primary care physician for screening, evaluation, and treatment of other potential age-related disorders is often indicated.

Stretching

The current national trend is toward stretching as a health-based activity. There is significant concern regarding the validity of general stretching as a rehabilitation tool. The general question is why an individual would want to move a joint farther than he or she could control the motion actively. There is a novice tendency among therapists, coaches, physicians, and the lay public to think that if a certain muscle length and range of motion is desirable, then more is better. This belief can lead to overstretching, which can result in instability and weakness [68]. Excessive stretching over a prolonged period of time can elongate muscle fibers and the surrounding fascia beyond a desirable range. This increase in passive flexibility has been shown to lead to an increase in injuries [69,70]. No evidence exists to show that stretching improves performance [71].

This is not to say that tissue-specific stretching is not indicated after appropriate evaluation. Muscle tightness has been shown to correlate with muscle injury because of the shortening of soft tissue elements and the inability of tissue to comply with elongation forces applied during activity [72]. The increased tension applied to tendons of adaptively shortened tissues has been correlated to joint injures and the development of faulty movement patterns, which might lead to inappropriate stress being applied to joint surfaces [73]. The shortened tissue also causes increased tension at the osseoustendinous insertion and potentially leads to tendonitis [74].

Stretching also has been reported to help decrease delayed-onset muscle soreness [75]. Stretching is often used after work as a preventive measure, especially after a strenuous activity. Several studies have addressed this question and have found no short- or long-term correlation between stretching and delayed-onset muscle soreness [76,77]. This is not to say that there is no value in active range of motion or dynamic warm up that might increase flexibility before activity or work. The warming up of muscular and connective tissue is important in preparation for competition, training, or work activities. Increased tissue temperature through dynamic activity increases the metabolic process and decreases tissue viscosity, which results in less resistance with muscle contraction, increases oxygen uptake, increases neuromuscular transmission, and improves the elasticity of collagen [78–80].

When muscle and soft tissue elongation issues are encountered in the clinic setting, dynamic range-of-motion activities have been shown to cause a greater degree of muscular relaxation than other stretching activities, and they demonstrate faster and more efficient increases in range of motion and strength [81].

Summary

Upper extremity disorders in the workplace continue to be an economic strain on society. Physical and occupational therapy plays a crucial role in the management of the disorders. Medical providers should use therapists whose treatments demonstrate improvement in function and provide superior outcomes. Skilled therapy intervention requires that a therapist be able to identify and treat an injured worker in a holistic manner by looking at the whole individual, including issues that involve mechanical dysfunctions, psychosocial issues that include job satisfaction, and other age-related organic comorbidities. Therapists who work with injured employees must be highly skilled in identifying behavioral and organic disorders and must be confident in communicating these findings to various members of the health care team to help facilitate further medical testing.

References

[1] Fox S, Borba P, Liu T. Return-to-work outcomes of injured workers: evidence from California, Massachusetts, Pennsylvania and Texas. Cambridge (MA): Workers' Compensation Research Institute; 2005.

[2] Courtney T, Webster B. Disabling occupational morbidity in the United States: an alternative way of seeing the Bureau of Labor Statistics. J Occup Environ Med 1999;41(1):60–9.

[3] Hashemi L, Webster B, Clancy E. Trends in disability duration and cost of workers' compensation low back pain claims. J Occup Environ Med 1988;40:1110–9.

[4] Feuerstein M, Miller V, Burrell L, et al. Occupational upper extremity disorders in the federal workforce: prevalence, health care expenditures, and patterns of work disability. J Occup Environ Med 1998;40:546–55.

[5] Monitor. Texas: Research and Oversight Council on Workers' Compensation. Volume 7, No. 2, Special edition; 2002. p. 4–9.

[6] Walsh N, Dumitru D. The influence of compensation on recovery form low back pain. Occup Med 1988;3:109–21.
[7] Hawkins R, Saddemi S, Moor J, et al. Arthroscopic subacromial decompression: a 2-year follow up study. Arthroscopy 1992;8(3):409.
[8] Misamore G, Ziegler D, Rushton J. Repair of the rotator cuff: a comparison of results in two populations of patients. J Bone Joint Surg 1995;77-A(9):1335–9.
[9] Hadler N. Coping with arm pain in the workplace. Clin Orthop 1998;351:57–62.
[10] Roye R, Grana W, Yates C. Arthroscopic subacromial decompression: two to seven year follow-up. Arthroscopy 1995;11:301–6.
[11] Nicholson G. Arthroscopic acromioplasty: a comparison between workers' compensation and non-workers' compensation populations. J Bone Joint Surg 2003;85-A(4):682–9.
[12] Deyo R, editor. Back pain in workers. OccupMed 1988;3:vii.
[13] Savoie F. Cost analysis of successful rotator cuff repair surgery in workers' compensation patient. J Shoulder Elbow Surg 1996;5:S10.
[14] Cook A, Szabo M, Birholz S, et al. Early mobilization following carpal tunnel release: a prospective randomized study. J Hand Surg [Br] 1995;20B(2):228–30.
[15] Nathan P, Meadows K, Keniston R. Rehabilitation of carpal tunnel surgery patients using a short surgical incision and an early program of physical therapy. J Hand Surg [Am] 1993; 18A(6):1044–50.
[16] Kadsan M, June L. Returning to work after a unilateral hand fracture. J Occup Med 1993; 35:132–5.
[17] Johnson K. Psychological evaluation of patients with industrial hand injuries. Hand Clin 1986; 2(3):567–75.
[18] Pilowski I. Aspects of abnormal illness behavior. Psychother Psychosom 1993;63:62–74.
[19] Martin F. Co-morbidity of depression with physical illness: a review of the literature. Ment Health Care 2001;4(12):212–25.
[20] Pope D, Croft P, Pritchard C, et al. Occupational factors related to shoulder pain and disability. Occup Environ Med 1997;54:316–21.
[21] Peterson M, Wilson J. Job satisfaction and perceptions of health. J Occup Environ Med 1996; 38(9):891–8.
[22] Bongers P, de Winter C, Kompier M, et al. Psychosocial factors at work and musculoskeletal disease. Scand J Work Environ Health 1993;19:297–312.
[23] Swaen G, van Maeisvoort L, Bultmann U, et al. Psychosocial work characteristics as risk factors for being injured in an occupational accident. J Occup Environ Med 2004;46(6):521–7.
[24] Derebery V, Tullis W. Disability prevention with work compensable injuries. Phys Med Rehabil 1988:165–76.
[25] Brewer B. Adherence to sport injury rehabilitation regimens. In: Bull S, editor. Adherence issues in sports exercise. Chichester, UK: Wiley; 2001. p. 145–68.
[26] Brewer B, Daly J, Van Raalte J. A psychometric evaluation of rehabilitation adherence questionnaire. Journal of Sports and Exercise Psychology 1999;21:167–73.
[27] Johnson R. Attitudes don't just hang in the air: disabled people's perceptions of physiotherapists. Physiotherapy 1994;79:619–27.
[28] Ford J, Gordon S. Social support and athletic injury: the perspective of sports physiotherapists. Aust J Sci Med Sport 1993;25(1):17–25.
[29] American Academy of Orthopedic Manual Physical Therapist. Orthopedic manual physical therapy: document describing advanced clinical practice. Biloxi (MS): American Academy of Orthopedic Manual Physical Therapist; 1998. p. 29.
[30] Paris S. Mobilization of the spine. Phys Ther 1979;49(8):988–95.
[31] Lewit K. The muscular and articular factor in movement restriction. Manual Medicine 1985; 1(1):83.
[32] Stokes M, Young A. The contribution of reflex inhibition on arthrogenous muscle weakness. Clin Sci 1984;67:7–14.
[33] Schiable H, Grubb B. Afferent and spinal mechanisms of joint pain. Pain 1993;55:5–54.

[34] Abbott J, Patla C, Jensen R. The initial effects of an elbow mobilization with movement technique on grip strength in subjects with lateral epicondylagia. Man Ther 1993;17(4):172–6.
[35] Davis T, Hulbert J, Kassak K, et al. Comparative efficacy of conservative medical and chiropractic treatments for carpal tunnel syndrome: a randomized clinical trial. J Manipulative Physiol Ther 1998;21(5):317–26.
[36] Hill Jr J, Bogumill H. Manipulation in the treatment of frozen shoulder. Orthopedics 1988;11(9):1255–60.
[37] Kaufman R, Bird J. Manipulative management of post-Colles' fracture weakness and diminished active range of motion. J Manipulative Physiol Ther 1999;22(2):105–7.
[38] Kushner S, Reid D. Manipulation in the treatment of tennis elbow. J Orthop Sports Phys Ther 1986;7(5):264–72.
[39] Labelle H, Guibert R, Joncas J, et al. Lack of scientific evidence for the treatment of lateral epicondylitis of the elbow: an attempted meta-analysis. J Bone Joint Surg Br 1992;74(5):646–51.
[40] Lee D. Tennis elbow: a manual therapist's perspective. J Orthop Sports Phys Ther 1986;14(8):134–42.
[41] Roubal P, Dobritt D, Placzek J. Glenohumeral gliding manipulation following interscalene brachial plexus block in patients with adhesive capsulitis. J Orthop Sports Phys Ther 1996;24(2):66–77.
[42] Schultz K, Middendorp J, Meyer V. Ulnodorsal impingement syndrome: meniscus lesions of the wrist. Handchir Mikrochir Plast Chir 1996;18(2):98–104.
[43] Struijs P, Damen P, Bakker E, et al. Manipulation of the wrist for management of lateral epicondylitis: a randomized pilot study. Phys Ther 2003;21(7):448–53.
[44] Vicenzino B, Collins D, Wright A. The initial effects of a cervical spine manipulative physiotherapy treatment on the pain and dysfunction of lateral epicondylalgia. Pain 1996;68(1):69–74.
[45] Vicenzino B, Wright A. Effects of a novel manipulative physiotherapy technique on tennis elbow: a single case study. Man Ther 2000;1(1):30–5.
[46] Vicenzino B. Lateral epicondylalgia: a musculoskeletal physiotherapy perspective. Man Ther 2003;8(2):66–79.
[47] Vicenzino B, Paungmali A, Buratowski S, et al. Specific manipulative therapy treatment for chronic lateral epicondylalgia produces uniquely characteristic hypoalgesia. Man Ther 2001;6(4):205–12.
[48] Backstrom K. Mobilization with movement as an adjunct intervention in a patient with complicated DeQuervain's tenosynovitis: a case report. J Orthop Sports Phys Ther 2002;32(3):86–97.
[49] Kochar M, Dogra A. Effectiveness of a specific physiotherapy regimen on patients with tennis elbow. Physiotherapy 2002;88(6):333–41.
[50] Clarkson P, Tremblay I. Exercise induced muscle damage, repair and adaptation in humans. J Appl Physiol 1988;65(1):1–6.
[51] Sargeant A, Dolan P. Human muscle function following prolonged eccentric exercise. Eur J Appl Physiol 1987;56:704–11.
[52] Gibala M, MacDougall J, Tarnopolsky M. Changes in human skeletal muscle ultrastructure and force production after acute resistance exercise. J Appl Physiol 1995;78:702–8.
[53] Nosaka K, Clarkson P. Muscle damage following repeated bouts of high force eccentric exercise. Med Sci Sports Exerc 1995;27(9):1263–9.
[54] Kannus P, Jozsa L. Histopathological changes preceding spontaneous rupture of a tendon: a controlled study of 891 patients. J Bone Joint Surg Am 1991;73:1507–25.
[55] Kannus P. Tendon pathology: basic science and clinical applications. Sports Exercise and Injury 1997;3:62–75.
[56] Kahn K, Cook J, Maffulli N, et al. Where is the pain coming from in tendinopathy? It may be biochemical, not only structural, in origin. British Journal of Sports Medicine 2000;34:81–4.
[57] Stanish W, Rubinovich R, Curwin S. Eccentric exercise in chronic tendonitis. Clin Orthop 1986;65(1):1–6.

[58] Ehmer B. Orthopadische erkrankungen des ellengbogengelendes. In: Verlag FE, editor. Orthpadie und traumatologie für physiotherapeuten. 9th edition. Stuttgart: Fredinand Enk Verlag; 1998. p. 251–5.
[59] Golvochinsky V. Relationship between damage of cervical nerve roots or brachial plexus and development of peripheral entrapment syndromes in upper extremities (double crush syndrome). Journal of Neurological and Orthopedic Medicine and Surgery 1995;16(2):61–9.
[60] Elvey R, Hall T. Neural tissue evaluation and treatment. In: Donatelli R, editor. Physical therapy of the shoulder. 3rd edition. New York: Churchill-Livingstone; 1997. p. 131–52.
[61] NIOSH. Occupational disease surveillance: carpal tunnel syndrome. MMWR Morb Mortal Wkly Rep 1989;39:485–8.
[62] Ferry S, Hannaford P, Warskyj M, et al. Carpal tunnel syndrome: a nested case-control study of risk factors in women. Am J Epidemiol 2000;151:566–74.
[63] Macfarlaine G, Hunt I, Silman A. Role of mechanical and psychosocial factors in the onset of forearm pain: prospective population based study. BMJ 2000;321:1–5.
[64] Nathan P, Wilcox A, Emerick P, et al. Effects of an aerobic exercise program on median nerve conduction and symptoms associated with carpal tunnel syndrome. J Occup Environ Med 2001; 43:840–3.
[65] Nathan P, Keniston R. Carpal tunnel syndrome and its relation to general physical condition. Hand Clin 1993;9:253–61.
[66] Stalling S, Kasden M, Soergel T, et al. A case control study of obesity as a risk factor for carpal tunnel syndrome in a population of 600 patients presenting for independent medical examination. J Hand Surg [Am] 1997;22:211–5.
[67] Must A, Spandano J, Coakly E, et al. The disease burden associated with overweight and obesity. JAMA 1999;282:1523–9.
[68] Iashvilii AV. Active and passive flexibility in athletes specializing in different sports. Teoriy I Prakita Fizicheskoi Kultury 1987;7:51–2.
[69] Ekstrand J, Gillquist J. The frequency of muscle tightness and injuries in soccer. Am J Sports Med 1982;10:75–8.
[70] Ekstrand J, Gillquist J. The avoidability of soccer injuries. Int J Sports Med 1983;4:124–8.
[71] Dintiman G. Effects of various training programs on running speed. Res Q 1964;35:456–63.
[72] Murphy D. The neglected nervous system: its role in the pathophysiology of the subluxation complex. J Chiro 1990;27(12):36–40.
[73] Janda V. Pain in the locomotor system: a broad approach. In: Glasgow EF, Twomey L, Scull E, et al, editors. Aspects of manipulative therapy. New York: Churchill-Livingstone; 1986. p. 148–51.
[74] Saal J. Flexibility training. Phys Med Rehabil 1987;1(4):537–54.
[75] deVries H. Prevention of muscular distress after exercise. Res Q 1961;32:177–85.
[76] McGlynn G, Laughlin N, Rowe V. Effect of electromyographic feedback and static stretching on artificially induced muscle soreness. Am J Phys Med 1979;58(3):139–48.
[77] Buroker K, Schwane J. Does postexercise static stretching alleviate delayed muscle soreness? Phys Sportsmed 1989;1:350–7.
[78] Schultz P. Flexibility: day of the static stretch. Phys Sportsmed 1979;7(11):427–48.
[79] O'Neil D. Preventing injuries in young athletes. J Musculoskel Med 1989;6(11):21–35.
[80] Safran M, Seaber A, Garret W. Warm up and muscular injury prevention: an update. Sports Med 1985;2:21–3.
[81] Guissard N, Duchateaus J, Hainaut K. Muscle stretching and motor neuron excitability. Eur J Appl Phys 1988;58:47–52.

ELSEVIER
SAUNDERS

Clin Occup Environ Med
5 (2) 483–490

CLINICS IN
OCCUPATIONAL AND
ENVIRONMENTAL
MEDICINE

Worker's Compensation Litigation of the Upper Extremity Claim

Walter E. Harding, JD

Boehl Stopher and Graves, LLP, 2300 Aegon Center, 400 West Market Street, Louisville, KY 40202, USA

Claims that involve alleged work-related upper extremity injuries represent one of the largest areas of workers' compensation litigation. Traditionally, these claims have involved soft tissue injuries, fractures, crush injuries, problems with bone healing, and management of patients who have diabetes. Over the last 20 years, however, there has been a dramatic increase in injuries allegedly derived from "repetitive" or "cumulative" trauma-type injuries. These injuries principally include pronator teres syndrome, thoracic outlet compression, and carpal tunnel syndrome.

Many studies have shown that there is a demonstrable difference between workers' compensation cases and cases in which litigation is not an issue. From a practical standpoint, the workers' compensation patient has become a major financial factor in many medical practices. In many situations, a physician can make more money if work is identified as the cause. The advent of managed care, insurance adjuster oversight, increased competition between medical practices, and the growing willingness of physicians to critique each other publicly have altered the litigation landscape significantly.

This article focuses on problems that face the litigator and the physician in developing and presenting a workers' compensation claim for litigation and conclusion.

Overview

Workers' compensation intersects in an interesting way with medicine: The law, in fact, tends to lead the science. As of the time of this writing, many of the

E-mail address: wharding@bsg-law.com

doi:10.1016/j.coem.2005.11.005 *occmed.theclinics.com*

alleged work-related so-called repetitive or cumulative injuries seem to be actually media driven and scientifically unsupportable. State legislatures have stepped in, embraced many of these conditions, and found them compensable.

There is a danger that the sheer volume of claims may corrupt medicine and law in their respective rigors and, presumably, their search for the truth. The most obvious examples include that of cost shifting, the medicalization of ordinary aches and pains, and the apparent epidemic of carpel tunnel syndrome, thoracic outlet compression, pronator teres syndrome, reflex sympathetic dystrophy, myofascial pain, and fibromyalgia. There seems to be an ignorance of the nocebo effect, with the all-too-frequent harmful labeling of patients with a syndrome, which reinforces in their minds that they have an actual disability and a consequent entitlement to benefits because of a perceived inability to partake fully in life [1].

The workers' compensation act

Workers' compensation is the statutory remedy available to employees for injuries that arise out of the workplace. It is available in all 50 states, territories, commonwealths, and, on the federal level, in several specific acts, such as the Long Shore and Harbor Workers' Compensation Act. The principles of workers' compensation are fairly uniform across the United States. Most statutes are based on and interpreted in accordance with the authoritative 12-volume work "Larson's Workers' Compensation Law" [2].

In workers' compensation, an employee is relieved of having to confront the issue of negligence and generally is given an expectation of a considerably more prompt resolution of the claim than in the exercise of a civil remedy. Employers' liability is restricted to that of income benefits, which is determined as a percentage of actual wages as multiplied by a functional impairment rating derived from a statutorily accepted guideline; reasonable and necessary medical care, and vocational rehabilitation. Civil litigation remedies, such as actual wage loss, pain and suffering, loss of consortium, and punitive damages, are not available.

Workers' compensation recognizes three types of disability: temporary partial or total disability, which contemplates payments to the injured worker until maximum medical improvement and a return to work is obtained; permanent partial disability, whereby the claimant's permanent condition after the reaching of maximum medical improvement is then quantified and compensated through a payment of indemnity benefits; and permanent total disability, which compensates employees who are unable to return to employment as a result of an industrial injury. These benefits are all based on various formulas applied to two thirds of the claimant's average weekly wage up to a statutory maximum. In considering permanent partial disability, an award to a claimant is based on taking the aforementioned two thirds of their average weekly wage up to the state maximum and multiplying it times the functional impairment as set out by a recognized guideline, such as the "AMA Guides for Evaluation of Permanent Partial Impairment" [3]. That result then may be multiplied by various factors, depending on the jurisdiction, that reflect an ability to return to employment, education, or other variables.

The requirements for compensability are set out in the state and federal statutes, and they make it clear that not all work-related harmful changes are compensable. In many jurisdictions, only physical injuries and their residuals that can be measured objectively by standardized methods are compensable, including a worsening of condition caused by medical malpractice.

The injured worker bears the risk and burden of persuasion as to each and every element of the prima facie case. The worker must be able to show that arising out of and in the course of employment within a certain statutorily determined period of time, he or she has given "due and timely" notice that he or she has suffered a physically traumatic or cumulative event, which is the proximate cause of a harmful change in the human organism as evidenced by objective medical findings confirmed by a functional impairment rating from a guideline such as the "AMA Guides for Evaluation of Permanent Partial Impairment" [3]. An industrial injury that arises from a sudden, unexpected, impact and results in a broken bone, crush injury, amputation, or dislocation easily fits within this paradigm. The more difficult question presented is when the allegations of a work-related injury derive from what are colloquially known as cumulative or repetitive trauma.

These claims are presented to either an administrative law judge or adjudicative board, sitting in lieu of a jury, who sifts through the evidence and evaluates which expert opinion is to be believed. Like most lawyers, the adjudicator may have no background in science. The adjudicator applies the relevant statute and case law, making findings of fact and conclusions of law. Appeals are generally available to higher boards and courts with regard to legal error or only the most egregious factual conclusions.

The adjudicative process

Unlike medicine, the legal process is concerned not with the "exhaustive search for a causative understanding, but for the particularized resolution of legal disputes" [4]. Law, unlike the sciences, attempts to obtain finality of conflicts. The legal system, in assessing expert medical or scientific testimony, has its own priorities. In *Daubert v Merrell Dow Pharmaceuticals, Inc.* [4], the Supreme Court held that,

> It is true that open debate is an essential part of both legal and scientific analyses. Yet there are important differences between the quest for truth in the court room and the quest for truth in the laboratory. Scientific conclusions are subject to perpetual revision. Law, on the other hand, must resolve disputes finally and quickly. The scientific project is advanced by broad and wide-ranging consideration of a multitude of hypotheses, for those that are incorrect will

> eventually be shown to be so, and that in itself is an advance. Conjectures that are probably wrong are of little use, however, in the project for reaching a quick, final, and binding legal judgment, - - often of great consequence - - about a particular set of events in the past. We recognize that in practice a gatekeeping role for the judge, no matter how flexible, inevitably on occasion will prevent the jury from learning of authentic insights and innovations. That, nevertheless, is the balance that is struck by rules of evidence designed not for the exhaustive search for cosmic understanding but for the particularized resolution of legal disputes.

Consequently, the court found that the trial judge must analyze offered scientific evidence so as to determine

> . . .whether the reasoning or methodology underlying the testimony is scientifically valid and whether that reasoning or methodology properly can be applied to the fact at issue.

The court emphasized that the focus of the trial judge's inquiry must be on principles and methodology rather than conclusions. It should investigate whether there were any attempts to falsify the theory or hypothesis underlying the offered scientific methodology, whether there was any peer review or publication, the potential rate of error of the offered theory, and its general acceptance in the scientific community. Although this is the recognized standard in federal and state courts, it has only imperfectly filtered down to the level of the workers' compensation adjudication, where it is still in the process of being adopted. This process is further complicated by the fact that the administrative law judge is the gatekeeper and the trier of fact. Consequently, assessing the quality of expert testimony is a significant ongoing problem in workers' compensation litigation.

Accordingly, the traditional rules of substantial evidence in many jurisdictions allow an adjudicator, who is considered to be in a unique position to hear the testimony and analyze the evidence, to take the opinion of an individual in family practice over that of a board certified specialist with several fellowships. In many jurisdictions, the adjudicator is allowed to pick and choose parts of medical evidence from single or different witnesses, even if contradictory, in arriving at a single conclusion [5]. One is tempted to agree with Justice Oliver Wendell Holmes of the United States Supreme Court, who once observed (paraphrases), "The law is whatever judges say that it is." The unstated policy has been to give the adjudicator enough latitude so that it is difficult, if not impossible, to overturn these findings of fact on appeal. The interest of the court is, again, in finality.

The expert witness

The physician is the only one who can address adequately the elements of the claimant's prima facie case. He or she is asked as the treating physician or evaluating expert to make a diagnosis and prognosis, assess residual restrictions, determine causation, render a functional impairment rating, relate when the disabling condition was communicated to the patient, and outline reasonable and necessary medical care. This information can be assembled only after a thorough medical examination that involves the taking of a complete history, a clinical examination, the review of past medical records, and appropriate diagnostic testing.

This expert opinion is entered into the court record through a medical report or deposition, the purpose of which is either to elicit testimony for purposes of later impeaching the witnesses' testimony or present to the court in lieu of a formal appearance by the physician. Depositions should be taken seriously because the contents contained therein can last forever. Sworn testimony pursuant to a deposition can follow a physician throughout his or her career.

What is expert opinion? How does a judge determine what is a valid scientific opinion and what is an opinion based on nothing more than personal or anecdotal experience (junk science)? This is an important question. We have sport coaches who tout open-sided MRI facilities, hospitals setting up expensive areas for Native American faith healers, natural medicines being consumed by a significant number of people, physicians in specialties such as orthopedics failing their board certification examinations multiple times but still being allowed without supervision to diagnose and perform multilevel fusions with instrumentation. The utter lack of an enforced, standardized credentialing system that could determine a physician's specialization and parameters of practice magnifies the problem.

In assessing a physician's testimony, a lawyer first should attempt to determine the quality of medical judgment underwriting the diagnosis. In other words, is the diagnosis merely a medicalization of ordinary aches and pains by the use of frightening sounding Latin and Greek terms? What about the nocebo effect [1]? Is the doctor actually an expert or practicing beyond his or her professional qualifications? Does the physician hold any certifications or added qualifications or memberships in specialized societies that involve surgery of the upper extremity? Are these certifications recognized by the American Board of Medical Specialties? Who is the adjudicator, and how persuasive is this evidence before that individual?

The legal system recognizes that the term "diagnosis" refers to the process whereby a physician analyzes the nature and cause of a patient's harmful change or injury and develops the working differential for a logical basis for treatment and prognosis. One arrives at the likely diagnosis from several possibilities: noting the symptoms that the patient reports, physical examination, history taking, observation, and evaluating the significance of the results of objective or standardized testing. The ultimate diagnosis must be stated within a degree of medical probability, however, or it is useless to the adjudicator. In their testimony, many physicians use the terms "certainty," "probability," and "possibilities" interchangeably. These terms each have specific legal effect, which is a critical point.

Physicians frequently testify in the sense of medical certainty, which means without any reasonable doubt, absolute certitude. There is no certitude in science, however. There are probabilities and possibilities. Possibilities are usually a physician's working differential. They are potential—but not necessarily probable—causes. Physicians often testify that various types of potential causes are possible; however, anything could be construed as possible. In general, a mere possibility is not construed as representing substantial evidence and is generally insufficient before an adjudicative proceeding. Conversely, probability means that there is a likelihood—more than a 50% chance—of occurrence or a relationship. This is the accepted standard for the admissibility of evidence in worker's compensation.

Much of the workers' compensation prima facie case that alleges upper extremity repetitive or cumulative trauma revolves around the question of epidemiology. Does the physician actually understand epidemiology? What other reason could there be for many medical practices allowing a determination of work relatedness based solely on a clerk or a nurse asking a patient whether the injury occurred at work? Cost shifting? It is one thing to render a diagnosis, another to determine causation. How has the physician concluded that there is a work-related condition in all medical probability? Was the doctor's conclusion based on comparison of the instant case with the available scientific knowledge (ie, the syllogism used by the physician)? The courts have recognized that this is the essential method by which a physician reaches an opinion on matters of causation. The recognized scientific knowledge of the alleged hazardous exposure constitutes the "major" premise; the facts in the current case surrounding the claimant's alleged exposure constitute the minor premise. From this information, the expert forms an inference regarding the issue of work relatedness or causation [6].

At the time of this writing, in so-called "cumulative trauma" litigation, there is no recognized scientific relationship between activities described as repetitive and the development of carpal tunnel syndrome, pronator teres, or thoracic outlet compression. The only risk factors, which have been identified with increased incidences of carpal tunnel syndrome, are those that include age, gender, obesity, thyroid problems, diabetes, and various neuropathic disorders. This requires the physician to substitute what is, in essence, an untested hypothesis—perhaps anecdotal experience—for the basis of his or her opinion. In workers' compensation, this may be sufficient.

General questions of the physician include those concerning professional qualifications to actually testify as an expert in causation; articles, chapters, or books that one has published that qualify a physician to testify as an expert in causation; what epidemiologic studies can be cited and what scientific methodology was used to show that the claimant's place of business is dangerous and causes a risk for carpal tunnel syndrome; whether the physician can show notes concerning the patient's job description that fit within this methodology; what peer review papers the physician has presented that qualify one to testify as to causation; what peer reviewed articles can be cited that prove that the work this patient did caused the diagnoses; what meetings the physician has attended in the last 3 years on this subject (proof of registration and program); whether the physician holds a certificate of added qualification in hand surgery and what the certificate number is; and whether the physician took the examination to qualify for the American Society for Surgery of the Hand?

The minor premise (ie, the facts of the instant case) also may not be fully developed by the physician. Did the physician take a thorough history, including past medical, family, social, psychiatric, and work histories? Did the work actually cause the condition, worsen it, or simply cause what could be best described as symptoms? In this latter regard, symptoms may not necessarily create a compensable injury. In many states, to be compensable, an injury must cause a harmful change in the human organism. Causation of symptoms is not enough. If a person has an ongoing condition, work could aggravate that condition and cause symptoms, which does not mean that the work actually causes a harmful change, however.

How has the physician established that the worker had a sufficient exposure so as to develop the condition? Is the injurious exposure temporally related to the employment? If the claimant had not engaged in the activity, would that individual have avoided the harmful exposure? Could avoidance of that activity have prevented the development of the condition? Are any of the symptoms actually specific for that condition? How sensitive are the tests that have been conducted to substantiate the condition clinically? Has the physician actually obtained an employment history and viewed the work? How many Newtons of force are involved with the suspected offending activity? What about past work activities? Has the physician taken an adequate social and psychiatric history? Could there be a factitious disorder? Have any tests for malingering been performed?

The diagnosis of an upper extremity problem is clinically subtle and relies in large part on a patient's subjective responses as the physician puts the affected extremity through various positions to elicit a certain level of symptoms. These findings are usually verified through electrical studies, such as an electromyographic/nerve conduction velocity (EMG/NCV) study. Were specialized tests, such as an electromyographic or nerve conduction study, administered by a competent specialist in accordance with the protocol of the American Electrodiagnostic Society (ie, someone who is board certified in neurology or certified by the American Board of Electrodiagnostic Medicine)? Did the specialist hold a certificate of added qualification for the performance for this test? What was the technique? Were the hands warmed or cooled? Were the distances in the palm measured? Were the measured latencies realistic? Were the nerves adequately shocked? What was the temperature of the patient? Was it set out on the report? Does the laboratory wherein these studies were performed meet the guidelines of the American Association of Electrodiagnostic Medicine?

The lawyer should question the physician and obtain an opinion as to the mechanism of the offending injury and how it constitutes a proximate cause of the impairment. For example, if multiple nerves were involved, how did the physician rule out a systemic condition? Were any tests conducted to rule out diabetes, thyroid dysfunction, or some other systemic or neuropathic condition? What about a vascular disorder? Was this investigated?

Finally, are there any objective medical findings? This term can mean different things to the legal and medical community. The fact that a particular diagnosis is made in a manner acceptable to physicians for treatment does not necessarily render it a legally acceptable objective medical finding on which an award of benefits could be based. In general, objective medical findings are defined as information gained by direct observation and testing, applying objective or standardized methods. A harmful change based solely on complaints of symptoms may constitute a valid diagnosis for the purposes of medical treatment by a physician as evidence of a harmful change. A patient's complaints of symptoms clearly are not objective medical findings as the term is defined by many statutes, however. A diagnosis based on a worker's complaints of symptoms but not supported by objective medical findings can be insufficient to prove an injury for the purposes of workers' compensation [7].

Summary

For the foreseeable future, workers' compensation will remain a major source of interest, income, and frustration for legal and medical practitioners. Many physicians find themselves placed in the dubious position of asserting that there is—or is not—a recognized scientific relationship between repetitive activities at work and the development of a particular pathology (ie, carpal tunnel syndrome) and that the exposure in the instant case would allow one to conclude that the claimant did or did not have a work-related condition. The continuing politicalization of our sciences and lack of public scientific education will only compound these conflicts.

References

[1] Kasdan M, Lewis K, Bruner A, et al. The nocebo effect: do no harm. J South Orthop Assoc 1999;8:108–13.
[2] Larson A, Larson LK. Larson's workers' compensation law. New York: M. Bender; 1997.
[3] American Medical Association. Guides to the evaluation of permanent impairment. 5th edition. Chicago (IL): American Medical Association; 2000.
[4] *Daubert v Merrell Dow Pharmaceuticals, Inc,* 125 L.Ed.2d 469; 113 S. Ct., 2786 (1993).
[5] *Caudill v Maloney's Discount Stores,* Ky., 560 S.W.2d 15 (1977).
[6] *Porter v Whitehall Labs, Inc.,* 790 Fed Sup. 1335 (SD Ind. 1992) affirmed 9 Fed 3rd 607 (7th Circuit 1993).
[7] *Gibbs v Premier Scale,* Ky., 40 S.W.3rd 754 (2001).

ELSEVIER
SAUNDERS

Clin Occup Environ Med
5 (2) 491–500

CLINICS IN
OCCUPATIONAL AND
ENVIRONMENTAL
MEDICINE

Index

Note: Page numbers of article titles are in **bold face** type.

1526-0046/06/$ – see front matter
doi:10.1016/S1526-0046(06)00032-X

G

H

I